Becoming a Reflective Practitioner

Fifth Edition

Edited by

Christopher Johns
Visiting Professor at Christ Church Canterbury and University of Bedfordshire

WILEY Blackwell

Registered Offices
John Wiley & Sons, Inc., 111 River Street, Hoboken, NJ 07030, USA
John Wiley & Sons Ltd, The Atrium, Southern Gate, Chichester, West Sussex, PO19 8SQ, UK

Editorial Office
9600 Garsington Road, Oxford, OX4 2DQ, UK

For details of our global editorial offices, customer services, and more information about Wiley products visit us at www.wiley.com.

Wiley also publishes its books in a variety of electronic formats and by print-on-demand. Some content that appears in standard print versions of this book may not be available in other formats.

Library of Congress Cataloging-in-Publication Data

Names: Johns, Christopher, editor. | Preceded by (work): Johns, Christopher.
    Becoming a reflective practitioner.
Title: Becoming a reflective practitioner / edited by Christopher Johns.
Description: Fifth edition. | Hoboken, NJ : John Wiley & Sons Inc., 2017. |
    Preceded by Becoming a reflective practitioner / Christopher Johns ; with
    contributions from Sally Burnie ... [et al.]. 4th ed. 2013. | Includes
    bibliographical references and index.
Identifiers: LCCN 2016059300 (print) | LCCN 2016059908 (ebook) | ISBN
    9781119193920 (paperback) | ISBN 9781119193937 (Adobe PDF) | ISBN
    9781119193944 (ePub)
Subjects: | MESH: Philosophy, Nursing | Models, Nursing | Thinking
Classification: LCC RT84.5 (print) | LCC RT84.5 (ebook) | NLM WY 86 | DDC
    610.73–dc23
LC record available at https://lccn.loc.gov/2016059300

Cover Design: Wiley
Cover image: © Matt Anderson Photography/Gettyimages

Set in 10/12pt, SabonLTStd by SPi Global, Chennai, India.
Printed by CPI Group (UK) Ltd, Croydon CR0 4YY

10 9 8 7 6 5 4 3 2 1

Contents

Notes on Contributors

Christopher Johns

Formerly Professor of Nursing at University of Bedfordshire, where I continue to supervise PhD students using reflexive narrative. I am also Visiting Professor at Christ Church Canterbury. My academic work is focused on developing reflective practice from clinical, educational and research perspectives reflected in many journal, book and chapter publications, conference presentations and performances. I have convened the International Reflective Practice Conferences since 1993. In 2011 I convened the first Reflective Practice Gathering as a more congruent approach to reflective conferencing through dialogue. *Becoming a reflective practitioner* was first published in 2000. My latest book is *Mindful leadership* published by Palgrave in 2015. My other books are: *The Burford NDU Model: caring in Practice* (1994); *Being mindful, easing suffering* (2004); *Transforming nursing through reflective practice*, second edition with Dawn Freshwater (2005); *Engaging reflection in practice: a narrative approach* (2006); *The good, the wise, and the right clinical nursing practice*, with Charlotte Delmar (2008); *Guided reflection: a narrative approach for advancing practice*, second edition, 2010.

I live in Cornwall with my wife, Otter, and Jerry, our Labrador Retriever. We offer bespoke workshops and consultancy for those interested in developing reflective practice and leadership from any perspective.

c.johns198@btinternet.com

Otter Rose-Johns

My background is in nursing, community and hospice, the latter developing an art room for patients to use for expression. My interests are reflective and mindful practice and using art as a means of discovery, teaching and learning. I have exhibited and performed widely including in Sweden, the United States and Japan. I have recently finished a year-long mentoring course at the Newlyn School Of Art, Cornwall and I have been working with another 14 artists in a group called Drawing Down The Feminine, a travelling show, next due to exhibit in Plymouth. I work with mixed media and intuition, and my work includes wrapping, scratching, covering and scraping. I peel back the layers, almost like getting rid of the ego to find the core of the art and enhance meaning to the piece on which I am working.

Margaret Graham

I am a qualified nurse and lecturer at the Department of Nursing and Midwifery Education and Health Sciences, Faculty University of Limerick, Ireland. I lead and coordinate reflective practice within undergraduate programmes. Exploring how we create dialogical learning spaces with students through reflection, fostering transferable learning to practice is central to my work. I have been a member of a community of inquiry with Professor Chris Johns as Guide in constructing my doctoral thesis. Insights gained through my journey of self-inquiry and transformation, sustain my commitment to the potential of developing practice through reflexive narrative methodologies.

Adenike Akinbode

I am currently working in a university school of Education. My first career was teaching in primary schools and a secondary school after completing my PGCE. Reflective practice has been a research interest for some years. I conducted research for my masters degree into supporting student teachers' reflective practice development. I then went on to self-inquiry through reflective practice for my doctoral research.

Gerald Remy

I am a 53-year-old Afro-Briton who was raised with six siblings in a deprived neighbourhood in southeast London. I grew up with Catholic teachings in a black ghetto environment of crime and violence. I was educated by the code of the streets; the school curriculum lacked cultural competence, so I was inspired by black antisocial leaders in my neighbourhood. My father was hard-working, honest and charismatic. My mother was a strict disciplinarian, but she was my main motivator. As a youth, optimism was stifled because the power of the ghetto gripped and rendered me powerless to achieve. On becoming an adult I was almost lost to every tender feeling until I met my wife and, with our five children, life began to have meaning and purpose. I was energised by a spiritual calling and underwent a transformation to the amazement of my friends and family, turning to Christianity. This prompted me towards self-improvement and I re-educated myself to university degree level in the sciences. Fortunately, I was able to evade the stereotype of black delinquency and became a medical professional in the NHS and am now I am now a respectable State Registered Dietitian in my twentieth year of dietetics. I moved from London to Buckinghamshire in 2004 and became a manager and therapy lead, responsible for a large team of medical professionals in a large public organization, and completed a master's degree in leadership with distinction. The masters gave me insight into the world of reflective practice, which has influenced me ever since and impacted on my team, who now see reflective enquiry as a meaningful requirement for great quality care.

Jill Jarvis

Jill worked as a hospice staff nurse at the time of writing her story as part of her BSc Nursing Studies.

Clare Coward

Clare worked as a psychiatric staff nurse at the time of writing her story as part of her BSc Nursing Studies.

Preface

There are no facts, only interpretations.
Friedrich Nietzsche[1].

Imagine. Otter visits her father in intensive care following a triple heart bypass. A staff nurse is attempting to put some TED compression stockings on his legs. The nurse does not introduce herself. Otter, who is a trained community nurse, anxiously asks 'What are you doing?' 'All patients have them,' the nurse responds. 'That's not how to put them on,' Otter says, 'Here let me show you. But wait, Dad's legs are so swollen and he has arterial disease. I don't think he should have them anyway.' Leaving the nurse, Otter approaches a doctor who confirms Dad should not have the TED stockings applied. Later a ward sister when challenged says 'All staff are taught to apply TED stockings.'

You can draw your own conclusion about this experience but clearly a case of poor professional artistry. Facts aren't enough. Every situation requires interpretation.

Healthcare professions are practice disciplines in changing times. As such, professional education must be primarily concerned with enabling practitioners to develop professional artistry – that knowing necessary to practice. In the uncertain world of practice such knowing is largely intuitive, informed as appropriate by theory or technical rationality. Indeed, theory has always to be applied to inform the particular situation within an organisational context with its own particular mores and resources. Professional practice is a string of experiences, with each experience as a potential learning opportunity. Reflection on experiences is the gateway to developing professional artistry. Such learning ultimately leads to mindful practice and the development of wisdom.

However, education and clinical practice are dominated by a technical rational approach that seeks certainty, predication and control. Hence, as Schon (1983) has illuminated, a tension exists between technical rationality and professional artistry. Whilst reflective practice within curriculum has become normal, it is usually accommodated from a technical rational perspective, thus limiting its learning impact. This book explores this tension and advocates that professional artistry must be the focus of professional healthcare education through a truly reflective approach.

In her introduction to the exhibition catalogue 'Drawing down the feminine' Kate Walters writes – *'this world which seems to me to focus on the surface of things. So I became more alert and looked about myself'.*

These words resonate in relation to education: *this education which seems to me to focus on the surface of things.* No depth. This *surface* is grounded in the technical and rational that fails to value or nurture the intuitive. Take nursing as an example. It is fundamentally concerned with the relationship between nurse and patient. Nothing about this relationship can be assumed to be certain or predictable. Everything is an interpretation depending on context. As such the practitioner's response to the patient is largely intuitive gleaned through understanding the patient's experience and needs and informed as appropriate by the technical, that is unless the patient is viewed as an object to do things to. Then the patient is no more than of technical interest. Disembodied. Education must radically shift to ways of learning and knowing that value and nurture the intuitive rather than skid along the technical surface of things. We need to create opportunity to learn through experience to reveal the very depth of professional artistry. This is the way of reflective practice. And yet, if we are not *alert,* reflective practice too can skid along the surface of things.

Like previous editions, this fifth edition has been extensively scrutinised, revised and developed:

- I have moved to an edited book with guest authors to give wider perspectives on reflective practice;
- I focus more on the idea of *guiding* reflection and in doing so acknowledging that skilled guidance is a necessary for effective reflective learning;
- Linked to the previous point I give greater emphasis to the idea of the 'reflective curriculum' and utilising performance narrative as a curriculum approach;
- I introduce skill boxes through the book to guide and engage readers in reflection and action making the book a more engaging and practical text.

The book is constructed in 25 chapters. Chapter 1 opens the dialogue with a broad gaze at the nature of reflective practice. Reflective practice is at risk of being a cliché with its multiple interpretations that raise the question, what exactly is reflective practice? Of course this concern reflects a technical rationale to know it. If known, it can be applied with prediction and control. Everyone knows what we are talking about. However, this perspective misses the point that reflective practice is fundamentally an ontological quest to know self rather than an epistemological quest to know something, which, whilst important, is a secondary issue.

I have always viewed reflective practice as practical rather than theoretical, as something learned through doing. Indeed, this is true for my own description of reflective practice through the six dialogical movements.

In Chapters 2–6 I develop the artistry of reflective practice through six dialogical movements, commencing with *bringing the mind home* and *writing self.* The idea of bringing the mind home is to learn to pay attention to experience. Paying attention is also a highly significant clinical skill. It is simply learned using the breath.

Writing self is the raw data of experience and sets up the reflective encounter using the Model for Structured Reflection [MSR]. I have revised the MSR, now in its 17th edition, to better appreciate the essence of reflective practice. From global feedback, I get the impression that many people think that simply using the MSR *is* reflective practice. Worse they view a model of reflection as a prescription. It isn't! It is a heuristic, a means to an end towards gaining insight. I urge readers to dwell with the MSR, to feel the depth of the cues rather than view it superficially and skid along the surface of reflection. If approached superficially, reflection looses its vitality. It can become a chore and waste of time. It must be taken seriously. In Chapter 5 I explore dialogue between insights and an informing literature. This is the value of technical rationality: to inform rather than control knowing. No theory is accepted on face value but is always critiqued for its value to inform. I also explore the art of guiding reflection, arguing that guidance is imperative for learning through reflection. In Chapter 6 I explore the expression of insights in a reflexive narrative form. Insights are the manifestation of learning and yet they are not easy to articulate, given that much knowing in practice is tacit. Insights often emerge over time, recognised reflexively within subsequent experiences. Perhaps it is easier to ask someone what was significant about an experience rather than what insights were gained from it. Significance points the finger at insights.

The word 'narrative' has seeped into everyday speak. I wonder, does this seepage indicate that we have moved beyond the technical rational to value experience and anecdote? Or is *narrative* simply a word that means 'the story' or 'vision'. Whatever, it does suggest a valuing of context and subjectivity; that people are not machines. People are human and their experience is human and unique. And that no matter the difficulty, learning through reflection is dynamic. Narrative is creative and cannot be prescribed, even though academic institutions will nevertheless impose criteria about how it should be expressed.

In Chapter 7, I advocate a poetic approach, not simply for its aesthetic value and expressive pleasure but as a way of opening up language to reveal and communicate insights. In Chapter 8 Otter and I explore storyboard as a visual approach to reflection and narrative that may offer an alternative to language approaches and hence may benefit visual reflectors. Like poetry, breaking narrative into visual scenes aids the revelation of insights. Poetry and art are expressive forms that open up the neglected right brain, moving away from rational thought to nurture imagination, perception and ultimately intuition.

In Chapter 9, I contemplate the reflective curriculum. It is fascinating to look back at the two immediately preceding editions to see this chapter's reflexive development. It is the most vital chapter because the health discipline curriculum is so entrenched in a technical rational modus that reflection is viewed as just another technical rational approach. If so, its real value is lost. The reflective curriculum views professional artistry and identity as its education aim, and reflective practice as its primary approach, re-orienting theory to inform this process. In other words, it turns the traditional relationship between practice and theory on its head. Easier said than done.

In Chapter 10, I give an example of my reflective thinking in preparing for a teaching session on reflective practice. It shows the problem of falling between two stools, of wanting to be in control of a session and yet wanting it to be open and dialogical.

In Chapter 11, I offer an example of reflective writing and explore how reflective academic writing can be meaningfully graded from a professional artistry perspective in contrast to a technical rational perspective.

Chapter 12 offers a further example of reflective writing for readers faced with setting and writing reflective assignments. Students must feel free to express themselves rather than have stringent criteria imposed on the way they write. The imposition is resented, resisted, and its value diminished.

In Chapter 13, Margaret Graham reflects on using story in her teacher teaching and its learning significance through evaluating student response. Teaching becomes alive through relevant story because students can easily relate to it through their own experiences, especially in addressing difficult topics such as family abuse where stories are often hidden through fear and shame.

Chapters 14 and 15 open a dialogical space to contemplate guiding nursing students. The two situations – Michelle finding a woman upset about her breast biopsy and Hank's complaint – are real situations that were shared with me in clinical supervision (Johns 2013). I have transposed these situations into how they could be explored within first-year and third-year student guided reflection groups. As you would expect, the first-year group is more directed whilst the third-year group is more open, reflecting the curriculum agenda and experience of the student both in reflective learning and the topics being explored.

In Chapter 17, I imagine how two teachers with differing teaching methods educate nursing students about stroke. John takes a theory-driven line typical of the dominant technical rational approach. Jane takes a reflective approach that embraces performance and with it, cross-discipline teaching. At Bedfordshire I involved drama and dance teachers as co-supervisors for reflexive narrative doctoral students. Their involvement opened up the performance potential as a profound learning space. Performance engages and empowers people. It is an embodied learning that is necessary for practice disciplines where the body has to learn rather than the mind simply think.

Much reflective practice teaching in universities is carried out by people who are not reflective. As a consequence they apply inappropriate technical rational approaches to the teaching of reflection. This whole book is itself a treatise on the need to create reflective learning environments if we are to practise reflective practice critically rather than as a superficial problem-solving technique. Of course, it has value even at that level if it enables practitioners to pause and reflect on what they are doing in terms of best practice. But much of what we do and the way we think about what we do is culturally prescribed. So, if the value of reflective practice to develop professional artistry is to be more than a technical rational approach to the doing of reflection, the reflective teacher, like the reflective practitioner, must lift this cultural veil to understand and shift the norms that govern teaching of teachers.

In Chapter 17, Adenike, herself a teacher of teachers, relates the classroom to chaos theory – that nothing is certain or predictable despite previous experience, and that order evolves around meaning. In other words, order is inherent and unfolds. This means the teacher does not have to worry about 'controlling' the classroom. Indeed the more she tries to control the classroom the more difficulty she will have with control. It is the same with the clinical health environment: order manifests itself around meaning. Hence, the attempt to control the healthcare environment is counter-productive. Things work just fine or even better when left to unfold naturally around meaning such as the intention to care.

So when Adenike writes – 'I view the idea of teacher as "strange attractor" as a valuable way to understand what takes place in the classroom' we can see its parallel - 'I view the idea of nurse as "strange attractor" as a valuable way to understand what takes place in the clinical environment.' Hence, the way the nurse teacher performs role models how the nurse might perform. Reflection lifts this dynamic into mindfulness, hence processes become more significant than outcomes or, put another way, get the process right and the outcomes naturally emerge. In Chapter 18 Adenike explores a range of issues that face her as a reflective teacher, notably emotional ethical issues. It is so easy to get caught up in the classroom tension – mindfulness falls away and the teacher resorts to learned ways of dealing with her anxiety. Hence the pivotal idea of poise as clinician or teacher and as a hallmark of mindful practice.

In Chapter 19, I turn my attention to creating the reflective clinical environment in which reflective practitioners can flourish. This is based on my work developing the Burford NDU Model of nursing: caring in practice. Experience, such as depicted in 'People are not Numbers to Crunch' (Chapter 23), illuminates the mechanical approach to assessment based on set questions, an approach that is insensitive and unreflective. Applying a person-centred vision, practitioners need to tune into the person to identify and focus on his or her health needs. Unequivocally, this must be the basis for care. Reflective systems of quality, staff development and communication are designed to support this focus against a background of leadership and learning culture.

In Chapter 20, I pick up the idea of a reflective quality system through developing standards of care, imagining an actual standards group. Setting standards may be time-consuming yet its value is immense, begging the question, how much effort should be devoted to ensuring quality as something lived rather than having quality judgement imposed through systems such as CQC? Surely any professional should be actively involved in ensuring quality of her performance? In Chapter 21 I examine the idea of clinical supervision as both a quality and developmental process through my supervision of Trudy over six sessions. In doing so I endeavour to portray its reflexive movement.

In Chapter 22, Gerald Remy reflects on his leadership. The need for strong leadership is acknowledged with the NHS Forward Review[2] at a time of radical change. However, it needs to be the right type of leadership. Gerald was part of a learning community of ten aspiring healthcare leaders. I emphasise community for at least five reasons. Firstly, from a leadership perspective, creating community is fundamental requirement for any leader. Secondly, I believe that learning through community whereby others in a similar aspiring boat are available to each other through a period of time (in this case 28 months) enhances learning through reflection. Community creates the conditions for dialogue for a group of learners aspiring to similar goals. This idea permeates many of the chapters in the book and reinforces the need for guides to be themselves leaders and skilled at guiding others to learn through reflection. Indeed this ability to guide learning in others is a prime quality of leadership.

Thirdly, there is the question of whether learning can be sustained without guidance, especially in a hostile culture that puts constant pressure on the practitioner to conform to organizational norms that are previously learned ways of being. The ability to sustain learning, against the grain so to speak, is reflected in the extent to which reflection has become inculcated within the practitioner's community rather than being merely an individual thing. Gerald suggests he has achieved that to some extent, although it remains precarious as he continues to holds creative tension. Of course, in terms of the efficacy of reflective learning, this issue of sustained learning at depth of is of vital concern; it underlines the necessity of, first, a clear understanding of the nature of reality (organizational norms that govern everyday ways of relating]) and, secondly, being able to detach self from the anxiety of transgressing these norms. Living this tension is akin to playing a subversive and dangerous game of survival where guidance is vital.

Fourthly, Gerald's chapter opens up a dimension on expressing learning through metaphor. Gerald, like all NHS staff, has been socialised into the transactional culture that governs healthcare organisations. Hence the idea of being a servant-leader or a transformational leader is immediately at odds with this culture. It raises the question 'How can one come to appreciate and separate self from this culture whilst being immersed within it, a culture where one's every action has been socialised towards being transactional from either a subordinate or managerial perspective?' Gerald used the metaphor of David and Goliath to see and work with this tension. If the tension is not addressed then learning is limited, and yet one can see how difficult it is to unlearn learned ways of knowing (embodiment) to begin to respond differently and without coercive fear.

Fifthly, Gerald highlights the significance of one's background in shaping the person. To become a leader from a servant-leader or transformational perspective required Gerald to look back at his upbringing in order to understand how his background influences who he is now and whom he seeks to become. He recognises the tension between a Goliath within and a David within, and accepts the need to vanquish his Goliath through his David. Anybody learning through reflection will need to consider their background – perhaps using the Influences Grid in Chapter 3, Table 3.4 (how does my background influence the way I respond within this particular situation/ experience?).

Chapters 23, 24 and 25 offer three performances. Performances are stylised narrative written to intentionally open a dialogical space towards social action. By focusing on unsatisfactory situations they intend to disturb an audience into action. 'People are not Numbers to Crunch' is my reflection on accompanying Otter for an angiogram. Here, performance intends to expose the unsatisfactory behaviour of nurses who do not introduce themselves and treat Otter as if she is an object and myself as an outsider beyond their gaze. The performance is set against a CQC report of care at this particular hospital. Hence, I reflect not so much as a clinician but as a relative. 'Smoking Kills' was initially written as an educational performance for young people based around my care for three men dying of lung cancer in a hospice. The performance has many themes that can be adapted for different audiences. I developed the performance to focus on the way that tough men dying can problematise the hospice approach. Later I added the supervision scenario to illustrate unsatisfactory guidance. 'Anthea: An Inquiry into Dignity' is based on an experience shared by a staff nurse in guided reflection (personified as 'Kate' in the actual performance). I then developed the performance based on Anthea's discharge home raising controversial issues for audience to discuss. All these performances are powerful teaching tools. They can involve students in their performances and give teachers and students pointers to constructing their own, as I suggested in Chapter 16.

Throughout the book I usually refer to practitioners rather than specific healthcare practitioners. An exception is the particular focus on teaching nurses in Chapters 14–16. I generally use 'her' to represent people. I also use a different referencing format for performance-related chapters.

Endnotes

1   Wicks, Robert, "Friedrich Nietzsche", *The Stanford Encyclopedia of Philosophy* (Fall 2016 Edition), Edward N. Zalta (ed.), URL = http://plato.stanford.edu/archives/fall2016/entries/nietzsche/ .

2   https://www.england.nhs.uk/wp-content/uploads/2014/10/5yfv-web.pdf

Reference

Schön D (1983) *The reflective practitioner*. Avebury, Aldershot.

About the Companion Website

This book is accompanied by a companion website:

www.wiley.com/go/johns/reflectivepractitioner

The website consists of:

Powerpoint images for chapters 24 and 25

Chapter 1

Imagining Reflective Practice

Christopher Johns

Experience is a creative encounter

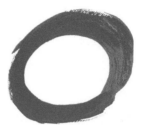

Hi, I'm beady eye. I'm called beady eye because I like to keep my eye on what's going on the quality of healthcare.

I was sitting in the train the other day
When a woman hobbles on
Finds a seat to put her leg up
She says to her mate
'They just don't care anymore
She didn't look properly at my foot
She wasn't interested
Told me it was probably a corn
Wasn't listening to me
Told her the pain was in me 'eel
In the end she said
'Your 10 minutes are up
Got to see someone else.'
Her mate rolls her eyes
'Bloody awful ain't it
Chiropody on the NHS.'

Becoming a Reflective Practitioner, Fifth Edition. Edited by Christopher Johns.
© 2017 John Wiley & Sons Ltd. Published 2017 by John Wiley & Sons Ltd.
Companion Website: www.wiley.com/go/johns/reflectivepractitioner

Such experience reminds me of the fragile quality of health care. I wonder how the chiropodist would recall the event? Bet she isn't a reflective practitioner!!

You'll meet me again in some later chapters. Until then enjoy the book.

O'Donohue (1997: 26) writes, 'Everything that happens to you has the potential to deepen you.' This potential is actuated through reflection as a self-inquiry into experience to find meaning, gain insight and prompt action that will deepen you.

Reflection enables you to understand yourself and, on that basis, to take leadership of your professional life. By leadership I mean the action towards realising your values or vision about your practice.

Recall a situation when you were last at work and ask yourself – 'Did I respond in tune with my values?' which, of course, raises the question 'What are my values?' I assume as a healthcare practitioner you hold a set of values or a vision that is important in guiding your individual and collective practice. Now, ask yourself – 'Did I respond in the most effective way?' Be open and curious about that. Did you choose to respond in that way or was it your normal practice? How do you know if you were effective? Perhaps there are more effective ways? Think about what factors influence your response. What interferes with realising effective practice? As a consequence of this self-inquiry, you become more sensitive to your values and the notion of your effective practice. As such, you step along a reflective road.

Reflective Practice

Reflective practice has become a normal requirement within professional curriculum and, as such, demands serious consideration. However, the words *reflection* and *reflective practice* are often used glibly in everyday discourse, as if reflection is simply a normal way of thinking about something that has happened and which requires little skill or guidance. Smyth (1992: 285) writes:

> Reflection can mean all things to all people ... it is used as a kind of umbrella or canopy term to signify something that is good or desirable ... everybody has his or her own (usually undisclosed) interpretation of what reflection means, and this interpretation is used as the basis for trumpeting the virtues of reflection in a way that makes it sound as virtuous as motherhood.

Smyth's words are both salutary and provocative. They remind us to be careful about defining reflection in an authoritative way and yet, on the other hand, practitioners do need something to grasp, a conceptual grasp on reality.

Turning to the *Compact Oxford English Dictionary* 3rd edition (2005: 86), it defines 'reflect' as:

> throw back heat, light, sound without absorbing it
> [of a mirror or shiny surface] show an image of
> represent in a realistic or appropriate way
> bring about a good or bad impression of someone or something [on]
> think deeply or carefully about

Interpreting this array of definitions, reflection can be viewed as a mirror to see images or impressions of self in the context of a particular situation in a realistic way. It is an awareness of the understanding about the way the person thinks and feels about whatever he is experiencing. It is also judgemental, distinguishing between good and bad. If healthcare is concerned with understanding and responding to the experiences of people who require care then it is first necessary for the practitioner to understand herself.

My description of reflection is always evolving –

> Being mindful of self, either within or after experience, as if a mirror in which the practitioner can view and focus self within the context of a particular experience, in order to confront, understand, and become empowered to act towards resolving contradiction between one's vision of desirable practice and one's actual practice to gain insight within a reflexive spiral towards realising one's vision of practice as a lived reality and developing professional identity and artistry.

Contradiction

The learning potential of reflective practice is the contradiction between one's vision of practice and one's actual practice as recalled. Contradiction is usually experienced as a 'disturbance' that things are unsatisfactory in some way. However, because contradiction is so normal, it may not be noticed, or simply shrugged off. As such, much of experience is unexamined.

To explore contradiction it is necessary for the practitioner to have a vision of her practice. A vision gives purpose and direction to clinical practice. It is constructed from a set of values that are ideally constructed and shared with colleagues. In this way everyone pulls in the same direction. The practitioner must inquire into her vision. For example, if the vision states words such as 'caring', 'holistic' or 'excellent', then what do these words mean as something lived? Vision is thus a moveable feast.

Yet, It is one thing having a vision of practice it is another thing to realise it as something lived (Rawnsley 1990).

The practitioner must first seek to understand the nature of the contradiction. Only when practitioners truly understand themselves and the conditions of their practice can they begin to realistically change and respond differently. To understand, the reflective practitioner creeps 'underneath his habitual explanations of his actions, outside his regularized statements of his objectives' (Pinar 1981: 177).

The practitioner must then act towards resolving the contradiction. If people were rational they would change their practice on the basis of evidence that supports the best way of doing something. However, we do not live in a rational world. There are powerful barriers that limit the practitioner's ability to respond differently even when they know there is a better way to respond. Fay (1987) identifies these barriers as tradition, authority or force, and embodiment. These barriers govern the fabric of our social world. Their influence lies thick within any experience. They are evident in patterns of talk that reflect deeply embodied and embedded relationships that serve the status quo (Kopp 2000). Reflections are stories of resistance and possibility; chipping away at resistance and opening up possibility; confronting and shifting these barriers to become who we desire to be as health care practitioners.

Barriers to rational change (Fay 1987)

- Tradition: a pre-reflective state reflected in the assumptions and habitual practices that people hold about the way things should be.
- Force: the way normal relationships are constructed and maintained through the use of power/ force.
- Embodiment: the way people have been socialised to think, feel and respond to the world in a normative and pre-reflective way.

Fay (1987: 75) writes from a critical social science perspective,

> The goal of a critical social science is not only to facilitate methodical self-reflection necessary to produce rational clarity, but to dissolve those barriers which prevent people from living in accordance with their genuine will. Put in another way, its aim is to help people not only to be transparent to themselves but also to cease being mere objects in the world, passive victims dominated by forces external to them.

In other words, reflection is concerned with empowerment. The language of a critical social science may be intimidating with its rhetoric of oppression and misery, yet it can be argued that nursing's largely female workforce has been oppressed by patriarchal attitudes that renders it docile and politically passive, and thus limits its ability to fulfil its therapeutic potential. If so, then realising desirable practice would require an overthrow of oppressive political and cultural systems. The link between oppression and patriarchy is obvious, considering nursing as women's work, and the suppression of women's voices 'knowing their place' within the patriarchal order of things. Images of 'behind the screens' where women conceal their work, themselves, and their significance (Lawler 1991) and images of emotional labour being no more than women's natural work, therefore unskilled and unvalued within the heroic stance of medicine (James 1989), are powerful signs of this oppression.

Maxine Greene (1988: 58) writes,

> Concealment does not simply mean hiding; it means dissembling, presenting something as other than it is. To 'unconceal' is to create clearings, spaces in the midst of things where decisions can be made. It is to break through the masked and the falsified, to reach toward what is also half-hidden or concealed. When a woman, when any human being, tries to tell the truth and act on it, there is no predicting what will happen. The 'not yet' is always to a degree concealed. When one chooses to act on one's freedom, there are no guarantees.

Reflection opens up a clearing where desirable practice and the barriers that constrain its realisation can be *unconcealed* and understood, where action can be planned to overcome the barriers whatever their source, and where the practitioner is empowered to take necessary action to resolve contradiction. No easy task, for these barriers are embodied, they structure practice and patterns of relating. Fear is a powerful deterrent to being different. It suppresses practitioners from speaking their truth. The commitment to the truth is evident in Greene's words. Yet how comfortable are people in their illusions of truth? Is it better to conform than rock the boat? Is it better to sacrifice the ideal for a quiet life and the patronage of more powerful others? Better to keep your head down than have it shot off above the parapet for daring to reveal the truth?

As such, reflection is always in context. Context is the background against which experience is positioned. 'Context refers to the grand societal narratives, those clusters of beliefs and cultural norms that give shape and meaning to the human cultures within which we live' (Dawson (2015: 25). All too often, when people reflect, the background is ignored or alluded to in a superficial way. Hence, reflection can help the *loosening of authority*. Dawson continues

> Within this context, personal narratives of becoming, whatever the focus of that becoming, can be viewed as 'a loosening of the authority' of the grand narratives of science and education where the dominant construction of the learning self is the receptor of knowledge.

Of course we can passively accept the grand narratives as our truth. Yet even to passively accept suggests we have become aware of the narratives, and such awareness begins to change them. We would always be restless knowing about them and knowing we were unable to shift them. It is hitting a reality wall that frustrates and gives headaches. Perhaps ignorance is bliss. Better to swim in the shallow waves than drown in the rip currents of critical reflection? Taking reflection seriously leads to these considerations from a critical reflection stance. From a technical rational perspective, reflection is no more than problem-posing and problem-solving.

Empowerment

To reiterate, reflection is concerned with empowerment. This may require guidance as explored through subsequent chapters. Empowerment is enhanced when practitioners are committed to and take responsibility for their practice, have strong values, and understand why things are as they are. However, empowerment is not easy for practitioners socialised into norms that render them docile.

Kieffer (1984: 27) noted that the process of empowerment involved

> reconstructing and re-orientating deeply engrained personal systems of social relations. Moreover they confront these tasks in an environment which historically has enforced their political oppression and which continues its active and implicit attempts at subversion and constructive change.

The truth of the situation is stark – if practitioners truly wish to truly live their visions of practice then they have no choice but to become political in working towards establishing the conditions of practice *where that is possible*. The practitioner must come to realise a new reality for herself, rather than have this reality explained to her. For example, many experiences that practitioners reflect on are concerned with conflict that has a fundamental power inequality at their root that manifests itself through different attitudes, beliefs and behaviours. This is not difficult to see or understand providing it is sought, and not just taken for granted as part of the 'natural' background of the experience.

Empowerment reflects integrity. It is not easy to be silent when faced with injustice or uncaring. Yet so many practitioner voices are silent or suppressed for fear of sanction.

They lack agency to formulate and attain their goals. They depict their lives as out of their control, shaped by events beyond their control. Others' actions determine life outcomes, and the accomplishment or failure to achieve life goals depends on factors they are unable to change. To view self as a victim is to experience a loss of personhood and to project the blame for this loss onto others rather than take responsibility for self. Victims are oriented towards avoiding negative possibilities than to actualising positive possibilities.

Bruner (1994: 41) notes that persons construct a victimic self by

> reference to memories of how they responded to the agency of somebody else who had the power to impose his or her will upon them, directly or indirectly by controlling the circumstances in which they are compelled to live.

In theory, reflection would enhance the core ingredients of personal agency; self-determination; self-legislation; meaningfulness; purposefulness; confidence; active-striving; playfulness; and responsibility (Cochran and Laub, 1994 cited in Polkingthorne 1996).

Through reflection, the practitioner creates a plot out of a succession of actions, as if to direct to her in the midst of action. Locating ourselves within an intelligible story is essential to our sense that life is meaningful. The practitioner tries to make certain things happen, to bring about desirable endings, to search for possibilities that lead in hopeful directions. Kermode (1966: 813) writes,

> Because we act with the sense of an ending, we try to direct our actions and the actions of others that will bring the ending about.

The idea that reflection can help the individual practitioner turn this scenario around is fraught with difficulty. Reflection can so easily be like swimming in the shallow end of a deep swimming pool, literally splashing about with surface issues rather than tackling the deeper political and systems issues necessary to support best practice. However, that is not to say that tackling surface issues is not important, as indeed is developing reflective skills and understanding deeper issues even if they are not amenable to change on an individual level. The need for collective reflection and action becomes vital for organisational change.

Reflexivity

Reflexivity is the practitioner 'looking back' to see self becoming in the sense of realising desirable practice set against an analysis of forces that have constrained her, evidenced through a chain of experiences whereby one link of the chain leaves a thread that is picked up and developed by the next link (Dewey 1933). It is a review of one's journey of learning through reflection whereby the threads are weaved into a coherent pattern expressed as narrative (see Chapter 6).

Span of Reflective Practices

Reflection and reflective practice can be interpreted in different ways. As Smith (2011: 212) writes,

> Despite widespread and long standing commitment to the notion of critical reflection across the health and social care professions, it can be difficult to assimilate into teaching because the language is complex, and the same terminology is used in different ways in different contexts so carries different nuances.

Reflective practices span a number of approaches (Table 1.1):

- From *doing* reflection towards *being* reflective.
- From a technical rational to a professional artistry perspective.
- An increasing criticality.

Doing reflection reflects an epistemological approach, as if reflection is a tool or device. *Being* reflective reflects an ontological approach concerned more with 'who I am' rather than 'what I do'. Bulman, Lathlean and Gobbi (2012), in their investigation of student and teacher perspectives on reflective practice, revealed that a focus on being rather than doing was significant. The ontological approach subsumes the epistemological, as if the way we think about and do things must involve we who are to think about things in the first place. Doing reflection reflects a technical rational approach whereas being reflective reflects a professional artistry approach. Criticality reflects the depth of inquiry into the background that frames experience.

Table 1.1 Typology of reflective practices

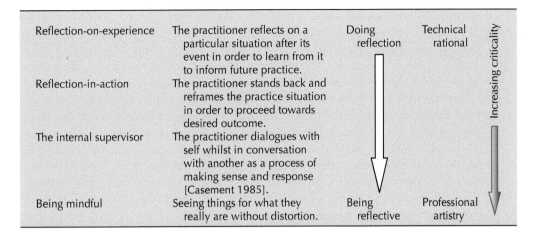

Reflection-on-experience	The practitioner reflects on a particular situation after its event in order to learn from it to inform future practice.	Doing reflection	Technical rational	
Reflection-in-action	The practitioner stands back and reframes the practice situation in order to proceed towards desired outcome.			Increasing criticality
The internal supervisor	The practitioner dialogues with self whilst in conversation with another as a process of making sense and response [Casement 1985].			
Being mindful	Seeing things for what they really are without distortion.	Being reflective	Professional artistry	

Reflection-on-experience

When people refer to reflection, they usually refer to reflection-on-experience. Indeed, most theories of reflection are based on this idea of looking back on 'an experience'; something done after the event. Experience can be thinking, feeling or doing something. As a verb, 'experience' is 'something I encounter and which leaves an impression on me' (*COED* 3rd edition 2005: 349). If experience doesn't make an impression presumably it is not significant in any way, or just routine practice.

Reflection-in-action

Schön (1983, 1987) distinguished reflection-*on-action* with reflection-*in-action* as a way of thinking about a situation whilst engaged within it, in order to reframe it as necessary to overcome some impediment. The practitioner naturally adjusts to minor interruptions within the smooth flow of experience because the body has embodied knowing. However, the practitioner is sometimes faced with situations that require her to stop and reframe the situation in order to proceed. This requires a shift in thinking and contemplating new ways of responding. As such it is problem-solving yet recognising that old ways of thinking are inadequate. Reflection is the practitioner's unique encounter and conversation with a situation through which, as Schön (1983: 163) puts it 'he shapes it and makes himself part of it'.

Schön (1987) drew on exemplars from music and architecture, situations of engagement with inanimate forms. His example of counselling is taken from the classroom not from clinical practice. The classroom is a much easier place to freeze and reframe situations in contrast with clinical practice grounded within the unfolding human encounter. It is easy to misunderstand reflection-in-action as merely thinking about something whilst doing it.

The Internal Supervisor

Casement (1985) coined the expression the 'internal supervisor' as a continuous dialogue the practitioner has with herself in response to the unfolding situation, 'What is going on here?' 'How am I responding?' etc. The practitioner is also mindful of intent – 'What am I trying to achieve?' It is a more dynamic form of reflection-in-action.

Being Mindful

Being mindful is an extension of the internal supervisor. Being mindful, the practitioner is aware of her pattern of intention, thinking, feeling and actions moment by moment without distortion. Goldstein (2002: 89) writes, 'Mindfulness is the quality of mind that notices what is present without judgment, without interference. It is like a mirror that clearly reflects what comes before it.'

Goldstein writes from a Buddhist perspective whereby being mindful is being aware moment by moment of things and the world around us, of our body, our feelings and thoughts, of self in relationship with others, and of ultimate reality. Ultimate reality can be viewed on two levels: the mundane level being concerned with holding and intending to realise a vision of practice; the transcendental level concerned with spiritual growth. Realising the mundane is inevitably a movement towards the transcendental. Being mindful, I know myself in what I am doing and why I am doing it, and aware of any contradiction with my intention.

Wheatley and Keller-Rogers (1996: 26) write,

> The more present and aware we are as individuals and as organisations, the more choices we create. As awareness increases, we can engage with more possibilities. We are no longer held prisoner by habits, unexamined thoughts, or information we refuse to look at.

Being mindful I am vigilant against unskilful actions and negative mental events that constantly try to distract the mind, for example anger, arrogance, resentment, envy, greed and the suchlike (Sangharakshita 1998). In Buddhism, this quality of mind is called *Apramada* – the guard at the gate of the senses ever watchful for those negative mental events that cloud the mind.

Becoming mindful is the ultimate goal of reflective practice and essence of professional artistry. It is that quality of being clearly aware of self within the moment and what self needs to do.

A Brief View of Reflective Theories

When I first explored reflective theories I discovered the work of Mezirow (1981), Schön (1983, 1987), Boyd and Fales (1983), Boud, Keogh and Walker (1985), and Gibbs (1988). Although these references are dated, they remain key contributions, although the work of other theorists is significant, especially in the field of education. It is not my intention to review this work in any depth. The reader is directed to the primary sources to explore these theories more deeply.

Boyd and Fales (1983)

These authors write,

> We define reflection as the process of creating and clarifying the meaning of experience (present or past) in terms of self (self in relation to self and self in relation to the world). The outcome of the process is changed conceptual perspective. The experience that is explored and examined to create meaning focuses around or embodies a concern of central importance to the self. (p. 101)

From their research with counsellors they extrapolate reflection through six components (p. 106):

- a sense of inner discomfort;
- identification or clarification of the concern;
- openness to new information from internal and external sources, with ability to observe and take in from a variety of perspectives, and a setting aside of an immediate need for closure;
- resolution, expressed as 'integration', 'coming together', 'acceptance of reality', and 'creative synthesis';
- establishing a continuity of self with past, present and future;
- deciding whether to act on the outcome of the reflective process.

In relation to stage 6, Boyd and Fales note 'the new insight or changed perspective is analyzed in terms of its operational feasibility (p. 112) involving the practitioner's sense of rightness, values and potential acceptance by others'.

I generally agree that reflection is triggered by 'inner discomfort' for practitioners first engaging with reflection. However, as the practitioner becomes more mindful, then all experience, not just 'inner discomfort' becomes available for reflection. I equate the idea of changed conceptual perspective with insight (see Chapters 4 and 5).

Boud, Keogh and Walker (1985)

These authors posit reflection as moving through three key stages:

- returning to experience;
- attending to feelings: utilizing positive feelings, removing obstructing feelings;
- re-evaluating experience: re-examining experience in light of the learner's intent, associating new knowledge with that which is already possessed, integrating this new knowledge into the learner's conceptual framework, and appropriation of this knowledge into the learner's repertoire of behaviour

Appropriation is akin to gaining insight; the practitioner has changed through the reflective process, so that when faced with a similar situation she will respond differently. This differs from Boyd and Fales's approach, in that the practitioner makes a choice whether to respond differently in light of learning. Boyd and Fales (1983: 112) write, 'The need to test one's self-changes [insights] against the mirror of others is an essential component of all growth.' These words emphasise that all individual learning must be set within its context.

Gibbs (1988)

Gibbs offers a reflective circle moving through six stages:

- description (of the situation);
- feelings (What were you thinking and feeling?);
- evaluation (What was good and bad about the experience?);
- analysis (What sense can you make of the situation?);
- conclusion (What else could you have done?);
- action plan (If it arose again what would you do?).

Feedback from students using this model suggests that stages 3 and 4 are similar and hence confusing to distinguish. The same with stages 5 and 6. Gibbs lacks an intellectual edge evident in Boud and Keogh and Walker's approach, notably the process of 're-evaluating experience'. However stage 6 has a practical element that can lead into a new cycle of reflection.

Mezirow (1981)

Mezirow offers a radically different perspective. He viewed reflection as a process leading to emancipatory action. He posited a depth of reflection through seven levels of reflectivity spanning from consciousness, the way we might think about something, to critical consciousness where we pay attention and scrutinise our thinking processes. Thinking is inherently problematic. Hence our thinking is a focus for reflection. Hence I need to think differently to perceive the situation differently, and in doing so, to unearth those assumptions that govern thinking. If reflection is viewed merely as a problem-solving, and we used the same thinking to solve the problem that caused the problem, then we wouldn't get very far. Our solutions would quickly break down. He conceptualised the outcome of reflection as *perspective transformation,*

> the process of becoming critically aware of how and why the structure of psycho-cultural assumptions has come to constrain the way we see ourselves and our relationships, reconstituting this structure to permit a more inclusive and discriminating integration of experience and acting upon these new understandings. (1981: 6)

Mezirow's focus on understanding assumptions takes reflection into what is generally regarded as a 'critical' domain. The focus on emancipatory action is to rewrite one's own and collective assumptions to govern a more satisfactory state of affairs, however that might be framed.

Balancing the Winds

The above theories all stem from a rational Western cognitive tradition reflected in their words, ideas and language. Put another way, they all come from one direction or 'wind'. My engagement with and exploration of Buddhism and Native American lore gave me wider perspectives and different winds that give a balance between knowing and wisdom (Johns 2005). It is not enough to 'know' reflection. It is deeper than that – it is about developing wisdom, something beyond rational thinking that is not easily defined. Certainly, the idea of mindfulness stems from Buddhism as I view reflection as a contemplative and meditative form tending towards seeing reality clearly. From a native American wind I suggest reading *Earth Dance Drum* to view reflection as a way to connect with all things, gain respect, inner strength and to realise one's vision as reflected in the idea of *bimadisiwin*.
    Jones and Jones (1996: 47) write,

> Bimadisiwin is a conscious decision to become. It is time to think about what you want to be. The dance cannot be danced until you envision the dance, rehearse its movements and understand your part. It is demanding, for every step needs an effort in becoming one with the vision. It takes discipline, hard work and time. It is freeing, for its frees the spirit. It releases you to become as you believe you must.

Such words stir the imagination. Bimadisiwin is reflection. It is a ritual dance of becoming.

> Listen to the drum!
> Believe in the vision of you
> Practice the vision
> Become the vision.

Prerequisites of Reflection

Fay (1987) identifies certain qualities of mind that are prerequisites to reflection: curiosity, commitment and intelligence. These qualities of mind are significant to counter the more negative qualities of mind associated with defensiveness, habit, resistance and ignorance.

Commitment

Commitment is energy that sparks life. Yet, for many practitioners, commitment to their practice has become numb, or blunted through working in non-challenging, non-supportive, and generally stressful environments, where work satisfaction is making it through work with minimal hassle. These practitioners do not enjoy reflection. They turn their heads away from the reflective mirror because the reflected images are not positive. They do not want to face themselves and accept responsibility for their practice. Things wither and die if not cared for. When those things are people, then the significance of commitment is only too apparent. Commitment harmonises or balances the conflict of contradiction – it is the energy that helps us to face up to unacceptable situations. The small child is ambivalent about learning to walk; he stumbles and falls, he hurts himself. It is a painful process. Yet the satisfaction of developing his potential far outweighs the bumps and bruises (Rogers 1969).

van Manen (1990: 58) writes,

> Retrieving or recalling the essence of caring is not a simple matter of simple etymological analysis or explication of the usage of the word. Rather, it is the construction of a way of life to live the language of our lives more deeply, to become more truly who we are when we refer to ourselves [as nurses, doctors, therapists].

Curiosity

Curiosity is self-inquiry, questioning who I am and what I do. It is the opening up of possibility. Gadamer (1975: 266) writes,

> The opening up and keeping open of possibilities is only possible because we find ourselves deeply interested in that which makes the question possible in the first place. To truly question something is to interrogate something from the threat of our existence, from the centre of our being.

Curiosity is fundamental to the creative life and yet many practitioners are locked into habitual patterns of practice. Often, when things get overly familiar, we take them for granted and get into a habitual groove.

O'Donohue (1997: 122–3) writes,

> People have difficulty awakening to their inner world, especially when their lives become familiar to them. They find it hard to discover something new, interesting or adventurous in their numbed lives.

Curiosity is turning over pebbles, wondering what lies on the other side, while open to the possibilities of viewing the same thing from different perspectives.

Intelligence

Being intelligent, the practitioner is open to self in response to new ideas, keen to explore their value for practice rather than be defensive in viewing new ideas as a threat. Intelligence moves beyond abstract knowledge into a deeper awareness of self that Krishnamurti terms intuition.

Krishnamurti (1996: 89) writes,

> There is an intelligent revolt [against environment] which is not reaction but comes with self-knowledge through the awareness of one's own thought and feeling. It is only when we face experience that we keep intelligence highly awakened; and intelligence highly awakened is intuition, which is the only true guide in life.

Put another way, reflection nurtures intelligence and intelligence nurtures intuition, the very essence of professional artistry.

The Significance of Reflective Practices for Professional Practice

Reflective practice is the gateway to appreciating and developing the nature of professional identity and artistry. For a practice discipline nothing can be more significant. These issues are not theoretical, they can only be gleaned within practice. Take the example of caring. Frank (2002: 13) writes,

> Caring is one of those activities that people know only when they are involved in it. From within, and only from within, caring makes sense. To try and explain care leads to the circularity expressed in statements such as 'caring for this person requires doing this, and I do this because I care for this person'. Philosophy teaches that, for some activities, there is only practice.

It follows that if we accept Frank's position, we can only know caring from within caring – the professional artistry perspective. Caring is therefore not a thing that can be known as an abstract idea. The practitioner knows herself as caring only within the moment.

Through reflection the practitioner comes to understand the nature of reality, the background against which she practices, and to empower her to take action, by herself or with others, to transform the background as necessary to realise desirable practice. It is the quest of any professional who takes herself seriously.

Consider

- What does it mean to be a nurse or any other health professional?
- What vision of your practice do you hold? Is it valid?
- What knowledge/ knowing is significant to being an expert nurse, or any other health professional?
- Identify one thing you would change in your practice environment to help realise desirable practice? Is that possible?

Clearly for anyone aspiring to be a nurse or to enable others to become nurses, these are vital questions to consider. So, as we mindfully practice and as we reflect on our practice we ask these questions. It becomes the focus for our inquiry and learning.

The nature and significance of knowledge and knowing is contestable. Schön (1987: 1) writes,

In the varied topography of professional practice, there is the high, hard ground overlooking the swamp. On the high ground, manageable problems lend themselves to solution through the application of research-based theory and technique. In the swampy lowland, messy, confusing problems defy technical solution. The irony of this situation is that the problems of the high ground tend to be relatively unimportant to individuals or society at large, however great their technical interest may be, while in the swamp lie the problems of greatest human concern. The practitioner must choose. Shall he remain on the high ground where he can solve relatively unimportant problems according to prevailing standards or rigor, or shall he descend into the swamp of important problems and non-rigorous inquiry?

Schön posits two types of knowledge – technical rationality (research-based theory) and professional artistry (knowing in action). He suggests that professional artistry is the more significant type of knowing because it is the knowing with which the practitioner responds to the situations of everyday practice. However, both types of knowledge are important for the practitioner to draw on. Indeed, through reflection, technical rationality is critiqued for its value to inform and subsequently assimilated into professional artistry.

Every experience is different. We may have had similar experiences but not this particular one. We draw parallels but they are not the same. Subtle differences between this experience and previous experiences demand subtle shifts of response that cannot be known outside the unfolding moment. We have to be mindful, to read the particular signs or we may get it wrong. These signs are often subtle, requiring perception, imagination and intuition. There are no prescriptive solutions. Knowing in action is intuitive drawing on tacit knowing. The practitioner might not be able to say exactly why she responded as she did, yet she can attempt to articulate it as a story. In doing so, she makes her tacit or intuitive knowing more explicit. It is this intuitive knowing that reflection feeds and accelerates with its focus on the whole picture and encouraging the practitioner to become integral to the experience rather than outside it (Dreyfus and Dreyfus 1986; Dreyfus 2004)[1]. The Dreyfus model of skill acquisition offers a reflective framework for practitioners to mark their growth of expertise (see Table 1.2).

King and Appleton (1997) and Cioffi (1997) endorse the significance of intuition within decision making and action following their reviews of the literature and rhetoric on intuition. They note that reflection accesses, values and develops intuitive processes.

Table 1.2 The expert in the Dreyfus and Dreyfus model of skill acquisition

Pattern recognition	A perceptual ability to recognize relationships without pre-specifying the components of the situation
Similarity recognition	An amazing human ability to recognise 'fuzzy' resemblance despite marked differences
Common sense	A deep grasp of the language culture so that flexible understanding in diverse situations is possible
Skilled 'know how'	The practitioner can respond without resorting to rule-governed behaviours
Deliberate rationality	The expert practitioner has a web of different perspectives that cases them to view a situation in terms of past situations

[1] See also Benner 1984; applying the Dreyfus model to nurse education.

Aristotle drew a distinction between practical wisdom and theoretical wisdom. Practical wisdom does not result in knowledge which is determinate and universal; indeed, it does not result in propositional knowledge at all but in discriminations and actions.

Technical rationality (or evidence-based practice) has been claimed as necessary for nursing's disciplinary knowledge base because it can be observed and verified (Kikuchi 1992). Historically, professions such as nursing have accepted the superiority of technical rationality over tacit or intuitive knowing (Schön 1983, 1987). Yet, a technical rational mentality is likely to lead to stereotyping; fitting the patient to the theory rather than using the theory to inform the situation. As Visinstainer (1986: 37) writes,

> Even when nurses govern their own practice, they succumb to the belief that the 'soft stuff' such as feelings and beliefs and support, are not quite as substantive as the hard data from laboratory reports and sophisticated monitoring.

People are not objects. It is unimaginable for any nurse to face clinical practice with a technical rational mindset simply because each clinical moment is a unique human-human encounter.

In a culture of 'evidence-based practice' practitioners are exhorted to 'evidence their practice'.

Consider

- What research-based theory do you use in practice?
- Do you consider its authority to inform the situation or do you take its authority on face value?

Since the Briggs Report (DHSS 1972) emphasised that nursing should be a research-based profession, nursing has endeavoured to respond to this challenge. However, the general understanding of what 'research-based' means has followed an empirical pathway, reflecting a dominant agenda to explain and predict practice. This agenda has been pursued by nurse academics seeking academic recognition that nursing is a valid science within university settings. Whilst abstract knowledge has an important role in informing practice it certainly cannot predict and control, at least not without reducing the patient and nurses to the status of objects to be manipulated like pawns in a chess game. The consequence of this position in nursing has been the repression of other forms of knowing that has perpetuated the oppression of nurses through neglect of or refusal to acknowledge their clinical nursing knowledge (Street 1992). Has it improved in the past 20 years? I see no evidence to support that. We who plough the professional artistry field reap poor reward in academic acclaim. Professional artistry is subjective and contextual, yet is often denigrated as a lesser form of knowing, even dismissed as 'mere anecdote' by those who inhabit the hard, high ground of technical rationality. People get locked into a paradigmatic view of knowledge and become intolerant of other claims because such claims fail the technical rationality injunction as to what counts as truth.

Evaluating Reflection

Reflective practice has been criticised for its lack of definition, modes of implementation and for its unproven benefit (Mackintosh 1998: 556). Mackintosh singled out the Burford reflective model for criticism. She writes,

> The benefits of reflection are largely unaddressed by the literature [*that is, beyond unsubstantiated claims*], and instead the underlying assumption appears to be that reflection

will improve nursing care or the nursing profession in some intangible way. This is demonstrated by Bailey (1995), who, although describing the introduction of reflection into a critical area and claiming that an improvement in problem-solving skills occurred, gives no evidence that the quality of care was improved in any way. These failings can also be found in much of the literature describing the Burford reflection in nursing model (Johns 1996a, b, c), which attempts to integrate reflective practice into a clinically grounded nursing model through use of a series of 'cues'. Much of the published evidence regarding the model's impact on clinical practice appears to be based on personal anecdote, and again, evidence in support of its impact on patient care is of a mainly qualitative and descriptive nature. [italics, my inclusion]

Mackintosh's words pointedly address the tension of knowing the impact of reflective practice on practitioner performance. The accounts within the Burford NDU model: caring in practice (Johns 1994) were not cited in the above references. Yet in this book there are four collaborating accounts from Burford practitioners and accounts from four other nursing units besides Burford, accounts that testify to the impact of the Burford model on clinical practice. In other words Mackintosh reviews the literature with her own partial eye, seeing or interpreting what she wants to read to support her prejudice against subjective accounts and methodologies. Without doubt, there is a strong prejudice within healthcare research and education against what Mackintosh pejoratively describes as anecdote.

Attempt to evaluate the impact of reflective practice on patient outcomes from a technical rational perspective is fraught with difficulty given the variables of healthcare. It is trying to measure the wrong thing using the wrong approach.

As one practitioner wrote[2]

Reflection is transforming my practice in so many meaningful and profound ways.... I have never felt so free to care and to be true to what I consider to be ideal practice.... Reflection had enabled me to contextually refocus on the individual. My interactive skills are being sharpened and I am rediscovering the therapeutic value of establishing a close relationship with clients. Until now I have never been able to find an approach to nursing which recognises the true potential of this unique relationship.... My first few reflections were triggered by a feeling that I had failed to achieve my goals in some way ...guided reflection had enabled me to make use of the creative energy of conflict. I have been challenged to stoke up a far more challenging style of practice. I have become empowered to provoke and maintain the contradictions I feel between my goals of desirable practice and actual practice. Just as there are no limits to my expanding consciousness ...

If you were to look at this practitioner's reflexive narrative, you would clearly see an evaluation of reflective practice on her development and subsequent impact on patient care. But would you believe it? The narrative's claim for truth is *authenticity* (Wilber 1998). Authenticity is revealed in the reader's identification with the experience. It rings true! Such narratives offer genuine evaluation of the impact of reflective practice on practitioner development and patient outcome.[3]

Doctoral level reflexive narrative research reveals practitioner journeys of becoming a reflective practitioner across diverse practice and teaching environments (Jarrett 2010, 2015; Fordham 2012; Foster 2013; Akinbode 2015, Graham 2015). Reflexive narratives have been published (Johns 2010; Johns and Freshwater 2005) that demonstrate the impact of guided reflection on practitioner development and the consequential impact on clinical practice.

---

[2] MSc dissertation, Leadership in healthcare.
[3] For example, see the narratives of becoming a leader in Mindful Leadership (Johns 2015).

Narratives inform and influence organisational practice. Fordham (2012) writes of the influence of taking her experiences of working with homeless people into the executive meetings and disturbing the gathered professionals with the reality of homelessness, in contrast with a view of homelessness through statistics. Maddex (2002: 21) writes,

> I found that the more I journaled, the more I started to use narratives in my teaching, in meetings – telling stories of experiences with patients to make my points more real.

Some Studies

In one study spanning 12 years, leaders were required to construct a reflexive narrative of becoming a leader as the dissertation methodology of an MSc course on Leadership in healthcare. Ninety narratives were constructed, enabling a meta-analysis to understand the tensions of becoming a leader within transactional organisations (Johns 2015). The programme was constructed as a collaborative inquiry where learning and research became the same endeavour.

A number of studies use art and poetry to help practitioners find meaning in their experiences of being with patients (Vaught-Alexander 1994; Begley 1996; Eifried, Riley-Giomariso and Voight 2000; Brodersen 2001; Parker 2002). These studies reflect the way humanities open a reflective space where practitioners can express their experiences.

The six Dialogical Movements

The reflexive process of self-inquiry and transformation through reflection can be viewed as comprising six dialogical movements within the hermeneutic circle of interpretation (Figure 1.1). It commences with the practitioner pausing from her unreflective pattern of experience to pay attention to a particular experience. Paying attention, the practitioner then writes a story about the particular lived experience with the intention of gaining insight through reflection, dialogue and narrative as explored through subsequent chapters.

The Hermeneutic Circle

Hermeneutics is the interpretation of text (Gadamer 1962) stemming from a particular philosophic tradition. From this perspective, the practitioner's reflection written as a story is the text. Having written the story, the practitioner must stand back from their text in order to see it more objectively, with the intent to gain insight through interpretation towards development of professional identity and artistry (however that is most appropriately appreciated).

The insights gained from one experience are always in dialogue with insights gained from previous experiences – leading to a deepening of insights and personal knowing. Hence, subsequent experiences are set against a background of the collective of previous experiences. Thus there is a continuous dialogue between the whole unfolding narrative and new experiences, each informing each other in an ever deepening circle of interpretation in which meaning is always fluid. This movement forms the practical foundation of reflexive narrative. It is like throwing a stone into a pool. It makes a splash and sends

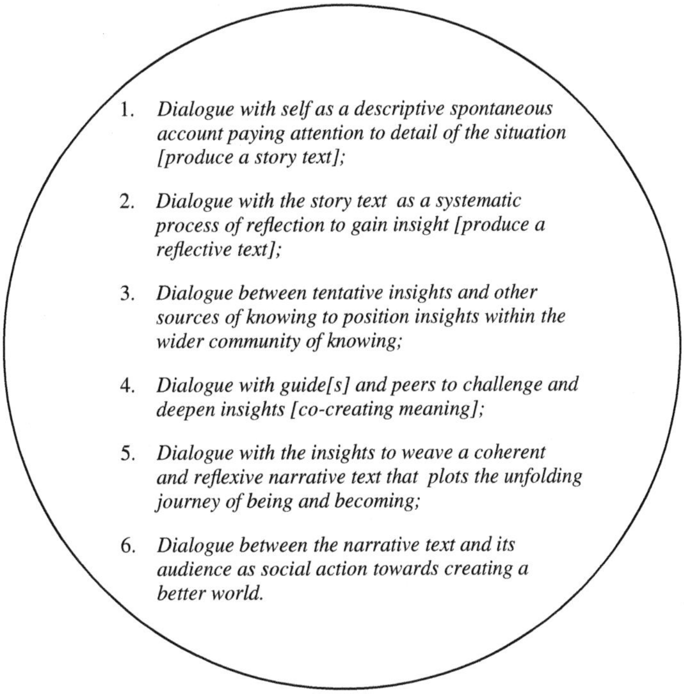

1. *Dialogue with self as a descriptive spontaneous account paying attention to detail of the situation [produce a story text];*

2. *Dialogue with the story text as a systematic process of reflection to gain insight [produce a reflective text];*

3. *Dialogue between tentative insights and other sources of knowing to position insights within the wider community of knowing;*

4. *Dialogue with guide[s] and peers to challenge and deepen insights [co-creating meaning];*

5. *Dialogue with the insights to weave a coherent and reflexive narrative text that plots the unfolding journey of being and becoming;*

6. *Dialogue between the narrative text and its audience as social action towards creating a better world.*

The hermeneutic circle

Figure 1.1   The six dialogical movements of reflexive narrative construction.

out ripples over the whole surface of the pool. The pool represents the whole of one's understanding and informs the splash whilst at the same time the splash provides new information to deepen the whole pool's understanding in an every increasing deepening of the pool's understanding. Whilst this learning process may seem complex at first glance, I shall review it as one movement at a time commencing with the ideas of bringing the mind home and writing self.

Summary

Reflection has generally been accommodated into educational and practice organisations from a technical rational perspective with little evidence of its efficacy in terms of better practice or more competent practitioners. As such, it is an awkward fit. As I shall explore, reflective practices need compatible environments in which to flourish. It is a chicken and egg situation. Can reflective practices cultivated against the grain turn the grain to create compatible environments? Or can compatible environments be created beforehand? I suspect it is a mixture of the two, whereby reflective practices by their nature quickly realise the paucity of the environment to support it and hence begin to turn the grain.

In Chapter 2 I explore the first dialogical movement of writing self.

References

Akinbode, A. (2014) Transforming self as reflective teacher: journey of being and becoming a teacher and teacher educator. Unpublished PhD Thesis. University of Bedfordshire.

Bailey, J. (1995) Reflective practice: implementing theory. *Nursing Standard* 9.46, 29–31.

Beauchamp, C. (2015) Reflection in teacher education: issues emerging from a review of current literature. *Reflective Practice* 16.1, 123–141.

Begley, A.-M. (1996) Literature and poetry: pleasure and practice. *International Journal of Nursing Practice* 2, 182–188.

Benner, P. (1984) *From novice to expert.* Addison-Wesley, Menlo Park.

Boud, D., Keogh, R. and Walker, D. (1985) Promoting reflection in learning: a model. In D. Boud, R. Keogh and D. Walker (eds.), *Reflection: turning experience into learning.* Kogan Page, London.

Boyd, E. and Fales, A. (1983) Reflective learning: key to learning from experience. *Journal of Humanistic Psychology* 23.2, 99–117.

Brodersen, L. (2001) Creatively capturing care: poetry and knowledge in nursing. *International Journal for Human Caring* 6.1, 33–41.

Bulman C, Lathlean J, and Gobbi M. (2012) The concept of reflection in nursing: qualitative findings on student and teacher perspectives. *Nurse Education Today* 32 (2012), e8–e13.

Bruner, J. (1994) The remembered self. In U. Neisser and R. Fivush (eds.), *The remembering self: construction and accuracy in the self narrative,* Cambridge University Press, Cambridge.

Casement, P. (1985) *On learning from the patient.* Routledge, London.

Cioffi, J. (1997) Heuristics, servants to intuition, in clinical decision making. *Journal of Advanced Nursing* 26, 203–208.

Cochran, L. and Laub, L. (1994) *Becoming an agent: patterns and dynamics for shaping your life.* State University of New York Press, Albany.

Dawson, J. (2015) *Resurgence and Ecologist* pp. 25–29.

Dewey, J. (1933) *How we think.* J. C. Heath, Boston.

Department of Health & Social Security (1972) *Report of the Committee on Nursing (Chairperson, Professor Asa Briggs)* HMSO, London.

Dreyfus, S. E. (2004) The five-stage model of adult skill acquisition. *Bulletin of Science, Technology & Society,* 24, 177–181.

Dreyfus, H. and Dreyfus, S. (1986) *Mind over machine.* Free Press, New York.

Eifried, S., Riley-Giomariso, O. and Voight, G. (2000) Learning to care amid suffering: how art and narrative give voice to the student experience. *International Journal for Human Caring* 5.2, 42–51.

Fay, B. (1987) *Critical Social Science.* Polity Press, Cambridge.

Finlay, L. (2008) Reflecting on 'Reflective practice'. A discussion paper prepared for PBPL CETL (PBPL paper 52) www.open.ac.uk/pbpl.

Fordham, M. (2008) Building bridges in homelessness, mindful of phronesis in nursing practice. In C. Delmar C and Johns C (eds.), *The good, the wise, and the right clinical nursing practice.* Aalborg Hospital, Arhus University Hospital, Denmark, pp. 73–92.

Fordham, M. (2012) Being and becoming a specialist public health nurse net weaving in homeless health care. Unpublished PhD thesis. University of Bedfordshire.

Foster, L. (2013) Narrative self-inquiry to capture transformation in mental health nursing practice. Unpublished PhD thesis. University of Bedfordshire.

Frank, A. (2002) Relations of caring: demoralization and remoralization in the clinic. *International Journal of Human Caring.* 6.2, 13–19.

Gadamer, H.-G. (1975) *Truth & method.* Seabury Press, New York.

Gibbs, G. (1988) *Learning by doing: a guide to teaching and learning methods.* Further Education Unit, Oxford Polytechnic, now Oxford Brookes University.

Goldstein, J. (2002) *One Dharma.* Rider, London.

Graham, M.M. (2015) Becoming available becoming student kind: a nurse educators reflexive narrative. Unpublished PhD thesis. University of Bedfordshire

Greene, M. (1988) *The dialectic of freedom*. Teachers College Press, Columbia University, New York.

James, N. (1989) Emotional labour: skill and work in the social regulation of feelings. *Sociological Review*, 37.1, 15–42.

Jarrett, L. (2008) From significance to insights. In C. Delmar and C. Johns (eds.), *The good, the wise, and the right clinical nursing practice*. Aalborg Hospital, Arhus University Hospital, Denmark, pp. 59–72.

Jarrett, L. (2009) Being and becoming a reflective practitioner, through guided reflection, in the role of a spasticity management nurse specialist. Unpublished PhD thesis, City University.

Johns, C. (ed.) (1994) *The Burford NDU Model: caring in practice*. Blackwell, Oxford.

Johns, C. (1996a) The benefits of a reflective model of nursing. *Nursing Times* 92.27, 39–41.

Johns, C. (1996b) Visualising and realising caring in practice through guided reflection. *Journal of Advanced Nursing* 24, 1135–1143.

Johns, C. (1996c) Using a reflective model of nursing and guided reflection. *Nursing Standard* 11.2, 34–38.

Johns, C. (2005) Balancing the winds. *Reflective practice* 5.3, 67–84.

Johns, C. (ed.) (2010) *Guided reflection: a narrative approach to advancing practice (second edition)*. Wiley-Blackwell, Oxford.

Johns, C. (2015) *Mindful leadership: a guide for the health care professions*. Palgrave Macmillan, London.

Johns, C. and Freshwater, D. (eds.) (2005) *Transforming nursing through reflective practice (second edition)*. Blackwell, Oxford.

Jones, R. and Jones, G. (1996) *Earth Dance Drum*. Commune-E-Key, Salt Lake City.

Kermode, F. (1966) *The sense of an ending*. Oxford University Press, New York.

Kieffer, C. (1984) Citizen empowerment: a developmental perspective. *Prevention in Human Services*, 84.3, 9–36.

Kikuchi, J. (1992) Nursing questions that science cannot answer. In Kikuchi, J. and Simmons, H. (eds.), *Philosophic Inquiry in Nursing*. Sage, Newberry Park.

King, L. and Appleton, J. (1997) Intuition: a critical review of the research and rhetoric. *Journal of Advanced Nursing* 26, 194–202.

Kopp, P. (2000) Overcoming difficulties in communicating with other professionals. *Nursing Times* 96.28, 47–49.

Krishnamurti, J. (1996) *Total Freedom*. Harper, San Francisco.

Lawler, J. (1991) *Behind the scenes: nursing, somology and the problems of the body*. Churchill Livingstone, Melbourne.

Mackintosh, C. (1998) Reflection: a flawed strategy for the nursing profession. *Nurse Education Today*, 18, 553–557.

Maddex, E. (2002) Shedding the armour: my leadership journey. Unpublished MSc Leadership in Health Care Dissertation. University of Bedfordshire.

Mezirow, J. (1981) A critical theory of adult learning and education. *Adult Education*, 32.1, 3–24.

Novelestsky-Rosenthal, H. and Solomon, K. (2001) Reflections on the use of Johns' model of structured reflection in nurse-practitioner education. *International Journal for Human Caring*, 5.2, 21–26.

O'Donohue, J. (1997) *Anam Cara: spiritual wisdom from the Celtic world*. Bantam Press, London.

Okri, B. (1997) *A Way of being free*. Phoenix House, London.

Parker, M. (2002) Aesthetic ways in day-to-day nursing. In D. Freshwater (ed.), *Therapeutic nursing*. Sage, London.

Pinar, W. (1981) 'Whole, Bright, Deep with Understanding': Issues in qualitative research and autobiographical method *Journal of Curriculum Studies* 13.3, 173–188.

Polkingthorne, D. (1996) Transformative narratives: from victimic to agentic life plots. *The American Journal of Occupational Therapy*, 50.4, 299–305.

Rawnsley, M. (1990) Of human bonding: the context of nursing as caring. *Advances in Nursing Science* 13, 41–48.

Rogers, C. (1969) *Freedom to learn: a view of what education might be.* Merrill, Columbus, OH.

Sangharakshita (1998) *Know your mind.* Windhorse, Birmingham.

Schön, D. (1983) *The reflective practitioner.* Avebury, Aldershot.

Schön, D. (1987) *Educating the reflective practitioner.* Jossey-Bass, San Francisco.

Smith, E. (2011) Teaching critical reflection. *Teaching in Higher Education* 16.2, 211–223)

Smyth, J. (1992) Teachers' work and the politics of reflection. *American Educational Research Journal,* 29, 267–300.

Street, A. (1992) *Inside nursing: a critical ethnography of clinical nursing.* State University of New York Press, Albany.

Vaught-Alexander, K. (1994) The personal journal for nurses: writing for delivery and healing. In D. Gaut and A. Boykin (eds.), *Caring as healing: renewal through hope.* National League for Nursing Press, New York.

Van Manen, M. (1990) *Researching lived experience.* State University of New York Press, Albany.

Visinstainer, M. (1986) The nature of knowledge and theory in nursing. *Image: The Journal of Nursing Scholarship* 18, 32–38.

Wilber, K. (1998) *The eye of spirit: an integral vision for a world gone slightly mad.* Shambhala, Boston.

Wheatley, M. and Kellner-Rogers, M. (1999) *A simpler way.* Berrett-Koehler, San Francisco.

Chapter 2
Writing Self

Christopher Johns

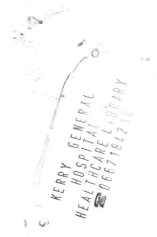

Writing self is the raw data of experience

Bringing the Mind Home

To write I find a quiet eddy out of the fast current of life, to pause, muse, to clear and let go of the mind and open the body to recall the experience, to create a space where I can get back into the experience with all my senses. Yet in the busy and material world in which we live this may not be easy. Our minds are often full of stuff that distract us. Like a juggler trying to keep eight plates spinning. Generally, people do not take time to slow down and press the pause button. Having the mind full of stuff also offers an excuse not to look at self in any deep way.

As Jones and Jones (1996: 90) write,

> We must slow down or we will miss all that has meaning. Meaning is revealed only when you pause, when you stop, when you pay attention. Learn the lesson of the tribal people. Put your busyness on pause, eliminate distractions, and allow the meaning of life and living to return to you. Slow down in order to connect to the meaning of life.

And yet, as Rinpoche (1992: 31) writes,

> how hard it can be to turn our attention within! How easily we allow our old habits and set patterns to dominate us! Even though they bring us suffering, we accept them with almost fatalistic resignation, for we are so used to giving into them.

Can we create the space in our crowded minds to bring the mind home?

Susan Brooks recognizes the value of bringing the mind home.

Susan writes (2004),

> *One of the most priceless skills learnt over the last two years of study on the MSc leadership programme[1] is 'bringing home my mind' – slipping out of the noose of anxiety, releasing all grasping and relaxing into my true nature. By relaxing in this uncontrived, open and natural state we obtain the blessing of aimless self-liberation of whatever arises (Rinpoche 1992). This*

has certainly been my experience and the joy of feeling able to distance myself from the daily pressures of work by bringing my mind home is immense and a practice that, I believe, will stay with me indefinitely. Hatha yoga has become an element of my daily practice as a means to 'bring my mind home' and to promote my own physical and mental well-being in a meditative context. Such practice has revealed to me that I do matter as a person and am not simply a faceless cog in the healthcare organisation. How many times have I said or heard the comment, 'I am just a nurse'? Nurses generally have not trusted their own sense of self-importance enough and yet the fact that nurses do matter is a fundamental truth (Tschudin 1993). Bringing my mind home focuses me on me, underpins my own sense of self-importance but also emphasises my crucial need, as a transformative leader, to recognise and encourage the development of the personhood and thoughts of others. Reflective thought has become a pleasure rather than a threat and as I sit to review the period of this study and my journey so far, I am contentedly aware that my mind is unshackled by the contradictory voices, dictates and feelings that usually fight for control over our inner lives (Rinpoche 1992). Being available to self in this way has implications for my leadership, support and development of others since I would argue that unless I am truly available and knowing to self, transference of such availability would be problematic.

Susan suggests that 'bringing the mind home' is a precursor to becoming mindful. It enables her to become focused on realizing her leadership vision by bringing her attention to her experience within practice. Of course, you do not have to do hatha yoga or formal meditation to bring the mind home.

Before you write your journal sit quietly and take your attention to your breath. Count each breath in and breath out. Count to ten and repeat. Notice the thoughts creep in. Just notice them and start counting again from one. Taking time out to reflect sounds easy, but when our lives are addicted to being busy, it may be hard to focus one's thoughts within rather than be scattered outside. Gradually, with practice, bringing the mind home becomes natural, achieved in seconds. Do you have the patience to wait till your mud settles and the water is clear? (Lao Tzu 571 BC[2]).

Skill Box

- *Learn to use your breath to bring yourself fully present to what you are doing, whether clinical practice or reflection. It will help you focus attention. It will help you tune into yourself and manage any emotions. It will help you think more clearly leading to better outcomes for both your patients and for yourself. It will make you healthier[3].*
- *Before going to see a patient or a meeting or teaching, pause before entering and use your breath to bring yourself fully present to this moment. Write about the impact of that.*

Writing Self: The First Dialogical Movement

To reiterate, bringing the mind home focuses us to pay attention. As Loori (2005: 74) writes – 'when we truly pay attention, we see each object or situation for the first time- and it always seems fresh and new, no matter how many times we've encountered it before. We break free of our habitual ways of seeing'.

Paying attention is liberating. It enables us to see. It enables us to write clearly. I write to capture the essence of my experience in order to create a canvass for reflection in my quest to realise my vision of practice as a lived reality, and in doing so develop my professional artistry. That is the plot that governs the pen stroke. In other words, writing is purposeful. Yet, what is my vision? Simply put, my personal vision as a healthcare practitioner is to ease suffering however that manifests itself in collaboration with my healthcare colleagues to enable the persons I care for to grow through their health–illness experience. Nice words but to what do they mean as something lived? 'Suffering' is a very complex word. Reflection becomes an exploration of vision. Visions are a moveable feast as 'we' seek to understand such words as suffering. I say 'we' because visions need to be owned by practice communities so that we pull purposively towards realizing the vision as a lived reality. I cannot state this strongly enough.

Of course, my vision is the heart or soul of my practice. Manjusvara (2005: 10) writes 'the practice of writing takes us to the heart of ourselves and makes it palpable how alive with possibilities we really are.' In other words writing wakes up the self to our human potential, a self that might have become deadened to the world for whatever reason, where potential has shrunk to virtually nothing.

At work, I carry a small notebook with me for making notes that I may later reflect on. These notes are usually facts about the situation or a record of actual dialogue. As I sit at the computer I reflect on what triggers my stories. Remembering a moment, the look on her face, a word said, a tear shed, frustration, joy, a sad smile, the smell of curry, the harsh word spoken, the ethical dilemma, a picture on the wall, the dance of the trees outside the window. Indeed, anything can trigger.

I prefer to write on the computer because I can move words around later as I construct narrative. I tend to write in a factual way, sometimes referring to the notes I scribbled earlier in my small notebook. I let the words come as a spontaneous flow in rich description, paying attention to as much detail as possible, pursuing signs, running off on tangents. I prefer to write in the present tense to better capture the moment.

Stories are the raw data of our experience. As Wheatley (1999: 143) writes, 'we paint a portrait of the whole, surfacing as much detail as possible'.

I write,

Peggy

A normal day at hospice day care. The usual suspects. Things go as normal that is until Peggy pulls me aside and says 'I'm first today'. Taken by surprise I am uncertain how to respond. After a momentary pause I say 'OK Peggy let's go'. I had not spoken with her beyond social niceties before even though I had been working here for the past six weeks. Others had grasped my attention. We walk to the therapy room and she talks about her life, losing her partner quickly to cancer and then her dog dying recently. She is sad. She likes to come to the centre for company but also feels she needs to be alone. She takes off her new walking boots and I give her reflexology. My base cream mixed with essential oils. She is relaxed and appreciative of the therapy. Afterwards I walk her back to the day room to rejoin the hungry throng – hungry in the sense of demanding my attention. Peggy smiles. She made her point and taught me a lesson about paying attention and taking nothing for granted. No such thing as a normal day when you pierce it rather than slide along its surface.

'Reflection is like opening the cover to the book of your own life, which up to now has been carefully closed' (Jones and Jones 1996: 22). Story is subjective and contextual, a rich descriptive account of experience that paints a broad reflective canvass. You might argue that my Peggy story is not very rich. Perhaps I could have written much more but in the moment of writing it seemed enough. Enough to pause and look at what I have written, opening the possibility of seeing myself in a different light, mindful that in writing 'I am changed by the process of writing it' (Flemons and Green 2002: 91). Knowing I am going to reflect on my experiences of the day prompts me to pay more attention to what is unfolding moment to moment. It always seems remarkable how much detail the body absorbs.

In writing, I draw on all my senses in spontaneous expression. What did things look like, smell like, sound like, even taste like, what did I sense? Paying attention to detail – the colour of the walls, what noises permeated the situation? What time of day? Such things may seem immaterial at the time of writing but on reflection may gain significance- hence the more detail the better. Holly (1989: 71–75) writes,

> It [keeping a reflective journal] makes possible new ways of theorizing, reflecting on and coming to know one's self. Capturing certain words while the action is fresh, the author is often provoked to question why … writing taps tacit knowledge; it brings into awareness that which we sense but could not explain.

At my reflective practice workshops I ask people to write a story about a recent experience for 20 minutes without taking the pen off the paper. It needn't be about clinical practice. *Without taking the pen of the paper* facilitates spontaneous expression. It seems when we write we think less, as if it is the body that speaks. When we lift the pen, we pause, and think and get stuck. Manjusvara (2005: 37) notes, 'as the hand begins to overtake the brain it is amazing how often there emerges a coherent statement of what I had previously been struggling to say'

Skill Box

- *Write for 15 minutes about a recent experience. Do not take your pen off the paper or finger off the keyboard. Be spontaneous and descriptive. Write in the present tense as if you are reliving the experience. Draw on all your senses.*
- *What senses did you draw on?*
- *Did you capture actual dialogue spoken?*

Journal Entry

One student asks 'How do I write?'
I respond 'Just do it. Let if come and flow as naturally as water flowing in a stream.'
'Give me a clue' the student asks.
'Were you at work yesterday? I respond
'Yes'
'Think of one patient you nursed- now write a story. For example 'Mr Smith is 46. He sits in his chair by the bed. He seems sad. I am frustrated that I do not have enough time to spend with him.'

The pen writes furiously for 20 minutes. Stemming from socialised patterns of learning based on technical rationality, practitioners are overly sensitive about doing it right, as if they will be judged. To dictate how to write and reflect reinforces an instrumental approach. The guide guides them to find their own way, knowing that this way will ultimately be the most productive way.

Practitioners are often surprised by what they have written. Often the writing has gone off on tangents to the extent that people did not write about what they had intended or hadn't yet come around to the specific point. They seem to enjoy this creative form of writing even though it may at first seem alien and difficult to start.

As one nursing student says '*I haven't yet got to the point of the experience.*'

She, like so many other participants, is astonished with the amount she has written. Revealing the storied self. Putting together the pieces of self, of life itself. It is a creative and restorative act.

Tufnell and Crickmay (2004: 41) write,

> We come to know more of what matters in our lives, less through an in-tuned search for self, than in conversation, in relationship to what is around us. We rarely know what currents flow beneath what we are doing and feeling. The impulses, instincts and intuitions that impel our thoughts and actions are as animals moving in the shadows of our everyday awareness. As we create we discover events, characters, places, sights and sounds, whose significance we cannot quite define, yet whose presence makes more visible what is moving through our lives. Creating is a way of listening and of trying to speak more personally from within the various worlds we inhabit. It is a way of discovering our own stories, refreshing and reawakening our language and giving form to the way we feel.

Writing is creative. It cannot be prescribed although teachers may try and impose some academic order on your writing (Woolf 1928/ 1945). Pay attention to everything no matter how tangential it is. Do not discard anything. Let the imagination run riot! Writing should be approached with a playful and creative spirit. IT is YOU! In writing, you are writing yourself, your body, nurturing your precious and unique self. In writing you change yourself on a subliminal level. As Ferrruci (1982: 42) says, 'it is like cutting a new pathway in a jungle'.

Some practitioners find writing story easy whilst others struggle as if some mind censor constrains the writing potential. If you have never written about self before it may feel strange, even threatening. The reflective mirror is not always kind, especially if we write about things we find difficult for whatever reason. Then we may subconsciously distort our recall and create false impressions of ourselves. Hence, writing is courageous. It requires effort, honesty, and perseverance.

Eleanor Gully (2005: 151) writes,

> Reflective practice is part of the way I work with others in my nursing practice. Journaling is both a professional and personal way of making sense of everyday living. It may be called a journey to wholeness and well-being. It is the process of journaling that is by far the most significant act in my practice, for it records the process of my evolving as a human being and connects me with the other in my nursing relationship; it is a journey from the 'I' to the 'we', the consciousness of the collective soul journey of each human being. The journey begins with the self, *the awakening to the self*, in relation to the spiritual path each of us is destined to follow.' [my italics]

Writing Rather than Telling

Some people like to tell their stories whilst others prefer to write them. I advocate writing because writing creates the reflective canvas. It is something substantial to work on. Some practitioners get stuck between telling their story and writing it. It is as if they hit a mental block. Perhaps telling stories is more spontaneous whilst writing is more considered, more cognitive, more self-conscious, even though I advocate spontaneous writing. I sense the presence of an internal censor at work in writing that tries to fit the description into learned ways of writing that denigrate feelings and imagination. Some people will always struggle to write despite advice to just let the words flow in a spontaneous stream.

Writing is confrontational and begins to loosen the self from its bondage. It is much more than a cognitive exercise of recall. It is as if I seek to dwell within the situation as a witness. In this way I tap into the right side of my brain and stir my perception and imagination. It is playful but I may have forgotten how to play, wrapped up as I am in reason and rationality.

Mimesis

The practitioner writes to capture something of the experience through rich description, paying attention to detail and drawing on all the senses in order to capture the reality of their experience as best they can. The attention to recall what actually took place, is the mimetic nature of reflective writing.

Boud, Keogh and Walker (1985: 27) suggest the value of mimetic writing as,

> one of the most useful activities that can initiate a period of reflection is recollecting what has taken place and replaying the experience in the mind's eye, to observe the event as it had happened and to notice exactly what occurred and one's reaction to it in all its elements, it may be helpful to commit this description to paper, or to describe it to others. By whatever means this occurs the description should involve a close attention to detail and should refrain from making judgments.

However, mimetic writing should not be naïve (Mattingly 1998). There is a distinction to be made between the actual lived experience and telling the story. The remembering of the story becomes distorted through perception and memory even when written shortly after the event. The reflective practitioner is aware that capturing the exact nature of the experience is elusive because of her subjective partial view. This is natural and is not a problem, not least because the practitioner's subjective partial view becomes a focus for scrutiny through reflection.

I do suggest people write about the experience soon after it happens. My own edict is to write within 24 hours of the experience. Although I have no hard evidence to support this, practitioners say this is useful advice. Of course, I don't always achieve this edict. Sometimes a week or even a month goes past and I haven't written about the experience for whatever reason. I can still recall it clearly and yet I wonder if my recall has become more distorted through time. It might suit some people to write at a later time when the immediacy of the experience has settled. Writing too soon after a situation may not be enough time for the emotional mud to settle and for things to become clearer.

Feelings

Reflection is often triggered by negative or uncomfortable feelings such as anger, guilt, sadness, frustration, and resentment (Boyd and Fales 1983). These emotions create a sense of drama in the mind. These feelings give access to our inner world, often a negative feeling or sense of discomfort about something that has happened during the day. Negative feelings create anxiety. As such, the practitioner may *naturally* reflect either consciously or subconsciously to defend against this anxiety. They may distort, rationalise, project or even deny the situation that caused these feelings. Pema Chodron (2000: 12) writes,

> Generally speaking, we regard discomfort in any form as bad news. But for practitioners or spiritual warriors – people who have a certain hunger to know what is true – feelings like disappointment, irritation, resentment, anger, jealousy, and fear, instead of being bad news, are

actually very clear moments that teach us where it is that we're holding back. They teach us to perk up and lean in when we feel we'd rather collapse and back away. They're like messengers that show us with terrifying clarity, exactly where we're stuck. This very moment is the perfect teacher and, lucky for us, it's with us wherever we are.

It seems natural to focus on negative experiences because it is these situations that present themselves to consciousness. Much of experience is not reflected on because it is unproblematic. In other words, much of practice is taken for granted. Paramananda (2001: 58] writes,

> Whenever we begin to feel frustrated in what we are doing, we should slow down and pay closer attention to it. Frustration takes us away from ourselves; we become alienated from our experience. When we feel this beginning to happen we need to pay more attention to our experience.

Senge (1990) argues that we need to deal with emotional tension before we can focus on creative tension, as if emotions smudge the mirror and distort rational thought. Boud, Keogh and Walker (1985) also suggest we need to remove obstructive feelings as part of the reflective process. Some practitioners may find writing helps them work through their feelings, but for other writers, reflecting on events, especially traumatic events, may be distressing. Gray and Forsstrom (1991: 360) write,

> The process of 'journalling' may sound simple and easy to execute, but at times it was extremely difficult. Mostly the incidents recorded were identified because there was an affective component. This may be related to feelings of personal inadequacy to cope with the demands of the situation. Alone, it was emotionally painful to journal events that were largely self-critical.

The idea of not being *alone* through guidance is explored in Chapter 5.

I might just write in my journal, 'I'm angry!!' A cathartic explosion to release the feeling. I can then add to this expletive at any time.

ANGRY!

I'm angry at Jane, the junior nurse, because I asked her to help a patient wash, but she ignored me and went to help someone else. I am puzzled why she did this. It made me angry but I couldn't challenge her. I didn't want to make a fuss. I'm still angry, angry at myself for letting her get away with it. Maybe I should have confronted her later. Grrghhhh! [Dog sound optional!]

For novice reflective practitioners, it is more natural to pay attention to things that haven't gone well than things that go well. As a consequence the practitioner may get into a pattern of negative thinking about self and practice. She may despair about her organisation and her colleagues. Not much fun. However, it is significant to experience our anger, our sorrow, our failure, our apprehension; for these feelings are all our teachers when practitioners do not try and defend against them. Then learning is not possible. That's not hard to understand, just hard to do (Beck 19997).

Whilst it may be natural to pay attention to negative feelings because they disturb us, practitioners can be guided to reflect on positive experiences. This is less likely because positive experiences are not viewed as problematic or dramatic enough. Such experiences are often taken for granted. However, I have discerned a pattern whereby practitioners, as they become more experienced with reflection, shift their focus from negative to affirming experiences.

Sylvia Plath (1975: 147) writes in one letter to her mother, 'the thing about writing is not to talk, but to do it; no matter how bad or even mediocre it is, the process and production is the thing, not the sitting and theorizing about how one should write ideally, or how one could write if one really wanted to or had the time.' Plath's words are a reminder about not getting caught up in technique.

Skill Box

- *Write two stories. One about a recent negative feeling and one about a positive feeling. See where this takes you. We will pick up and reflect on these stories in the next chapter.*

Susan Brooks (2004) reflects on writing a journal,

Having never attempted to keep a reflective journal before, the journey ahead seemed a little daunting as evidenced by the first recorded entry – 'Today I start my journal. What shall I write? I'm really worried about this whole thing – will I get time to do it – will I want to do it – will I do it right? If I'm honest in it will it matter if others read it? Reflective practice – what is it really? I think I know but I don't think I've ever really done it properly. I feel so uncertain about everything at the moment and a bit scared and threatened. I don't feel I know anything about myself really and I suppose I just do what I do to fit in. I need to get over this and get on with it – pull yourself together Sue – you know you can do it'.

This first journal entry reveals my initial uncomfortable reactions to the prospect of journal writing. I had doubts about my capacity to write, felt threatened by having to face myself on paper, questioned my ability to manage my internal censors that may inhibit complete honesty and held the naïve assumption that there is a correct way to keep a journal - all classic reactions to journaling (Street 1995). My initial fears were quickly dispelled as the value of my journal soon became evident. After I while, it seemed to become a powerful emancipatory tool in giving my innermost thoughts voice. I was the only person with access to the journal and, possibly because of this, it became a very cathartic experience to write. As the process continued, I soon recognised that I did not need to confront all the chaos of my personal or professional life at any one time and became more discriminatory about the events that I considered worthy of deeper reflection and subsequent action (Street 1995). The journal became, in a sense, my autobiography containing both positive and less than positive experiences - a non-hagiographic record of my daily life. My journal had, after just a few months on the course, become a silent but very powerful and challenging teacher – perhaps more persuasive and influential than any human embodiment that I had met. The following entry signifies just how my attitude had changed since that first entry at the start of the course. 'I read of a teacher today who got very excited about writing his journal. He wrote that he felt especially good about writing for himself instead of someone else. His written thoughts were entirely his own regardless of lack of style, format or academic expression. He had never written like this before and felt that he was really communicating with and understanding himself'. That's just how I feel now and I wish I had started writing like this ages ago. To be unrestricted by structural rigour, academic expectations and the approval of others is so liberating!'

From the practical aspect, a double entry technique was used with the factual account (data collection) of the experience written on the left of the page and the reflective thought (the analysis) on the right (Moon 2002). Both the ordinary and extraordinary events of every day practice were included to prevent selective inattention, particularly to the seemingly mundane, where habitual routinized practice is thought most likely to occur (Heath and Freshwater 2000). I considered myself to be the primary research tool here. If the journal was to accurately and consistently record my own experiential world I needed to maintain a strong sense of commitment to the task and demonstrate the skills necessary to the reflective cycle – self-awareness, description, critical analysis, synthesis and evaluation (Atkins and Murphy 1993). Keeping a journal enabled me to enter into a dialogue between my objective and subjective self and it transformed my feeling self into a spectator and analyst of my own personal professional drama (Street 1995). Street (1995) writes that journaling provides the reflector with a process for meta-theorising, that is thinking about the processes of thinking. This significantly developed not only my skills of reflection but also my skills as a learner in general, moving me away from my previously held attitude that knowledge (and not necessarily enhanced learning skills) was the goal to be achieved.

Susan extols the virtues of keeping a journal. Note her technique of dividing the page. And yet, at the beginning she felt daunted. It is a serious matter for the practitioner to enter into reflective practice. It requires commitment and responsibility. Perhaps this is why so many practitioners struggle to keep a reflective journal? They are tired at the end of the day, they want to switch off, they don't see the value, they do not have the discipline, they don't find it meaningful, they lack technique, or they don't see the point. Perhaps writing needs the stimulus of a specific purpose such as an educational course, clinical supervision or demand to keep a professional portfolio. Put another way, practitioners might need to do something with their writing. As such, it may need to be a means towards an end rather than just an end in itself. I found this true for myself as I wrote and reflected on my experiences with the intention of constructing a reflexive narrative, using my stories as a format for teaching, and analysing the learning process as an educational and research approach.

Tapping the Tacit

Writing may be difficult for practitioners because, as Schön (1983) suggests, much of our knowing is tacit and not easily explainable. In other words, they may struggle to write what they know. This can be frustrating. Schon (1983: 49) writes,

> When we go about the spontaneous intuitive performance of the actions of everyday life, we show ourselves to be knowledgeable in a certain way. Often we cannot say what it is we know. When we try to describe it we find ourselves at loss, or we produce descriptions that are obviously inappropriate. Our knowing is ordinarily tacit, implicit in our action and in our feel for the stuff with which we are dealing. It seems to right to say that our knowing is in our doing.

Spontaneous writing taps the tacit; it brings it to the surface like a bubbling underground brook. Holly (1989: 71) notes 'Writing taps the unconscious; it can make the implicit explicit, and therefore open to analysis.' It lifts feelings and thoughts to the surface where they can be looked at. Ferruci (1982: 41) writes 'writing can be much more powerful that we may think at first. We should not be surprised that unconscious material surfaces so readily in our writing'. It is these deeper reaches of the mind where old stuff lies buried, stuff that is fundamental to the assumptions we hold and which govern our practice. If we are to gain insight, then it is necessary to access and shake up these assumptions. If not, then we may merely scratch at the surface of our experience without meaning. No easy task and perhaps one reason why practitioners write superficially as a defensive ploy.

Table 2.1 Qualities of mind

Left brain (masculine)	Right brain (feminine)
Reason	Creativity
Logic	Imagination
Rationality	Perception
Analysis	Curiosity and wonder
	Intuition
	Spirit
	Wholeness

Opening the Reflective Space through the Humanities

I often write description as prose poetry, giving rein to my imaginative and creative side. This is in contrast with a more prosaic, factual and logical type of writing. Both types of writing are significant and reflect different sides of the brain (Table 2.1).

Virginia Woolf (1945: 97) writes, 'It is when this fusion takes place that the mind is fully fertilised and uses all its faculties.' The left brain, fed through education and practice processes, dominates modern life. It imposes logic over intuition, reason over imagination, observation over perception, technique over creativity, justice over care, outcome over process, science over art. The right brain has been neglected. It is as if everybody leans to the left! I have often heard that to succeed in a man's world women must become more manly then men. Look about your practice – is there a grain of truth in this idea? Pink (2005: 22) notes how, 'the left hemisphere analyses the details; the right hemisphere synthesises the big picture'. Imagine the neglected right side of the brain is like the dark side of the hill tucked away out of view, out of touch. To find balance, the feminine has to be nurtured. Letting go of the rational in order to play. Playing with the arts enables us to recover our imagination. Paramananda [2001: 71] writes,

> Of course, the sad thing, the tragic thing, is that many of us do get trimmed. We all start off with real heads full of space and imagination, but slowly, somewhere along the path that we call growing up, our heads get trimmed. We become caught up in the doings of this world, the realities of adult life, and we get down to size … without imagination the world loses its mystery and sense of depth in which we can find meaning.

Rather than words, practitioners may prefer to use prose poetry art or mixing words with art. In Chapter 7 I explore prose poetry and in Chapter 8 Otter and I explore how art can be used as a reflective means to directly access the right brain and nurture the creative spirit.

The Value and Therapeutic Benefit of Writing

Writing story has great value (Table 2.2). It is cathartic and healing. Without doubt, health care work is stressful, embracing suffering on a daily basis and working under conditions that do mot necessarily facilitate caring work. As such, it seems imperative that practitioners have a mode for expressing and sharing their feelings

Table 2.2 The value of writing a story[a]

Paints a rich descriptive canvas for reflection
Focuses attention on one's practice and recognising significance within the unfolding situation
Develops perception
Gives voice
Enables self to become aware of self and others within the context of the practice environment/ connection with self and with others (empathy)
Is cathartic/ healing/ transformative
Points to problems and contradictions with values
Others can relate to because of its subjective and contextual nature

[a] In Chapter 13 Margaret Graham reflects on the value of learning through story based on student feedback.

The subtitle of Rachel Remen's (1996) book *Kitchen Table Wisdom* is 'stories that heal'. She claims that in telling our stories we connect with something vital in us, something healing. She writes 'Whatever we have denied may stop us and dam the creative flow of our lives … avoiding pain, we may linger in the vicinity of our wounds … without reclaiming that which we have denied, we cannot know our wholeness or have our healing' (p. 70). The reclaiming is in telling or writing the story.

Writing is the creative flow of our lives. If we do this consistently then it washes away traumatic debris before it can accumulate into a dam. Then we have crisis. Jourard (1971) argues that self-disclosure of upsetting experiences serves as a basic human motive. As such, people naturally discuss daily and significant experiences with others. Talking through a trauma with others can strengthen social bonds, provide coping information and emotional support, and hasten an understanding of the event, the inability to talk with others can be unhealthy.

In reviewing the therapeutic benefit of telling and writing experience, the work of Pennebaker and his colleagues offers good evidence.[4] The title of his book – *Opening up: the healing power of confiding in others* tells his overall message – the idea of story as 'opening up'. And in opening up, letting go of the tension within.

Pennebaker (1989: 213) writes,

> When given the opportunity, people readily divulge their deepest and darkest secrets. Even though people report they have lived with these thoughts and feelings virtually every day, most note that they have actively held back from telling others about these fundamental parts of themselves. Over the past several years, my colleagues and I have learned that confronting traumatic experiences can have meaningful physiological and psychological benefit. Conversely, not confiding significant experiences is associated with increased disease rates, ruminations and other difficulties.

Pennebaker and his various colleagues (Pennebaker, Colder and Sharp 1990; Pennebaker, Mayne and Francis 1997) demonstrated the therapeutic benefit of therapeutic journaling in well-being, notably the benefit of connecting strong feelings to past traumatic events. Smyth et al.'s (1999) review of the literature suggested that emotional expression has a salutary health effect, whereas emotional inhibition has a detrimental health effect. Smyth cites Pennebaker et al.'s (1997: 175) claim that,

> Written emotional expression leads to a transduction of the traumatic experience into a linguistic structure that promotes assimilation and understanding of the event, and reduces negative affect associated with thoughts of the event.

Smyth and colleagues reviewed ten studies that demonstrated significant superior health outcomes in participants; psychological well-being, physiological functioning, general functioning, reported health outcomes, but not for health behaviours. Smyth noted that these studies demonstrated that short-term distress was increased but is thought to be related to long-term improvement.

Pennebaker et al. (1990: 536) write,

> The present experiment, as well as others that we have conducted, found that writing about transition to college resulted in more negative moods and poorer psychological adjustment by the end of the first semester. Our experiment may have effectively stripped the normal defences away from the experimental subjects. With lowered defences, our subjects were forced to deal with many of their basic conflicts and fears about leaving home, changing roles, entering college.

Indications from this study suggest that the power of confronting upsetting experiences reflects insight rather than cathartic processes. In follow-up questionnaires, for example, the overwhelming majority of the subjects spontaneously wrote that the value of the experimental condition derived from their achieving a better understanding of their own thoughts, behaviours and moods. The stripping away of defence mechanisms means that practitioners may benefit from guidance to support them through the consequences of the writing experience. Perhaps one way practitioners deal with negative experience is to avoid it, to bury it deeper into the subconscious. Writing opens the door to the subconscious with the threat of lifting these buried experiences into the conscious mind. Whilst this may be upsetting, burying experiences has a psychological impact that is not conducive to well-being and effective practice. In other words, health care practitioners have a responsibility to be fit for practice. However, writing about experience and disclosing these experiences are two different issues. Writing is an introvert activity whereas disclosure is a more extrovert activity perhaps more suited to different personalities. Having written the story the practitioner now stands back to reflect on it – the focus for the following chapter.

Skill Box

- *Think of the last time you were at work. Now think about one particular situation. It needn't be dramatic. It can simply be something mundane or ordinary, something you wouldn't normally give a second thought. Before going to see a patient or a meeting or teaching, pause before entering and use your breath to bring yourself fully present to this moment. Write about the impact of that.*
- *First, relax and bring your mind home. Now write a description of this situation for 15–20 minutes. Do not to take your pen off the paper. Do not stop and think about the why's of the situation. Just let the pen or keyboard flow spontaneously, in rich graphic description, paying attention to detail, drawing on all your senses. Just write.*
- *After 20 minutes, pause, and stand back. Read what you have written with an open and curious mind. Ask yourself – 'What is significant in what I have written towards becoming a more effective practitioner, towards realizing my vision of clinical practice as a lived reality?'*

As you do, you enter the reflective spiral. This is the focus for the following chapter.

Summary

Writing self is the raw data of experience. Hence, the richer the description the more data to reflect on. Through writing self the practitioner learns to pay attention, to become aware of self in context of her environment. Writing is also cathartic and healing. As such it is a vital learning medium in its own right. In chapter 3 we stand back from our stories and enter the reflective spiral.

Endnotes

1   MSc Leadership in healthcare programme [see Chapter **22**]
2   quote reflections.blogspot.co.uk
3   For example see - www.helpguide.org/harvard/benefits-of-mindfulness.htm. *Google health benefits of mindfulness for further information.*
4   See also DeSalvo L (1999) for a summary of Pennebaker's work.

References

Atkins, S. and Murphy, K. (1995) Reflective practice. *Nursing Standard 9.45*, 31–37.

Beck, C. Yoko (1989) *Everyday Zen*. Thorsons, London.

Boud, D., Keogh, R. and Walker, D. (1985) Promoting reflection in learning: a model. In D. Boud, R. Keogh and D. Walker (eds.), *Reflection: turning experience into learning*. Kogan Page, London.

Boyd, E. and Fales, A. (1983) Reflective learning: key to learning from experience. *Journal of Humanistic Psychology* 23.2, 99–117.

Brooks, S. (2004) Becoming a transformational leader. Unpublished Masters in Leadership dissertation, University of Bedfordshire.

Callahan, S. (1988) The role of emotion in ethical decision making. Hastings centre Report June/July pp. 9–14.

Chodron, P. (2000) *When things fall apart*. Shambhala, Boston.

De Salvo, L. (1999) *Writing as a way of healing: how telling our stories transforms our lives*. The Women's Press, London.

Ferrucii, P. (1982) *What we may be*. St. Martin's Press, New York.

Flemons, D. and Green, S. (2002) Stories that conform/ stories that transform: a conversation in four parts. In Bochner a & Ellis C (eds), *Ethnographically speaking*. AltaMira Press, Walnut Creek, CA.

Gadamer, H.-G. (1975) *Truth & method*. Seabury Press, New York.

Gray, G. and Forsstrom, S. (1991) Generating theory from practice: the reflective technique. In G. Gray and R. Pratt 9eds.), *Towards a discipline of nursing*. Churchill Livingstone, Melbourne, pp. 355–372.

Gully, E. (2005) Creating sacred space: a journey to the soul. In C. Johns & D. Freshwater (eds.), *Transforming nursing through reflective practice (second edition)*. Blackwell, Oxford.

Heath, H. and Freshwater, D. (2000) Clinical supervision as an emancipatory process avoiding inappropriate intent. *Journal of Advanced Nursing* 32, 1298–1306.

Holly, M. L. (1989) Reflective writing and the spirit of inquiry. *Cambridge Journal of Education* 19.1, 71–80.

Johns, C. (ed.) (2010) *Guided Reflection: a narrative approach to advancing practice (second edition)*. Wiley-Blackwell, Oxford.

Jones, R. and Jones, G. (1996) *Earth Dance Drum*. Commune-E-Key, Salt Lake City.

Jourard, S. (1971) *The transparent self*. Van Nostrand, Newark, NJ.

Loori, J. D. (2005) *The Zen of creativity: cultivating your artistic life*. Ballantine Books, New York.

Manjusvara (2005) *Writing your way*. Windhorse, Birmingham.

Mattingly, C. (1998) *Healing dramas and clinical ploys: the narrative structure of experience*. Cambridge University Press, Cambridge.

Moon, J. (2002) *Reflection in learning and professional development: theory and practice*. Routledge, London.

Moore, T. (1992) *Care of the soul*. HarperCollins, New York.

Paramananda (2001) *A deeper beauty: Buddhist reflections on everyday life*. Windhorse, Birmingham.

Pennebaker, J. (1989) Confession, inhibition and disease. *Advances in Experimental Social Psychology* 22, 211–244.

Pennebaker, J. (1990) *Opening up: the healing power of confiding in others*. Morrow, New York.

Pennebaker, J. Colder, M and Sharp, L (1990) Accelerating the coping process. *Journal of Personality and Social Psychology* 58; 528–537.

Pennebaker, J., Mayne, T. and Francis, M. (1997) Linguistic predictors of adaptive bereavement. *Journal of Personality and Social Psychology* 72; 863–871.

Plath, S. (1975) *Letters home*. Harper & Row, New York.

Pink, D. (2005) *A whole new mind: moving from information age to the conceptual age*: Riverhead Books, New York.

Remen, R. (1994) *Kitchen Table Wisdom*. Riverhead Books, New York.

Rinpoche, S. (1992) *The Tibetan book of living and dying*. Rider, London.

Schön, D. (1983) *The reflective practitioner*. Avebury, Aldershot.

Senge, P. (1990) The fifth discipline. *The art and practice of the learning organisation*. London: Century Business.

Smyth, J., Stone, A., Hurewitz, A. and Kaell, A. (1999) Effects of writing about stressful experiences on symptom reduction in patients with asthma or rheumatoid arthritis. *Journal of the American Medical Association* 281; 1304–9.

Street, A. (1995) *Nursing replay*. Churchill Livingstone, Melbourne.

Tschudin, V. (1993) *Ethics in nursing* (Second edition). Butterworth Heinemann, Oxford.

Tuffnell, M. and Crickmay, C. (2004) *A widening field*. Dance Books, Alton.

Tzu, Lao (1999) *Tao Te Ching* (trans S. Mitchell). Frances Lincoln, London.

Woolf, V. (1928/1945) *A room of one's own*. Penguin Books, London.

Chapter 3

Engaging the Reflective Spiral: The Second Dialogical Movement

Christopher Johns

Nothing happens because of a single thing

Having written my story text, I stand back from it to reflect and gain insight. I move into a more objective relationship with the text to see myself clearly. At first, this may prove difficult simply because I am wrapped up in my experience.

Standing back is a playful posture. Wheatley and Keller-Rogers (1999: 69) write,

> life is playful and life plays with us. The future cannot be determined. It can only be experienced as it is occurring. Life doesn't know what it will be until it notices what it has just become.

I move into a dialogue with the text guided by a model of reflection. I suspend any interpretation as to what the text means. I do not want to jump to hasty conclusions. We enter the reflective spiral, moving inwards to gain insight.

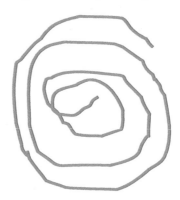

Becoming a Reflective Practitioner, Fifth Edition. Edited by Christopher Johns.
© 2017 John Wiley & Sons Ltd. Published 2017 by John Wiley & Sons Ltd.
Companion Website: www.wiley.com/go/johns/reflectivepractitioner

Models of Reflection

Models of reflection are guides for the practitioner to explore the breadth and depth of experience. There are many models on offer [see Chapter 1]. The practitioner should review all models of reflection for their value, rather than accepting the authority of any model on face value. Rather like the skilled craftsman, the practitioner will choose the tool that is most helpful. I am wary of cyclical or stage models of reflection because they suggest that reflection is an orderly progressive movement between different stages or cycles. It simply isn't like that.

Models are not prescriptions for reflection. They must always be viewed as heuristic, as a means to an end. In a technical rational society, reflective models are likely to be grasped as authoritative. The risk, from this perspective, is that practitioners will fit their experience to the model of reflection rather than use the model creatively to guide them to gain insight. It is easy to get wrapped up in the technology of reflection, especially in a learning culture dominated by technical rationality. It is a Western technological addiction (Rinpoche 1992). Reflection is complex, whereby the mind engages with all the cues or stages in dynamic flow.

However, it is natural for someone approaching reflection for the first time to ask certain 'technical' questions:

- What is reflection?
- How do I do it?
- How do I know if I am doing it properly?
- How do I learn through reflection?

Hold these questions as you read the text.

The Model for Structured Reflection [MSR]

I designed the Model for Structured Reflection [MSR] to enable practitioners to access the depth and breadth of reflection to facilitate learning through experience. The first edition of the MSR (Table 3.1) was constructed in 1991 through analysing the pattern of conversation between myself as a guide and practitioners in guided reflection relationships. I then framed this pattern within Strauss and Corbin's grounded theory paradigm model (Johns 1998). Since then, the MSR design has been reflexively developed based on insights gained in utilising it. In time, I utilised Carper's 'Fundamental ways of knowing in nursing' to frame learning through reflection. Table 3.2 sets out the 17th edition, which has some changes from the previous 16th edition (Table 3.3). The cues about feelings, ethics, knowledge, and past experiences have been incorporated within the *Influences Grid* (Table 3.4) linked to the cue – 'What factors influenced my response?' In doing this I give primary focus to the event itself and only then address the issue of feelings within the spectrum of influencing factors.

I have added two new cues:

'How does extant theory/ ideas inform and deepen my insights?'
'How does exploring with guides and peers challenge my insights?'

Table 3.1 The Model for Structured Reflection first edition

1 What was I trying to achieve?
2 Why did I intervene as I did?
3 What other choices did I have?
4 What would be the consequences of other interventions?
5 What were the consequences of my actions:
for the patient?
for myself?
6 How did I feel about the situation on reflection
7 How did the patient feel about it?
8 Could the situation have been better dealt with?

Table 3.2 The Model for Structured Reflection (Edition 17[a])

Reflective cue
Bring the mind home
Write a description of an experience
What in particular seems significant to pay attention to?
Why did I respond as I did?
Was I effective in terms of consequences for others and myself?
What factors influenced my response? (See Table 3.4 – 'Influences Grid')
Given the situation again, what are my options for responding more effectively?'
What are the potential consequences of responding differently?
How do those influencing factors need to shift so I can respond differently?
What tentative insights do I draw?
How does extant theory/ ideas inform and deepen my insights?
How does exploring with guides and peers challenge my insights?
How do I feel now about the situation?

[a] Christopher Johns, 17th edition. August 2015.

These two cues reflect the third and fourth dialogical movements concerned with deepening insights. As a consequence the MSR fits more coherently within the six dialogical movements. The cue 'How do I now feel about the situation?' guides the practitioner to reflect on any residual feelings especially if the experience felt negative in some way. In this way the practitioner can harness residual feelings as positive energy for taking action as a consequence of reflection.

Reflection can be viewed as five phases: preparatory, descriptive, reflective, anticipatory and insight. The cues remain arranged in a sequential order through these five phases, enabling a movement of thought through each cue and phase. They reflect a dynamic movement from recognising significance of the experience towards gaining insight. With repeated use, the reflective cues become embodied and focus the clinical gaze. The cues also have considerable value in developing clinical skills, as I indicate in my commentary on each cue in relation to my experience with Peggy in Chapter 2. As practitioners utilise them, the MSR cues inevitably become internalised. With use, the reflective practitioner will begin to use the cues spontaneously in her descriptive writing, breaking down the separation between the first and second dialogical movements.

Table 3.3 The Model for Structured Reflection (16th edition)

Preparatory phase
Bring the mind home

Descriptive phase
Focus on a description of an experience that seems significant in some way (balance between
    experiences that were affirming and experiences that were problematic)

Reflective phase
What issues seem significant to pay attention to?
How were others feeling and why did they felt that way?
How was I feeling & what made me feel that way?
What was I trying to achieve and did I respond effectively?
What were the consequences of my actions on the patient, others and myself?
To what extent did I act for the best and in tune with my values?
What knowledge did or might have informed me?
How does this situation connect with previous experiences?
What assumptions govern my practice and what factors influence the way I feel, think, and
    respond to the particular situation?

Anticipatory phase
How might I reframe the situation in order to respond more effectively?
What would be the consequences of responding differently for the patient, others and myself?
What factors might constrain me responding in new ways?
How do I feel NOW about this experience?

Insight phase
What insights have I gained? [framing perspectives]

Table 3.4 The Influences Grid

<ul><li>Conforming to 'normal practice'</li><li>Habit</li><li>Fear of sanction if I don't conform</li><li>Knowledge to act in a particular way</li><li>Ethics- doing what is right</li><li>My assumptions and values!</li><li>Past experience</li><li>Lack of support/ poor leadership</li></ul>	Expectations from others about 'how I should act'? What factors influenced my response? Expectations from self about 'how I should act' ?	<ul><li>How others were feeling</li><li>How I was feeling/ poise</li><li>Positive and negative attitudes/ prejudice</li><li>Emotional entanglement</li><li>Deeper psychological and socialisation issues</li><li>Need to be in control</li><li>Anxious about conflict</li><li>Time/ priorities/ resources/ busyness</li><li>Uncertain how to respond?</li><li>Transactional organisation</li></ul>

Preparatory and Descriptive Phases

The cues, 'Bring the mind home' and 'Write a description of an experience' have been
explored in Chapter 2. This description is the story text the practitioner moves into dialogue with in order to move towards gaining insight.

First, I repeat my description of working with Peggy, as set out in Chapter 2.

Peggy

A normal day at hospice day care. The usual suspects. Things go as normal that is until Peggy pulls me aside and says 'I'm first today'. Taken by surprise I am uncertain how to respond. After a momentary pause I say 'OK Peggy let's go'. I had not spoken with her beyond social niceties before even though I had been working here for the past six weeks. Others had grasped my attention. We walk to the therapy room and she talks about her life, losing her partner quickly to cancer and then her dog dying recently. She is sad. She likes to come to the centre for company but also feels she needs to be alone. She takes off her new walking boots and I give her reflexology. My base cream mixed with essential oils. She is relaxed and appreciative of the therapy. Afterwards I walk her back to the day room to rejoin the hungry throng – hungry in the sense of demanding my attention. Peggy smiles. She made her point and taught me a lesson about paying attention and taking nothing for granted. No such thing as a normal day when you pierce it rather than slide along its surface.

Why did I respond as I did?

Response is linked to intent, 'What was I trying to achieve?' All action is purposeful in response to perceived need through appreciating the particular situation and making judgment about how best to respond. In reality many decisions are made reactively or intuitively as if processing information takes place below the mind radar. Appreciating the situation with Peggy was not a rational thinking-out of my response. It was a reaction, essentially an emotional response to my guilt, rather like a naughty child being caught out. Intuitively I must have processed my emotion and recognised it as guilt, resulting in my response 'let's go' – meaning let's do it now. I lost my poise and control of the immediate situation. Wriggling on the hook so to speak! Hence my response intended to alleviate both Peggy's and my own suffering. Perhaps if I had paused and not reacted so quickly I would have had other options, as I explore later.

Response can be viewed as four movements that constitute clinical judgement: appreciation, judgement, response and evaluation (Figure 3.1). Through reflection, each movement is reviewed. I challenge my pattern of decision making, lifting it from a non-reflective to mindful mode. In terms of response, I know that practitioners tend to respond based on three inadequate criteria:

- Responses they have used before;
- Responses that have worked before;
- Responses they are comfortable using;

1. How I appreciated/ assessed the situation

4. Reflection on outcome – were the consequences of my responses the best they could have been? Could they have been better?

Effective action

2. How I made clinical decisions to meet desired outcomes, including weighing up consequences of alternative responses

3. How I responded to meet perceived outcomes in tune with my caring values

Figure 3.1   Model for clinical judgement.

These criteria reflect a habitual and unreflective practice that certainly does not lead to effective practice. Through reflection the practitioner constantly seeks to expand her ability to appreciate situations and her repertoire of responses to meet the patient's and family's needs.

Was I Effective in Terms of Consequences for Others and Myself?

All responses have consequences. On the surface such consequences may be quite obvious. Others less so. It is like throwing a pebble into a pond. The splash is the immediate consequence and the ripples spreading out are further consequences.

Considering effectiveness in terms of consequences enables the practitioner to develop foresight- to weigh up the likely consequences of actions as part of the decision-making process. It leads to the development of what Aristotle termed *phronesis* or practical wisdom – being mindful of the best way to respond within a particular situation considering the ethical consequences of such response.[1] Foresight is intuitive, for how can consequences be known given the uncertainty of life? Intuition in this sense suggests deeper embodied way of knowing. It is significant considering the impact of our actions not just for the patients we work with but more broadly towards creating better worlds for generations to come.

To ask the question – 'Was I effective?' requires me to have a grasp of what effectiveness would be like. For some situations this can be observed or measured – for example, wound healing and blood pressure. But most evaluation is subjective from the patient's perspective. Peggy's suffering, for example, is ineffable. Only Peggy can evaluate my effectiveness. She was satisfied with my response to her confrontation and appreciative of her therapy. Perhaps more than that, she was satisfied to have made her point. She felt that she had been heard, and this established a therapeutic relationship for the future. Any assumption I make that her suffering is eased is fraught with difficulty and yet necessary. In responding as I did I also alleviated my own sense of guilt, transforming this negative energy into positive action.

In reviewing whether my response was effective I review the way I appreciated the situation. Did I read Peggy's situation accurately? I let you, the reader, consider that.

One consequence of my response was to disrupt the pattern of the 'normal' day. Perhaps the other patients were left wondering where I was, possibly creating concern about getting their own therapies. This appreciation raises issues about managing time and setting priorities as a significant influencing factor, as is the busyness of the day with so many patients clamouring for attention. Then 'normal' becomes a defensive routine blown apart by Peggy.

Skill Box

- *Reflect on your decision making and response in light of any clinical experience (using Figure 3.1)*
- *Did you appreciate the situation correctly and see the 'bigger picture'?*
- *Justify the responses you made in light of its obvious and less obvious consequences.*

What Factors Influenced my Response?

How the practitioner responds to any situation is influenced by personal and cultural factors that have become embodied through socialisation. These factors are rooted in assumptions and attitudes that govern the practitioner's approach to practice, and which are reinforced within everyday patterns of relationships.

Assumptions are difficult to see because they are normal, deeply embodied, governing the way we perceive and respond to the world.

Bohm [1996: 69] writes,

> Normally, we don't see that our assumptions are affecting the nature of our observations. But the assumptions affect the way we see things, the way we experience them, and consequently the things we want to do. In a way we are looking through our assumptions; the assumptions could be said to be an observer in a sense.

The root of contradiction lies with a conflict of values. We might say 'we are caring' and believe this to be so, but failure to see a patient in their humanness may unwittingly lead to uncaring behaviours or the 'dark side of nursing' (Jameton 1992; Corey and Goren 1998). I say unwittingly because practitioners may inadvertently slip into uncaring behaviour as institutional practice, as evident in recent scandals, for example Mid-Staffs.

In Table 3.4 I organise influencing factors around the tension between 'expectations from self' and 'expectations from others'. The grid provides a systematic checklist for the reflective practitioner to review. The grid is imposing, identifying a range of factors that have become evident in my work with practitioners. Other factors can be added.

The reflective practitioner considers the way these factors have influenced her practice with a view to changing them as necessary to enable realising more desirable practice. However these factors are deeply embodied and rooted in cultural norms and as such may not be easy to perceive let alone change. Because these factors are often shared with colleagues changing them may incur resistance. 'Old habits die hard' simply because they are embodied and reinforced within everyday patterns of relationships. They need active and prolonged confrontation. It can be like hitting your head on a brick wall – what I term 'the hard wall of reality'. Collective action may be necessary to bring about deeper shifts in tradition and authority. And yet it does happen and quite dramatically as some of the stories within the book reveal. The reflective practitioner can open dialogue with her colleagues about some of these factors at opportune moments such as shift handovers. Using the influences grid is not necessarily easy. The practitioner may need guidance to see herself clearly within the grid.

How was I Feeling/poise

With Peggy, I felt a mixture of guilt and satisfaction. Guilt, because I had been caught out like a naughty boy, that I had passed her by as if I didn't care for her. Clearly my guilt influenced my response, reflecting the significant impact of feelings on my decision-making (Callahan 1988). This understanding challenges the idea that decision-making is a rational process where emotions are morally suspect and distort reason. As such, through paying attention to feelings the practitioner learns to know and manage her emotional self (Salovey and Mayer 1990).The risk is that I get swept along on an emotional tide anxious to resolve my discomfort rather than act in Peggy's best interests. As I become more mindful through reflection I learn to better monitor and focus my feelings within the moment, so as to make good clinical judgment or what I term as 'poise'.[2] As George Eliot wrote in *Daniel Deronda*, 'There is a great deal of unmapped country within us which would have to be taken into account in an explanation of our gusts and storms.'

Reflection is mapping, charting the unknown self, to better recognise, understand and control these gusts and storms in order to be more effective in our practice. It may not be easy to understand our negative emotions. They may stem from earlier unresolved issues in our lives. As Jones and Jones (1996: 56) write,

> When I fill up with negative thoughts, inside I am more worried and distracted. We cannot escape from our worrisome mind unless we unravel the mental fibre that we have erroneously woven. Take the time to reweave new patterns …

Reflection is reweaving. Through reflection we become aware of our fear and see the way it constrains our practice. Perhaps we see the fear as huge and immovable as if it was a boulder. As we reflect we can begin to accept the fear as our own rather than something that will destroy us. As we do, the boulder seems to crumble, loosen and fall away. We can learn to shift our images of fear and see fear as a cloud obscuring the blue sky. We can see that it is not permanent and will float away. Slowly our attachment to fear weakens and, as Rosenberg (1998) notes, *little by little, we're not so enslaved to things* (p. 145). At every point, reflection is freedom to become who we desire to be.

Jones and Jones (1996) offer words for reflection,

> Uncomfortable with the griever's uncertainty about life, deep sadness, encounter with death, and changed self, we turn away when we are needed most. Look at times when, perhaps, you have turned away – what were you avoiding? Most likely it was your own uncertainty, your own sadness, your own changes, your own mortality.

When we turn away we fail. Through reflection I work out and convert negative feelings such as pity, frustration, anger, hatred into to positive energy for taking action.

Moore (1992: 235) writes,

> Day by day we live emotions and themes that have deep roots, but our reflections on these experiences tend to be superficial … not only are our reflections often insufficient to account for intense feelings, but we may have been living from a place that is too rational and dispassionate. Rainer Maria Rilke advises the young poet to 'go deep into yourself and see how deep the place is from which your life flows'. We could all take note of this advice, go deep into ourselves and discover how deep is the source of our everyday lives.

Yet, what will *going deeper* reveal? Is it better to swim in the shallow end rather than risk of deep water? Exploration of feelings leads to deep insights into self and the development of therapeutic poise or equanimity.

Joko Beck (1997: 42/3) writes,

> for a time our life may feel worse than before, as what we have concealed becomes clear. But even as this occurs, we have a sense of growing sanity and understanding, of basic satisfaction. To continue practice through severe difficulties we must have patience, persistence and courage.… we learn in our guts not just in our brains.

Skill Box

• *When next in practice, consider the idea of poise when with a patient or student, especially where the person evokes strong feelings within you. Reflect on this experience.*

How were Others Feeling?

Peggy's outburst stopped me in my tracks. Imagine how she must have been feeling! Perhaps it can become a cliché to say to every patient 'How are you feeling?' Yet, beyond its social nicety it is important to inquire into feelings – what I term 'empathic inquiry'. It is the path to connect with the other and opens a gate to tune into the other's wavelength and talk about issues.[3] My experience with Peggy is about the consequence of failing to connect.

Peggy was frustrated at being passed by. I imagine Peggy seeing me each week waiting for me to offer her a treatment and her growing discomfort watching others week after week get treatment. But then, she may have not wanted a treatment; but then I should have known that, rather than assuming that because she didn't ask she didn't want. She was also sad and alone following the death of her partner and her dog. On my return to the sitting room with Peggy on my arm I sensed two of the more demanding patients were frustrated with me not following the normal pattern, anxious about their own turn in the schedule.

Skill Box

- *Reflect on an experience where the feelings of others were significant. Use empathic inquiry to consider why the other people felt as they did.*
- *How did you respond to the feelings of others? Consider the use of catharsis within the experience [see Heron's Six-category Intervention Analysis]*

Conforming to Normal Practice

Practitioners develop habits and routines that become normal and which are generally unexamined. The maxim is 'that's how we do it here'. It's as if practice is automatic. Indeed much of the practice environment is organised in this way.

As I wrote in the Peggy story, *it was a normal day*. I saw what I normally saw and responded in my normal way. In doing so I passed Peggy by. The experience was a wake-up call to become mindful of routine and habit that only serve my interests in managing my day, rather than the patients' best interests.

Skill Box

- *Next time you are at work, consider what aspects of your work might be labelled as 'normal', i.e. things you do unreflectively. Are these the most therapeutic ways for the patient or student? Reflection wakes us up and lifts us out of unreflective routine practices.*

How does this situation connect with previous experiences?

An experience is not an isolated moment in time. It is part of a continuous stream of unfolding experiences. How I respond today is influenced by how I responded previously. As Jones and Jones (1996: 78) write, 'If we don't stay connected and remember the lessons from the past, are we not doomed to repeat them?'

Reflection helps me appreciate links between my practices and see patterns of my behaviour grooved out over 30 years as a nurse. This is a disturbing cue for at least two reasons. Firstly, it pulls you out of autopilot and obliges you to think about what you do. Secondly, you may realise that learned patterns are not the best patterns and feel a deep sense of guilt. Two reasons why practitioners may shrink away from reflection?

With Peggy I cannot see obvious connection with previous experiences except that those who ask, get and those who don't ask are passed by simply because it is easier to manage workload from this perspective. Of course, this is ethically unsound practice, grounded in a task approach to practice rather than a patient-centred one, whereby Peggy and the other patients become merely task objects.

Skill Box

- *Return to any story you have written. Is there any connection between this story and previous experiences? Put another way, did you respond as you did because it was normal practice? Was that the most effective way?*

Values and Attitude

Values are enshrined in a vision. Values reflect the service we intend to offer the patient. As such, our values shape our attitude and manner towards the patient. Words such as respect, dignity and compassion easily roll of the tongue as prime values. Indeed there has been much media and professional attention to the lack of these values evident within practice. Negative attitudes lead to such phenomena as the 'difficult patient', the 'interfering relative' and racism. Emotional entanglement develops when practitioners get too involved. Indeed emotions can be an obstacle to caring (Ramos 1992). For example, issues surrounding racism continue to surface (Blackford 2003; Puzan 2003).

Puzan writes,

> There is so much familiarity in talking about the alleged racial differences of non-white people in public discourse and so little familiarity in talking about those racial properties attached to being white, that the concept of whiteness (or a recognition of racial formation) has little resonance within nursing (citing Jacobson 1998). While issues related to cultural difference are not ignored, they rarely include the difference specifically engendered by 'whiteness', which is structured to avoid and deflect interrogation or critical reflection (p. 194).

The Ethical Demand

Logstrup (1997: 18) writes,

> By our very attitude to one another we help to shape one another's world. By our attitude to the other person we help to determine the scope and the hue of his or her world; we make it large and small, bright or drab, rich or dull, threatening or secure. We help to shape his or her world, not by theories and views but by our very attitude to him or her. Herein lies the unarticulated and one might say anonymous demand that we take care of the life which trust has placed into our hands.

Logstrup suggests that our attitude is itself ethical, that we, who purport to care enter into a trust with our patients that they can expect us to care. Failure to care is a failure of trust. Failure to care is uncaring and causes suffering, a contradiction if our role is to be caring. I certainly hold patient-centred values. As such, my experience with Peggy reveals a contradiction between this value and my actual practice. It is easy to lose sight of values in the expediency of the moment. Reflection is a wake-up call to be careful.

Skill Box

- *As I have previously noted, our values or vision of practice sets up the creative tension between what is ideal and actual practice. This is the learning potential of reflective practice. Clarify your values in relation to a recent experience: think again about the cue – what was I trying to achieve in terms of values?*

Deeper Psyche Factors

The attitudes we hold are shaped by deeper psyche factors such as fear, dependency and insecurity. These factors are like emotional scars.

In his book *Awakenings*, Sacks (1976: 15) writes,

> In our study of our most complex sufferings and disorder of being, we are compelled to scrutinise the deepest, darkest, and most fearful parts of ourselves, the parts we strive to deny or not to see. The thoughts which are most difficult to grasp or express are those which awaken our strongest denials and our most profound intuitions.

Reading these words may give an impression that reflection is akin to therapy. Identifying these old patterns is a significant step in dealing with and healing them, as necessary with guidance. Jones and Jones [1996] describe these factors as crooked arrows that continue to hurt us. They advocate a focus on straight arrows that develop a strong sense of self-acceptance and love. Too often we get wrapped up in our negative parts of self and neglect strengthening the positive aspects. It is about the 'self' being fit for practice. With Peggy I sense my guilt stems from childhood where I had a strong aversion to 'being caught out'. I also view myself as a perfectionist and suddenly I fail! Not easy. I felt as if I was struggling to pick up the shattered pieces.

Skill Box

- *In relation to any experience – can you connect with the way you felt or responded with deeper psychological factors? This is an important aspect of self-understanding in order not to project these factors into the therapeutic relationship.*

Ethics – Doing What Was Right

Values and attitudes naturally lead into ethics. Every story is a moral story concerning the practitioner's intent to act for the good. Healthcare professionals are expected to practice within a code of professional ethics that set out their responsibility to act ethically at all times. Ethical principles often contradict each other. As such, *doing what was right* always needs to be interpreted within each moment (Parker 1990; Cooper 1991). This may be problematic if practitioners have different values, agendas and levels of authority to make decisions.

People want to be involved in decision-making about their health care. They are more informed – just Google any health condition to reveal an overload of information, challenging the idea of professional knowledge. Hence the role of health professionals shifts from doing things to, at, or for, patients to working with patients as far as they are able. The 'old' medical ethics of benevolence and non-malevolence are perhaps now less significant than a respect for the patient's autonomy (Seedhouse 1988). The other key ethical principle is utilitarianism – the idea of the greatest good that is explicitly concerned with finite resources – how do I use resources to the best effect, which, in an era of cash-strapped NHS, becomes very significant. It involves ideas such as establishing priorities and setting the need of the individual against the needs of many. This might strike tension between masculine and feminine moral development.

Gilligan (1982) argues that women and men have different criteria in judging 'moral goodness' – and that men, in a patriarchal society with moral claim to justice, is deemed higher than women's claim for caring and responsibility.

She (1982: 18) writes,

> the very traits that have traditionally defined the goodness of women, their care for and sensitivity to the needs of others, are those that mark them as deficient in moral development.'.

Other ethical values include integrity – acting within one's values, and confidentiality – as enshrined with the Data Protection Act (1998). To guide the practitioner in her explorations of *doing the right thing* I developed ethical mapping (Figure 3.2).

To use this map follow the ethical map trail – I have added my own responses based on working with Peggy to illustrate its use in action.

The Ethical Map Trail

1 *Frame the dilemma*
   Most ethical issues can be reduced into a dilemma.
   For example – should I give Peggy a therapy now or fit her in later?
2 *Consider different perspectives, commencing with the practitioner's own perspective*
   By considering the perspectives of people involved within the experience the practitioner challenges her own partial views and can come to see the wider perspective. These perspectives may be in conflict and are not necessarily motivated by 'the right thing to do' but by personal, professional or organisational interests. From a conflict perspective it helps to see where other people are coming from as the basis for any conflict resolution.
3 *Consider which ethical principles apply in terms of the best decision;*
   Having gained an understanding of different perspectives, the practitioner can consider what and how ethical principles might inform the situation. The major ethical principles to consider are:
   ○ Autonomy and advocacy
   ○ Beneficence and non-malevolence
   ○ Justice or utilitarianism
   ○ Integrity and virtue

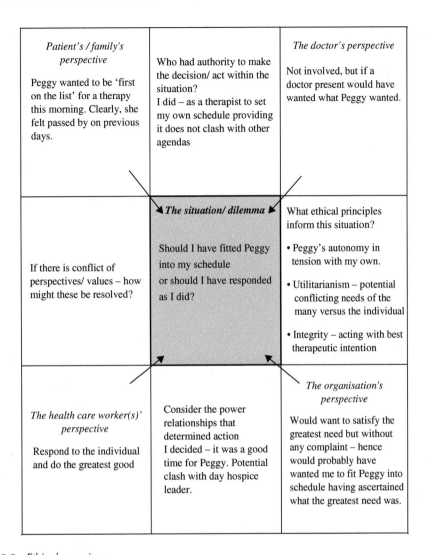

Patient's / family's perspective Peggy wanted to be 'first on the list' for a therapy this morning. Clearly, she felt passed by on previous days.	Who had authority to make the decision/ act within the situation? I did – as a therapist to set my own schedule providing it does not clash with other agendas	The doctor's perspective Not involved, but if a doctor present would have wanted what Peggy wanted.
If there is conflict of perspectives/ values – how might these be resolved?	**The situation/ dilemma** Should I have fitted Peggy into my schedule or should I have responded as I did?	What ethical principles inform this situation? • Peggy's autonomy in tension with my own. • Utilitarianism – potential conflicting needs of the many versus the individual • Integrity – acting with best therapeutic intention
The health care worker(s)' perspective Respond to the individual and do the greatest good	Consider the power relationships that determined action I decided – it was a good time for Peggy. Potential clash with day hospice leader.	The organisation's perspective Would want to satisfy the greatest need but without any complaint – hence would probably have wanted me to fit Peggy into schedule having ascertained what the greatest need was.

Figure 3.2   Ethical mapping.

Autonomy is the possession or right of self-government [*Compact Oxford English Dictionary* 2005: 58]. Seedhouse (1988) views autonomy as the highest ethical principle. Autonomy has two aspects; respecting the patient's right for self-determination and creating space for the patient to exercise their autonomy. Hence, Peggy might not assert her autonomy for many reasons, such as learnt passivity, fear of reprisal and such like. She may be happy for professionals to make decisions for her, although, as the story reveals, this was not in her best interests.

By contrast, professional autonomy is concerned with the practitioner's right for self-government, safeguarded with the ethics of beneficence and non-malevolence enshrined within the Hippocratic Oath: that doctors should do good (beneficence) and not do harm (non-malevolence). In the past, professional autonomy was universally accepted in a capitalist construction of healthcare whereby the patient gave up his rights in return for care (Talcott Parsons 1951). However, there is an ever-increasing recognition of the patient's right to be involved in decisions about their healthcare.

This creates a natural tension between professional and patient autonomy within which the practitioner must position herself.

professional autonomy 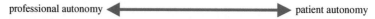 patient autonomy

Many patients, for whatever reason, are unable or reluctant to exercise their autonomy. From this perspective the health worker takes an advocacy role to act in the patient's best interests (beneficence). Acting on behalf of others is termed 'paternalism.' Benjamin and Curtis (1986) set out three criteria to legitimate such action:

o Harm – would the patient come to some harm if I don't act for them?
o Autonomy – is the patient able to act for themselves?
o Ratification – would the patient at a later time thank me for my actions?

Yet how easy is it to advocate for patients rather than respect their autonomy on the premise that we are the health professionals and we know what's best for the patient. The risk is that the patient becomes an object we do things to. We do not see the patient; we just see what needs doing to them.

Utilitarianism is based on the idea of 'the greatest good' whereby the needs of the individual are in tension with the needs of society as a whole due to available resources being finite.

needs of the individual 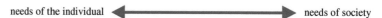 needs of society

As such, the way I use time (as a finite resource) and set priorities is a significant skill. I only have so many hours in the day. Who should I give therapy to? How long should a therapy take? Should I give less time to more patients so that more can benefit? Would the quality of my therapy suffer as a consequence? The fact that I am a volunteer means that the patients actually receive therapy even though there is no budget for it, despite it being valued by patients. An alternative would be to ask patients to pay for it, which goes against the ethos of the National Health Service.

Professional codes of ethics are constructed around the ethics of virtue or duty: the way the practitioner should conduct herself. An obvious example of this is that a nurse should always act in caring manner. This also means not causing suffering through careless action, as with me passing Peggy by. A further ethical principle is Kant's moral imperative – 'do as you would be done by'. In other words, imposing your own values into the situation – 'if that was my mother'. The problem with this principle is that the patient is not your mother and that imposing such values may be misguided.

4 *Consider what conflict exists between perspectives / values and how these might be resolved*
Having considered the different perspectives of people involved and ethical principles, the practitioner can consider the best decision to make or if there is conflict between professionals, how the conflict be resolved in the patient's best interest.

5 *Consider who had the authority for making the decision/ taking action*
This challenges the practitioner to consider her autonomy, authority, and accountability for making and acting on decisions. According to Batey and Lewis (1982), autonomy has two dimensions; legitimate autonomy as set out in the person's job description, and discriminant authority – the autonomy the person believes she has. However, job descriptions are often vague, and working in bureaucratic organisations may diminish discriminant autonomy, especially for professionals such as nurses, who may perceive themselves or be perceived by other professionals as a subordinate workforce. In this sense, reflection empowers practitioners to expand their field of autonomy and counter any sense of oppression.

6 *Consider the power relationships/ factors that determined the way the decision/ action was actually taken;*

In the real world, decisions are not necessarily made in terms of what's best for the patient or family, but in terms of the professional dominance that is implicit within normal patterns of relating between professionals.[4] However, dominance can be ethically challenged for its legitimacy in terms of the patient's best interests – what I refer to as the Achilles heel of medical dominance.

Loxley (1997) identifies a number of questions that are useful to inform stages 5 and 6:

- Who defines the problem?
- Whose terms are used?
- Who controls the domain or territory?
- Who decides on what resources are needed and how they are allocated?
- Who holds whom accountable?
- Who prescribes the activity of others?
- Who can influence policy-makers?

Skill Box

- *When you reflect on an experience apply ethical mapping to consider your ethical decision-making and practice.*
- *Did you respect the patient's autonomy?*
- *How do you balance the utilitarian tension between time and priorities?*
- *Who needed more time today you were unable to give? How did you rectify such tension?*
- *To what extent did you involve a patient in decision-making?*
- *Are you able to voice your opinion as necessary as an act of integrity?*

Stress and Anxiety

The tension between expectations from self and expectations from others, especially when the gap is wide, creates anxiety. Untreated stress accumulates and is debilitating. Neck and shoulder muscles ache giving headaches and sapping energy. Stress leaves us feeling heavy and drained. Morale plummets. Performance slackens.

I felt a wave of anxiety at Peggy's assertiveness as the guilt kicked in. I quickly adjusted and responded positively. On reflection I appreciate how I might have been 'stressed' commencing a new position and responding to the demand on my service.

Practitioners suffer more stress related to organisational issues and conflict than related to issues of patient care (Vachon 1988). Fear of sanction from more powerful others reflects how expectations from others can dominate the expectations tension when practitioners feel powerless to assert themselves and practice with integrity, especially within transactional organisations (Johns 2015). People become victims of the system.

There is little organisational sensitivity to the profound nature of caring work. There is a lack of recognition of emotional labour (James 1989; Bolton 2000), a prejudice that somehow emotional work is natural women's work and therefore is unskilled, doesn't need to be taught, and is not valued, when emotional work is the greatest gift nurses can offer patients. Yet if the organisation doesn't seem to care why should I? Yet the organisation's seeming not to care about the practitioner or the patient is a major stressor. Taylor (1992) noted a theme in the literature, remarking how nurses have been dispossessed 'of their essential humanness as human beings and as people, by emphasising their professional roles and responsibilities' (p. 1042). Taylor draws attention to the fact that nurses are human too and, as such, are vulnerable to the same issues that face their patients and their patients' families. The lack of recognition of humanness in nursing through a focus on roles and responsibilities has led practitioners to strive to be something they were clearly struggling to achieve. Consequently, they become alienated from themselves in their efforts to cope with and live with the contradictions in their lives. Jourard (1971) noted that such striving damages 'the self' and intensifies the struggle to cope in a vicious downward spiral of self-destruction towards burnout and a state of anomie.

Jade, one of the primary nurses at Burford Hospital said 'I don't come to work dressed in protective armour' (Johns 1993).

Dewey (1933: 30) observed,

> Unconscious fears also drive us into purely defensive attitudes that operate like coats of armour – not only to shut out new conceptions but even to prevent us from making new observations.

Dewey believed that anxiety limited the practitioner's ability to learn through experience. The professional is closed to protect self rather than open to possibility. 'Armour' is akin to professional detachment.

The reality of today's NHS is that nurse shortages are reportedly reaching crisis point; establishment shortfall is nationally 20 percent, one-third of all nurses are allocated no study time, and bed occupancy is running at 98 percent (Hall 2003). In such an environment, Wall et al. (1997) note that NHS staff suffer considerably more stress than any other workforce, with 28 percent recording levels above the symptom threshold. Wind the clock forward. BBC news reports that NHS Foundation Trusts need to resubmit their financial plans. Only essential posts should be filled. The news asks 'What will be the impact on patient care? What will be the impact on staff morale and stress?" I pick up my local newspaper and read that staff morale at RCHT is low.[5] As with all reflective activity, the practitioner must pay attention to her stress – it is part of *how am I feeling*?

At the end of your next shift, stop, reflect and mark how stressed you feel along the feeling fluffy–feeling drained visual analogue scale.[6]

I go home feeling light and fluffy	⟵						⟶	*I go home feeling totally drained*		
1	2	3	4	5	6	7	8	9	10

Then ask yourself

- What factors contribute to your sense of feeling drained?
- What factors contribute to your sense of feeling light and fluffy?
- What do you need to do to home feeling more fluffy and less drained?
- Use this scale over a period of time to monitor stress patterns and any improvement in your 'fluffiness'. See Table 3.5 for an applied example.

With Peggy, I scored 2 on the scale. I had converted my anxiety into positive action and felt satisfied with that. The rest of the day went without drama. I wouldn't want to go home with a score more than 4.

Table 3.5 Feeling fluffy–feeling drained scale

Week commencing	20 May 2002
Day	Wednesday
Average stress score	7
Range	[5-10]

Please score on the scale the extent you feel light and fluffy or drained at the end of the work day:		
I go home feeling light and fluffy ← →		*I go home feeling totally drained*
1 2 3 4 5 6 7 8 9 10		
What factors contribute to your sense of feeling drained?	*Arrived in the morning to a horrible phone call from a patient's relative who held me personally responsible for his wife's wait in A&E when I had already advised him that there were no beds in the hospital*	
What factors contribute to your sense of feeling light and fluffy?	*Did teaching session – I always enjoy teaching. Also put together a bid for further training in the hospital, Didn't think I would be able to do it this quickly.*	
What can you do to go home feeling more fluffy and less drained?	*I confronted the relative and listened to his worries. He apologised to me for being rude. Whilst I felt better because he apologised I need to learn not to take relatives' anger so personally.* *I recognise he was projecting his frustration – that I was in the firing line. Instead of defending myself I need to be more mindful and see the anger for what it was – this will help defuse it.*	

Stewing in our own juices is not healthy. Imagine your body is like a *water butt* – slowly filling with stress. As it fills we are more tired and more intolerant but we contain it. That is, until you feel you are drowning and then one of two things happens: either you blow up inside and have a breakdown, or else you snap and 'blow your top'. You rage at events or people (Wilkinson 1988; Parker 1990; Pike 1991).

Pike (1991: 351) writes,

> Moral outrage ensues when the nurse's attempts to operationalize a choice are thwarted by constraints. The outrage intensifies when these constraints not only block action, but also force a course of action that violates the nurse's moral tenets.

Many practitioners wear this T-shirt. However, the water butt does have a drainage tap. The practitioner can learn to monitor her stress levels and open her tap. She can then drain and convert the stress into positive energy necessary to take appropriate action to resolve the sources of stress (Hall 1964) just as the gardener draws water from the water butt to water the flowers and nourish their growth. However the tap might be blocked, requiring help to unblock it – again the value of guided reflection. If stress accumulates then the risk of burnout looms large on the horizon.

Cherniss (1980) describes burnout as a process in which 'the professional's attitudes and behaviours change in negative ways in response to job strain' (p. 5). Maslach (1976) suggested that the major negative change in those experiencing burnout in people-centred work was 'the loss of concern for the client and a tendency to treat clients in a detached, mechanical fashion'(p. 6).

McNeeley (1983) observed that when practitioners felt they had lost the intrinsic satisfaction of caring, they became focussed on the conditions of work, for example, off-duty rosters and issues, characteristic of bureaucratic models of organisation. McNeeley believes that bureaucratic conditions are antithetical to human service work and strongly advocated that such organisations needed to move to collegial ways of working staff in order to offset the risks of burnout. Burnout is a descent into a black hole when the caring self has been scrapped away on the uncaring sharp edges of systems.

And yet burnout can be a healing space, where the practitioner can recover/discover herself. It may be dark, lonely and painful but it can still be a necessary healing space. Such healing is a journey to discover rather than recover, because recovery suggests returning to what she was before, only for the hurting to start all over again.

Benner and Wrubel (1989) believe that the answer to stress and burnout is to reconnect to caring rather than the development of personal detachment as advocated by Menzies-Lyth (1988). Caring is a reciprocal relationship. If nurses and other healthcare practitioners are expected to care, then they need to work in caring environments. If the practitioner is suffering it is likely that other colleagues also suffer, sapping their energy and limiting their availability to be with patients. And yet, often, practitioners seem to need to cope, to not expose their vulnerability as if it were a weakness not to cope or admit to strain. They prefer a collusive silence. To care, we need ways to penetrate the silence to support each other and create a therapeutic team – a team whose members are actively and genuinely available to each other. As such, the reflective practitioner is mindful of her colleagues' well-being.

Consider the following questions:

- Are adequate support systems in place?
- Are people stressed or worse, burnt out?
- If so – why do you think that is?
- Do you see seeking help as a strength rather than weakness?
- Do you explore your anxiety as a learning opportunity?
- Are you truly available to support your colleagues?

The Need to be in Control

As I noted above, the tension between expectations of self and expectations from others, especially when the gap is wide, creates anxiety. The human response to managing anxiety is to control the environment, and with it, the source of anxiety. Unfortunately the mismatch of expectations within health care is wide, with a consequential impact on morale and patient care.

Returning to my experience with Peggy, consider – if I had interpreted Peggy's demand as a threat to my control, and reminded her that I was in control, not her, that I would determine my schedule, not her, what would have been the consequences? Ramos (1992) identified the need to be in control as an obstacle to developing therapeutic relationships. I can see the clamour of demand for my service each week and my response – that those who ask, get, and those who don't ask, don't get. I see that, in the crowded room, I only paid attention to those with the loudest voices. Is that my modus operandi? It is certainly the route of least resistance. Perhaps meeting so many new people in my new role, it make it easy for me to be approached as a way to control my anxiety. A loss of control leads to a loss of poise. Though not strictly a clinical skill, the ability to know and manage self or 'poise' is a vital attribute of the effective practitioner. In my experience very little education in practitioner training focuses on self-management, except perhaps an hour or two on stress management.

Knowledge to Act in a Particular Way?

This cue challenges the practitioner to identify relevant theory that informed, or might have informed, her experience. There is so much theory 'out there' to inform that it may seem an arduous task to keep abreast. It demands a curiosity. Just visit your university or hospital library to get a feel of the weight of theory. Of course, it then has to read and understood. I know that the evidence base for my choice of essential oils, or my approach to reflexology, is weak. Yet patients much appreciate both the aroma of oils and the relaxation effect of aromatherapy. Listening to Peggy's story is important – I wonder about the theories on 'listening'? Most practitioners I have worked with in guided reflection struggle to discern a theory to inform and back up their practice. Perhaps one reason for this struggle is the nature of human encounter work, where every situation is unique and where all knowledge must be interpreted for its value to inform. If knowledge is simply something to apply, then patients would be objects and practitioners, technicians. Without doubt, the effective practitioner is an informed practitioner. I explore this more deeply in Chapter 4.

Skill Box

- *Reflect on a recent experience and pedantically identify an informing theory. To what extent does this theory fit the situation?*
- *Do not be intimidated by the scope of the 'influences grid'. Use it pedantically as part of your reflection and come to appreciate the significance of each influencing factor. Be open, rather than defensive, to each factor. You will quickly begin to work towards resolving any negative impact of these factors on your practice, just as I did with Peggy. In particular consider the idea of 'control' and 'poise'.*

Anticipatory Reflection

The next reflective movement is to anticipate how I might respond given the situation again. Three cues guide me:

- What are my options for responding differently, more effectively and in tune with my values, given the situation again?
- What are the potential consequences of responding differently?
- How do those influencing factors need to shift so I can respond differently?

These cues open a creative learning space to play with possibility. It is an invitation to throw open the shutters of the mind to see things laterally, to get out of our normal frame of reference and challenge our habitual ways of perceiving and responding to practice. Patterns of thinking and behaviours become embodied as normal, often leading to habitual and unreflective practice. Practitioners carve out comfort grooves and then get stuck in them. We are creatures of habit and quickly become complacent.

As O'Donohue (1997: 163-4) writes,

Many people remain trapped at the one window, looking out every day at the same scene in the same way. Real growth is experienced when you draw back from that one window, turn and walk around the inner tower of the soul and see all the different windows that await your gaze. Through these different windows, you can see new vistas of possibility, presence and creativity. Complacency, habit and blindness often prevent you from feeling your life. So much depends on the frame of vision – the window through which we look.

Imagine going round your mind opening the shutters. It is a powerful metaphor for seeing any experience from new angles – challenging the normal and taken for granted aspects of your practice. Get curious!

Put yourself in my shoes with Peggy. Perhaps you can relate to a similar type of situation within your own practice. In either case- 'What might your options be for responding more effectively within this or a similar situation?' Put on your imaginative hat!

Revisiting Peggy

Perhaps a good place to start is to consider how I might respond differently to Peggy's demand 'I'm first on the list'? Just saying these words to myself confirms my suspicion that she would have liked a therapy on previous Mondays.

Perhaps I could have responded '*You should have asked, Peggy.*' But would that have put the onus on her when her natural inclination is not to ask, not to be a burden. I know from my hospice experience that women who care deeply for others, as she has for her partner, do not find it easy to ask for their own care. It would have increased the burden on her, to make it seem as if it was her responsibility to ask rather than mine to offer. Responding like this would be me projecting my anxiety at having been caught out, as if I were a naughty boy anxious to shift the blame.

Another option might be to say something like "*OK – I'll fit you into the schedule*". At first glance this response seems reasonable. It acknowledges that I plan a schedule of therapies for the day. Yet such a formulaic response might seem insensitive. It would not have acknowledged her desperate cry. It might have put her in her place, reminding her of her status and my authority.

Another possible response might be an act of apology '*I'm sorry Peggy I hadn't realised.*' In doing so I acknowledge my responsibility and that I can get it wrong. Humility. But by apologising, would I have burdened her with my guilt and made her feel she needed to care for me? The repentant child seeking forgiveness?

These alternative responses all seem feasible but in considering their potential consequences I reject them. Even so, exploring them is insightful, especially the child mode perspective as a response to guilt. Using Transactional Analysis (TA) as a framework, I believe it is vital to be in adult mode and to enable the other to respond likewise no matter the situation – unless it is therapeutically necessary to be otherwise. TA offers an excellent reflective framework for seeing patterns of communication and relationships.

My actual response to Peggy '*Let's do it now*' still feels the most appropriate because it acknowledged her desperate cry. It was intuitive, a response in the moment. I did not figure it out. You might argue that it was a reaction to my guilt, of having been caught out.

How could I have passed Peggy by? What had distracted me? I sense the way I plan my day is flawed. I need a schedule that is not at the beck and call of the loudest voices. What are my options?

1 Get people to put their name down for a therapy on arrival. I can then review and plan a schedule based on fairness, recognising I cannot give a therapy to everyone who wants one in one day.
2 We have two therapy rooms. If demand is greater than supply then perhaps seek a second volunteer therapist – explore at team meeting.
3 Shorten the time span of each therapy to enable more patients to have a therapy.
    I think option 1 is promising. But first I must speak with the hospice manager to get her viewpoint. I can also discuss option 2 with her.
    Option 3 *might* work but would the therapy benefit be compromised with shorter treatments? I sense my integrity as a therapist would be compromised.

I generated alternative options for responding to Peggy using Six Category Intervention Analysis (Heron 1975). Ideally I could have generated these options within the moment if I hadn't reacted as I did. Our responses tend to be learned and reactive to the moment. The value of anticipatory reflection is to plant seeds of possibility so that I might respond/ react differently given a similar situation (Margolis 1993). And this is the significant thing about this cue – the fuelling of inquiry and opening to other possibilities in the quest for expert professional artistry.

What Would be the Consequences of Alternative Actions for the Patient, Others and Myself?

Actions have consequences! In the above description I contemplated the consequence of responding differently. ~Both short-term and long-term consequences. Every action is a moral and political act towards creating a better state of affairs. For example, by responding to Peggy as I did, do I set a precedent that any patient can just grab me and demand a therapy now and then? Perhaps, if there were a book where patients could put their name down for a therapy I could ration my time to ensure everyone was dealt with fairly – the ethic of justice. This would also give me greater control over my use of time.

What Factors Might Stop me from Responding Differently?

Weighing up the consequences of different options leads the practitioner to choose the preferred option. Yet, can I actually respond as envisaged? Can I shift my embodied assumptions to reframe myself as necessary? Do I have the skills? Am I assertive enough? Can I overcome my natural inclination to avoid conflict? Can I shed my fear of sanction if I do so? It is scaling the hard wall of reality.

Skill Box

- *When you next reflect, consider alternative, more effective ways of responding. Think laterally. Open your imagination. Remember to consider the consequences of different options and whether you can actually act as you would like. If not, what constrains you?*

'How do I Now Feel About the Situation'?

Returning to the MSR the final cue asks '*How do I now feel about the situation?*'

Looking back at my experience with Peggy I feel somewhat amazed that a seemingly innocuous situation proved to be so insightful. It just goes to show the power of reflection in challenging my normal practice. I feel I have purged my guilt constructively. However, it wasn't easy facing up to my unsatisfactory performance and yet I have learnt so much from it especially the notion of becoming more poised, so that when faced with an uncomfortable situation I do not simply react, even though my reaction may be appropriate. I can respond to this cue in the knowledge that my practice day has been transformed in the way I 'book' appointments and see every person who attends day hospice as a suffering person. It feels as if someone wiped my mirror a little cleaner! I certainly feel more poised and more mindful about being poised. I feel the veracity of the idea that the more you try to control something the less you actually do so.

Summary

I have set out the reflective spiral structured by the MSR cues towards gaining insight that forms the second dialogical movement of narrative construction. The cues offer insight into the potential breadth and depth of reflection. Other models of reflection might be used, though always remembering that such models are heuristic cues rather than prescriptions.

In the following chapter I set out a framework for perceiving insights to respond to the MSR cue, '*What tentative insights do I draw?*'

Endnotes

1   Endnotes The 13th International Reflective Practice conference held in Aalborg was dedicated to the development of phronesis through reflective practice. Papers from this conference were collected in the book, *The good, the wise, and the right clinical nursing practice*, edited by Charlotte Delmar and Christopher Johns (2008).
2   Poise is an attribute of the Being Available template - see Table 4.3.
3   I explore the idea of wavelength in more depth in Chapter 19.
4   As I indicated in Chapter 1, power is a central tenet of critical reflection. See also pages 199-200 for a more detailed critique of power using French and Raven's framework.
5   *West Briton*, Thursday 12 March 2015.
6   See also Chapter 13.

References

Batey, M. and Lewis, F. (1982) Clarifying autonomy and accountability in nursing service: Part 1. *Journal of Nursing Administration* 12.9, 13–18.

Benjamin, M. and Curtis, J. (1986) *Ethics in nursing* (second edition). Oxford University Press, New York.

Benner, P. and Wrubel, J. (1989) *The primacy of caring*. Addison-Wesley, Menlo Park.

Blackford, J. (2003) Cultural frameworks of nursing practice: exposing an exclusionary healthcare culture. *Nursing Inquiry* 10.4, 236–42.

Bolton, S. (2000) Who cares? Offering emotion work as a 'gift' in the nursing labour process. *Journal of Advanced Nursing* 32, 580–86.

Callahan, S. (1988) The role of emotion in ethical decision making. Hastings Centre Report June/July, pp. 9–14.

Carper, B. (1978) Fundamental patterns of knowing in nursing. *Advances in Nursing Science*, 1.1, 13–23.

Cherniss, G. (1980) *Professional burn-out in human service organisations*. Praeger, New York.

Compact Oxford English Dictionary 2005: 58.

Cooper, M. (1991) Principle-orientated ethics and the ethics of care: a creative tension. *Advances in Nursing Science* 15.2, 22–31.

Corley, M. and Goren, S. (1998) The dark side of nursing: impact of stigmatizing responses on patients. *Scholarly Inquiry for Nursing Practice: An International Journal* 12.2, 99–121.

Delmar, C. and Johns, C. (2008) *The good, the wise and the right clinical nursing practice*. Aalborg Hospital, Arhus University Hospital, Denmark.

Dewey, J. (1933) *How we think*. J. C. Heath, Boston.

Elliott, G. (1876) *Daniel Deronda*. George Blackwood and Sons, Edinburgh.

Gilligan, C. (1993) *In a different voice*. Harvard University Press, Cambridge, MA.

Hall, L. (1964) Nursing – what is it? *Canadian Nurse*, 60.2, 150–54.

Hall, C. (2003) Nurse shortage in the NHS is near crisis point. *Daily Telegraph* 29 April.

Heron, J. (1975) *Six-category intervention analysis*. Human Potential Resource Group, University of Surrey, Guildford.

James, N. (1989) *Emotional labour: skill and work in the social regulation of feelings*. Sociological Review, 37.1, 15–42.

Jameton, A. (1992) Nursing ethics and the moral situation of the nurse. In E. Friedman (ed.), *Choices and conflict*. American Hospital Publishing, Chicago, pp. 101–9.

Johns, C. (1993) Professional supervision. *Journal of Nursing Management* 1.1, 9–18

Johns, C. (ed.) (1994) *The Burford NDU Model: caring in practice*. Blackwell, Oxford.

Johns, C. (1998) Becoming a reflective practitioner through guided reflection. PhD thesis. The Open University.

Johns, C. (1999) Unravelling the dilemmas of everyday nursing practice. *Nursing Ethics* 6, 287–98.

Johns, C. (2015) *Mindful leadership*. Palgrave Macmillan, Basingstoke.

Jones, R. and Jones, G. (1996) *Earth Dance Drum*. Commune-E-Key, Salt Lake City.

Jourard, S. (1971) *The transparent self*. Van Nostrand, Newark.

Logstrup, K. E. (1997) *The ethical demand*. University of Notre Dame Press, Notre Dame, IN.

Loxley, A. (1997) *Collaboration in health and welfare: working with difference*. Jessica Kingsley Publishers, London.

Margolis, H. (1993) *Paradigm and barriers: how habits of mind govern scientific beliefs*. University of Chicago Press, Chicago.

Maslach, C. (1976) Burned-out. *Human Behaviour* 5, 16–22.

McNeely, R. (1983) Organizational patterns and work satisfaction in a comprehensive human service agency: an empirical test. *Human Relations* 36.10, 957–72.

Menzies-Lyth, I. (1988) A case study in the functioning of social systems as a defence against anxiety. In *Containing anxiety in institutions: selected essays*. Free Association Books, London.

O'Donohue, J. (1997) *Anam Cara: spiritual wisdom from the Celtic world*. Bantam Press, London.

Parker, R. (1990) Nurses' stories: the search a relational ethic of care. *Advances in Nursing Science* 13.1, 31–40.

Parsons, T. (1951) *The Social System*. Free Press, Glencoe, IL.

Pike, A. (1991) Moral outrage and moral discourse in nurse–physician collaboration. *Journal of Professional Nursing* 7.6, 351–63.

Puzan, E. (2003) The unbearable whiteness of being (in nursing). *Nursing Inquiry* 10.3, 193–200.

Ramos, M. (1992) The nurse–patient relationship: themes and variations. *Journal of Advanced Nursing* 17, 496–506.

Rinpoche, S. (1992) *The Tibetan book of living and dying.* Rider, London.

Rosenberg, L. (1998) *Breath by breath.* Shambhala, Boston.

Sacks, O. (1976) *Awakenings.* Pelican Books, London.

Salovey, P. and Mayer, J.D. (1990) Emotional intelligence. *Imagination, Cognition and Personality* 9, 185–211.

Seedhouse, D. (1988) *Ethics: the heart of health care.* John Wiley and Sons, Chichester.

Taylor, B. (1992) From helper to human: a reconceptualisation of the nurse as a person. *Journal of Advanced Nursing* 17, 1042–9.

Vachon, M. (1988) Battle fatigue in hospice/ palliative care. In A. Gilmore and S. Gilmore (eds.), *A safer death.* Plenum Publishing, New York.

Wall, T.D., Bolden, R.I. and Borril, C.S. (1997) Minor psychiatric disturbance in NHS Trust staff. *British Journal of Psychiatry* 171, 519–23.

Wheatley, M. and Kellner-Rogers, M. (1999) *A simpler way.* Berrett-Koehler Publishers, San Francisco.

Wilkinson, J. (1988) Moral distress in nursing practice: experience and effect. *Nursing Forum* 23.1, 16–29.

Chapter 4

Framing Insights

Christopher Johns

> imagination is more important than knowledge
> Albert Einstein[1]

Having surfed the reflective spiral, I stand back and ask myself, 'What insights do I draw?' In standing back I create an objective space between myself and the text. In doing so I pull open the text to see it from a wider perspective, being open to what insights the text has to reveal but without forcing it.

Wheatley (1999: 118) writes,

> when we concentrate on individual moments or fragments of experience, we see only chaos. The complexity of our practice may seem like chaos – just how do I sort the wood from the trees to see clearly? But if we stand back and look at what is taking shape, we see order. Order always displays itself as patterns that develop over time.

Insights change practitioners. As a consequence they view their practice differently. Insights can be explosive moments of revelation or they may be subtle, and only revealed through subsequent reflections. They may not be easy to articulate.

However, as Subhuti (1985/2001:90) suggests:

> we need to make this attempt to describe the indescribable because words help us to reduce this cosmic complexity to a workable simplicity for the purposes of everyday functioning.

It is like trying to articulate tacit knowing – I know something but can't easily explain what it is I know (Polanyi 1958).

Single Lines

I break the reflective text into single lines and scroll down the text, reading between the lines where insights are often revealed. Scrolling down is like seeking the edges of the unfamiliar so I can pull away the veneer of normal practice and sense another world altogether less familiar (Winterson 2001).[2] Insights are like transitional points between old and new practice. It is an evolving process, as one thing leads to another – rather like a washing

Becoming a Reflective Practitioner, Fifth Edition. Edited by Christopher Johns.
© 2017 John Wiley & Sons Ltd. Published 2017 by John Wiley & Sons Ltd.
Companion Website: www.wiley.com/go/johns/reflectivepractitioner

machine going round and round, and spinning out something new with each revolution. Sometimes the insights are simply logical and rational. Of course! Like passing Peggy by! That sometimes we see something but only see it from a certain perspective because that perspective is so normal. In order to see something different we have to shift our perspective. Then discerning insights becomes a more imaginative, intuitive and creative process. Tuffnell and Crickmay (2004: 119) write,

> imagination is not a separate faculty, rather it engages all parts of the mind and intelligence – fusing or bringing together often surprising aspects of what we feel or know, imagination expands our seeing.

This means scrolling down the text in creative play; opening our right brains. Okri (1997: 21) writes,

> Creativity, it would appear, should be approached in the spirit of play, of foreplay, of dalliance, doodling, messing around — and then, bit by bit, you somehow get deeper into the matter. But if you go in there with a businessman's solemnity or the fanaticism of some artistic types you are likely to be rewarded with a stiff response, a joyless dribble, strained originality, ideas that come out all strapped up and strangled by too much effort.

The idea of dallying suggests giving the mind free rein to explore, allowing the imagination to wander and accept anything that comes up, laughing at our in-built censors that constantly seek to trim us, letting go of attachment to ideas to allow the imagination and creativity to flow until tentative insights rise to the surface. Be patient! Put aside the text and let it settle. Later, a new idea will dawn, perhaps as you sleep or walk, or indeed at any time of the day. It is as if the insight has been germinating within your body. Insights are not necessarily new, but a deepening of things already known or sensed to some degree. In this way insights reflexively build on each other.

Framing Insights

How might insights be framed? My endeavour to construct an adequate framework for learning through reflection has taken me through several learning frameworks. Initially, I used Carper's 'fundamental ways of knowing in nursing', an approach to nursing knowledge. However, it became apparent that practitioners struggled to frame their learning within these ways of knowing. I needed a more pragmatic mode. This led me to frame learning using the being available template (BAT) developed from my analysis of person-centred practice. In other words, how would a practitioner seeking to become person-centred know this? As such it was both a developmental and feedback format. However I felt this was too narrow an approach. Hence, I developed the framing perspectives as a more comprehensive approach to framing insights in which the BAT can be utilised from the perspective of 'developmental framing'. The framing perspectives span the breadth of knowing in health care. As with all reflective frameworks, the framing perspectives can be utilised, adapted or discarded.

Carper's Fundamental Ways of Knowing

I chose Carper's fundamental ways of knowing in nursing (1978) because it seemed to offer a comprehensive and authoritative approach to framing nursing knowledge (Figure 4.1). I viewed the *aesthetic* as the core way of knowing because it reflected the knowing the nurse used in practice (professional artistry) informed by the ethical, empirical and personal ways of knowing. More broadly, aesthetics is a branch of philosophy dealing with the nature of beauty, art and taste and with the creation and appreciation of beauty.[3] Here, I would include performance. Watch a nurse go about their practice and you witness a performance that integrates all aspects of that practice. Perhaps it flows with grace and perhaps it stutters awkwardly. Like dancers, they move about the patient. Like sculptors, they shape their practice. Like actors, they play out the drama. Like poets, they sense the poignancy within the unfolding moment.

I linked each MSR cue into the different ways of knowing. Indeed I was able to construct 'The model for reflective inquiry' (Figure 4.2) as an alternative MSR. Some practitioners found this interpretation of the MSR useful, with its primary focus on the event rather than on the self. It offers a useful clinical audit approach.[4]

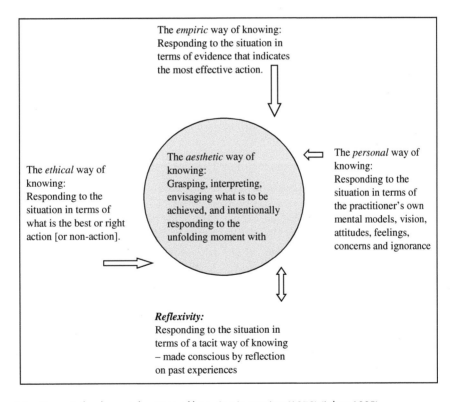

Figure 4.1   Carper's fundamental pattern of knowing in nursing (1978) (Johns 1995).

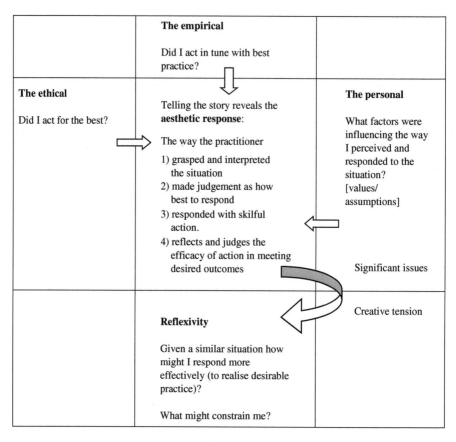

Figure 4.2   Model for Reflective Inquiry.

Other theorists had played with Carper's scheme and postulated other ways of knowing. White (1995) suggested the socio-political ways of knowing to contextualise the ways of knowing within societal norms, whilst Munhall (1993) suggested 'unknowing' as a way of knowing, that influences the clinical response. I too felt something was missing from this scheme, which led me to develop a fifth way of knowing that I labelled *reflexivity* to account for the insight feedback (Johns 1995).

The Framing Perspectives

Practitioners generally found Carper's approach to framing insights difficult to apply because it was too abstract. As such, I constructed the framing perspectives (Table 4.1). These reflect the MSR cues. It made sense that the approach to seeking insight is also the basis for framing them. They offer a perspective into the breadth of potential insights. As with all reflective frameworks, they are not offered as a prescription, but merely as an heuristic. In other words, they are at your discretion to use or disregard. But before you disregard them, play with them, and see if they are beneficial.

The first two perspectives, philosophical and role, provide an 'insight axis' because every reflection is implicitly an inquiry into values and role. Theoretical framing is evident throughout the book – the way I both use theory from literature and construct my own

Table 4.1 Framing perspectives

Philosophical framing:
How has this experience enabled me to confront and clarify my beliefs and values that constitute desirable practice?

Parallel process framing:
How has this experience enabled me to make connections between learning processes and my clinical practice?

Problem framing:
How has this experience enabled me to focus problem identification and resolution within the experience.

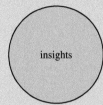

insights

Reality perspective framing:
How has this experience enabled me to understand the barrier of reality whilst helping me to become empowered to act in more congruent ways?

Theoretical framing/mapping:
How has this experience enabled me to draw on extant theory and research to inform my practice?

Temporal framing:
How has this experience enabled me to draw patterns with past experiences whilst anticipating how I might respond in similar situations in new ways?

Developmental framing:
How has this experience enabled me to frame becoming a more effective practitioner within 'whole' appropriate theoretical frameworks.

Role framing:
How has this experience enabled me to clarify my role boundaries and authority within my role, and my power relationships with others?

theory based on analysis of experience to construct reflective frameworks in which the practitioner can position self. Examples include transactional analysis, conflict management and assertiveness.

Developmental framing offers a whole picture of practice. So, for example, if my vision is to realise patient-centred practice, how might I know this? Similarly, if my vision is to become a transformational leader, how might I know this? Clearly, there are theories of patient-centred practice and transformational leadership that can be mapped as reflective frameworks, or if no adequate theory exists, one can be constructed through analysing patterns of insights emerging through guided reflection,[5] such as the being available template.

I write,

Peggy

Peggy threw out my schedule. Until then I didn't know I had a schedule. It wasn't written down. I had a flawed system of working. Next Monday I respond differently — the insight has changed me. I am now more aware of myself within the hospice. My attention has changed. I see a bigger picture. In fact I see everyone within the room with more attention. The room is transformed.

The hospice manager is enthusiastic about my schedule options. She agrees that getting people to sign up for a therapy is a good idea. She will think about recruiting a second therapist, but that goes against the grain, as the other days of the week are serviced by one therapist – so what makes me special? She respects the fact that I spend longer with each patient than other therapists, but the feedback from patients is very positive. We will start next week with the 'sign in' — she says she will organise it.

Table 4.2 Applying framing perspectives to my experience with Peggy

Framing perspective	
Philosophical	It reminds me of my vision of being 'patient-centred' and 'easing suffering' to reflect on what that means as something lived, notably the concept of 'paying attention'.
Role	Talking with the hospice manager helped me realise I need to attend staff meetings and be less marginal.
Reality perspective	How easy it was to assume that I was doing a good job. The experience was a loud wake-up call.
	Sharing my options with the hospice manager has enabled 'us' to review 'our' options for delivering a more effective therapy service. She has access to necessary resources and authority.
Theoretical	Reviewing the use of Six-Category intervention analysis within the moment to develop the range and skill of my communication responses.
	Theories of emotional intelligence (Goleman et al. 2002) in appreciating 'poise'.
Temporal	Exposing the idea that my routine may be flawed and considering other ways of organising my practice.
Problem	A number of problems that can be framed
	1 My reactive response
	2 My lack of consideration of the consequences of my response for other patients
	3 The limited extent I know patients and my lack of sensitivity to their predicament (which considering I am a therapist shocks me)
	4 My practice 'routine' is flawed with the consequence that I 'pass people by'.
	5 Lack of collaboration with my practice colleagues – perhaps reflecting how I tend to work alone as a therapist.
Parallel process	This perspective works in conjunction with guidance – this perspective is developed in Chapter 5.
Developmental	I ask myself 'to what extent was I available to Peggy?'
	The reader is referred to Tables 4.3 and 4.4 to consider the Being Available template as a framework for drawing insight.

I summarise the insights I gained through reflection on my experience with Peggy in Table 4.2. It is insightful in itself to list the number of problems that can emerge from just one experience, reflecting how an experience is a microcosm of the whole of my practice. My reflection on insights reinforces the idea of just how complacent practitioners can become, assuming that their practice is fine. It highlights the value of a 'vision' in revealing contradiction between our values and our actual practice.

So, reader, consider — to what extent are you patient-centred in your own practice (assuming that you intend to be patient-centred)?

The Being Available Template

To reiterate the question: how can practitioners know self as a patient-centred practitioner? My response was to construct the *Being Available* template. The idea of being available is a therapeutic posture that assumes that the core irreducible quality of patient-centred practice is the practitioner 'being available to work with the person[s] to enable the person

Table 4.3 The Being Available template*

Dimension	
1 The practitioner intends to realise a vision of practice	Holding intent, the practitioner is more likely to realise the vision in practice. Through reflection, vision is constantly scrutinised for its lived meaning in practice and value to frame practice.
2 The practitioner knows the other	Through empathic inquiry the practitioner appreciates the pattern of the person's wholeness and the meanings they give to health by tuning in and flowing with the unfolding pattern of the person's experience [wavelength].
3 The practitioner is concerned for the other.	Concern is an energy that creates possibility within the caring relationship. The greater the practitioner's concern for the other the more available the practitioner is.
4 The practitioner is effective in meeting the person's needs: the aesthetic response (Carper 1978)**	Four abilities constitute effective performance: 1 the ability to grasp and interpret the clinical moment, 2 the ability to make most appropriate and ethical clinical judgment in response to the patient's needs, 3 the ability to respond with appropriate skilful action, 4 the ability to evaluate one's efficacy.
5 Poise	The practitioner knows and manages self within relationship so their personal concerns do not interfere with being available to the person. It is the flip side of concern, whereas concern makes the practitioner vulnerable, so poise manages the vulnerability without diminishing concern. Poise is defined as: ● a graceful and elegant way of holding the body, ● calmness and confidence, ● ready and prepared to do something. All three aspects of this definition are relevant to my appropriation of poise. In being 'ready and prepared', I am mindful and in control of my emotional being.
6 Create and sustain an environment where being available is possible	Dimensions 1–5 above relate to the relationship between practitioner and patient. However, this takes place within a therapeutic environment. Hence the practitioner works towards: ● creating and sustaining collaborative and dialogical patterns of relationships with other health care workers towards realising a shared vision of practice, ● being political to maximise available resources to ensure availability to the patient and counter coercive patterns of management.

*The BAT is a living structure, constantly shifting in light of reflection on its relevance to represent the nature of patient-centred nursing. It can be adapted as appropriate by others.

to find meaning in their experience as the basis for negotiated decision making about their health and to assist them as appropriate to help them meet their health needs'.

The extent to which the practitioner can be available is determined by the pattern of six interrelated *influences*: holding and intending to realise a vision, concern for and knowledge of the person, aesthetic response, poise, and creating an environment where being available can be possible (Table 4.3). The first five influences concern the therapeutic relationship. The sixth influence positions the therapeutic relationship within the wider organisational and societal environment.

Table 4.4 Reflecting on the extent I was available to Peggy, I can draw some insights

Dimension	
1 The practitioner intends to realise a vision of practice	My vision is to ease suffering. Using the template draws my attention to suffering. Does this experience increase my sensitivity to the suffering person? Does it deepen my appreciation of the nature of suffering? Of course it does.
2 The practitioner knows the other	I know Peggy now as a person rather than as just another person attending day hospice. As a consequence I am more sensitive to all patients attending- seeing them more in their humanness than as cancer victims.
3 The practitioner is concerned for the other.	Developing relationship inevitably increases my concern for that person. It breaks through any detachment I may have inadvertently developed.
4 The practitioner is effective in meeting the person's needs:	Through reflection I can see better other ways I might have responded to Peggy's demand.
5 Poise	Poise is such a vital attribute of professional artistry and yet I found myself in an emotional and reactive situation. I mustn't confuse poise with detachment – it is about managing self within relationship!
6 Create and sustain an environment where being available is possible	I can also see myself more clearly within the practice environment and other ways of managing the environment. I am more aware of working with my colleagues to reflect on and create the most effective practice environment.

Attributes such as concern for the person and poise are two sides of one coin. They are also difficult to teach as a skill as they are part of someone's personal makeup. It is my view that such attributes can only really be nurtured through guided reflection. An example of this is Michelle and her peers (see Chapter 13).

Of course, the extent that I have embodied these insights will only become apparent through subsequent experiences. In working with others, I send out ripples of change that inevitably impact on the wider practice community. So others in contact also begin to respond, sending out further ripples of change through the community.

As Carson (2008 : 139) writes,

when you change the way an individual thinks of himself, you change the way he lives in his community and thereby you change the community in some way to a greater or lesser extent.

This is a vital idea about reflective practice – that whilst it is seemingly an individual learning process it inevitably impacts on the wider community.

Skill Box

- *Use the framing perspectives to enable you to explore the potential scope of insights emanating from your reflections.*
- *Consider whether the Being Available Template offers a reflective framework to both guide and monitor realising your vision of therapeutic nursing.*

Summary

Framing insights is a vital element of reflective learning. It enables the reflective practitioner to reflect deeper on and summarise learning. As with all reflective frameworks, the framing perspectives do not intend to impose a rigid framework that forces learning into arbitrary boxes. It isn't necessarily easy to summarise insights. However that shouldn't be an excuse not to do so.

Endnotes

1   Endnotes www.brainyquote.com/quotes/quotes/a/alberteins129815.html.
2   In Chapter 7 I break down my experience with Veronica into single lines and rewrite them as I do, until I emerge with the insight that perhaps it is I who is alone, seeking someone to give therapy to and hence make myself useful under the illusion of easing another's suffering.
3   http://www.merriam-webster.com/dictionary/aesthetics.
4   See Chapter 19.
5   See chapter **X** for examples of leadership reflective frameworks. In chapter **X** I set out the being available template as a reflective framework to know self as a patient-centred practitioner.

References

Carper, B. (1978) Fundamental patterns of knowing in nursing. *Advances in Nursing Science* 1.1, 13–23.

Carson, J. (2008) *Spider Speculations: a physics and biophysics of storytelling*. New York Theatre Communications Group.

Goleman, D., Boyatzis, R. and McKee, A. (2002) *Primal leadership: learning to lead with emotional intelligence*. Harvard Business School Press, Boston.

Heron, J. (1975) *Six-category intervention analysis*. Human Potential Resource Group, University of Surrey, Guildford.

Johns, C. (1995) Framing learning through reflection within Carper's fundamental ways of knowing. *Journal of Advanced Nursing* 22, 226–234.

Munhall, P. (1993) 'Unknowing': towards another pattern of knowing in nursing. *Nursing Outlook* 41.3, 125–128.

Okri, B. (1997) *A way of being free*. Phoenix House, London.

Polanyi, M. (1958) *Personal knowledge: towards a post critical philosophy*. Routledge and Kegan Paul, London.

Subhuti, D. (1985/2001) *The Buddhist vision: a path to fulfilment*. Windhorse, Birmingham.

Tuffnell, M. and Crickmay, C. (2004) *A widening field*. Dance Books, Alton.

Wheatley, M. J. (1999) *Leadership and the new science: discovering order in a chaotic world*. Berrett-Koehler, San Francisco.

White, J. (1995). Patterns of knowing: review, critique and update. *Advanced Nursing Science* 17.4, 73–86.

Winterson, J. (2001) *The powerbook*. Vintage, London.

Chapter 5

Deepening Insights (The Third And Fourth Dialogical Movements)

Christopher Johns

theory exists only to inform professional artistry

In the first dialogical movement the practitioner writes a description of her experience. In the second dialogical movement, she dialogues with the description to reflect and draw tentative insight. Now, in the third and fourth dialogical movements, the practitioner dialogues with an informing literature and with guides to challenge and deepen these insights. These two movements are not discrete but swirl together. The deepening of insight is reflexive, informing and being informed by previous experiences within the hermeneutic circle.

Third Dialogical Movement

The third dialogical movement is the dialogue between tentative insights and an informing literature prompted by the MSR cue 'How does extant theory/ideas inform and deepen my insights?' (see Figure 3.2) challenges the reflective practitioner to consider what theory might inform the practitioner's experience. This process of dialogue requires the practitioner to access critique and juxtapose appropriate relevant literature with her tentative insights.

One problem with a technical rational or theory-driven approach to practice is to encourage the practitioner to see the theory rather than the person. The risk is to reduce the person to some object to apply the theory to. From a reflective perspective, all theory is viewed through a skeptical eye for its authority to inform practice (Dewey 1933). It must always be interpreted in the context of the particular situation. It is never accepted at face value, reflecting how professional artistry assimilates technical rationality. Dewey (1933, cited by Tann 1993: 54) writes,

> Reflective action entails active and persistent consideration of any belief or supposed form of knowledge in the light of the grounds that support it and the consequences to which it leads.

Knowledge covers the whole spectrum of potential influence from nursing texts, science, philosophy, research and novels. The list is endless. It helps us identify and name things that have eluded our ability to conceptualise in any meaningful way. It helps us see and frame ideas.

Brookfield (1995: 36) writes,

> Theory can help us name our practice by illuminating the general elements of what we think are idiosyncratic experiences. It can provide multiple perspectives on familiar situations.

A recent example was reading Simon Woods's book *Death's Dominion* (2007) in which he explores Richard Dworkin's (1993) idea of coherence – that people need to die in a coherent way with the way they have lived, an idea that challenged the whole idea of hospices imposing a particular approach to death on patients. This informed my 'smoking kills' text (Chapter 24). I had picked up the book to explore autonomy. Hence this discovery was opportunistic.

Another example was reading *Of Mice and Men* by John Steinbeck (1937/2000). Reading about Slim, the jerkline skinner, gives the idea of 'poise' real substance in the sense of the way he moved, his expertise at his trade, the respect he received when he spoke, that he heard more than was said, of understanding beyond thought, his kindly gentle speech, the confidence he engendered in others and his acknowledgment of others' worth (34–6).

In Chapter 25 I show how Audre Lorde's words from her cancer journals (1980) both reflect and inform 'Anthea'. Indeed, Lorde's evocative words deeply enrich the narrative.

These examples suggest that the reflective practitioner reads broadly from a variety of texts, and there is potential in every text to inform. Through dialogue, theory comes alive because it is always explored in the context of practice. As such, it loses its eminence. It is cut down to size to simply inform, not to predict and control.

Skill Box

- *Enter into a dialogue between significant factors emerging from your reflection with a relevant literature. Open any newspaper or novel and read it with your experience in mind. Can you make any connection?*
- *Dialogue with at least one theory in relation to your experience for its value to inform your current practice.*

Finding Voice

Belenky et al. (1986) refer to the dialogue between extant theory and personal experience as the synthesis between the connected and separate procedural voices towards developing the constructed voice (see Table 5.1). Belenky et al. help us to view two types of knowing as significant. This understanding suggests that the dichotomy between technical rationality and professional artistry (as suggested by Schon 1987; see Chapter 1) is flawed because constructed knowing *is* professional artistry. Belenky et al.'s dichotomy between separate and connected voices links with the notion of left brain and right brain (see Figure 2.2) and Virginia Woolf's assertion about the great mind being androgynous; a fusion between the left and right brains, the masculine and the feminine. To reiterate: experience is the hat to hang theory on. Without experience theory has nothing to hold on to.

Table 5.1 Development of voice (Belenky et al. 1986)

	Connected voice Speaking with an informed and authentic voice	
Separate voice (left brain/ masculine) Connection with extant knowledge	**Procedural voice**	**Connected voice** (right brain/ feminine) Connection with experience of others an with self
	Subjective voice Finding the inner voice (opinion without substance)	
	Received voice Speaking through the voice of authoritative others	
	Silence	

Empowerment (arrow pointing upward on right side)

Belenky et al.'s theory of developing voice suggests that the writing and talking of experience, for example in writing, and verbally in guided reflection, can be the emergence of voice from the paucity of received knowing and silence. For practitioners socialised into subordinate roles, the emergence of voice is a vital stepping stone in developing professional artistry. It also suggests that the professional curriculum should focus on opportunities for students to express their voice rather than be viewed as receptacles for filling with knowledge which they then regurgitate without critical thinking.

Skill Box

- *What voice do you speak through?*
- *Does this voice vary depending on the situation?*
- *If so, why is that?*
- *Reflect on a sequence of experiences with the intent to develop your 'constructed voice'. What factors inhibit you? How can you overcome these?*

Guiding Reflection: The Fourth Dialogical Movement

In the fourth dialogical movement the practitioner is *guided* to challenge and deepen her tentative insights prompted by the MSR cue 'How does exploring with guides and peers challenge my insights?' (See Figure 3.2.)

Boud, Keogh and Walker (1985) suggest that, whilst reflection is something the student could do for themselves, 'the learning process can be considerably accelerated by appropriate support' (36).

Brookfield (1996: 36) writes,

Just knowing that we are not alone in our struggles is profoundly reassuring. Although critical reflection often begins alone, it is ultimately a collective endeavour. We need colleagues to help us know what our assumptions are and help us to change the structures of power so that democratic actions and values are rewarded, both within and outside our institutions.

Guided reflection is a testing place whereby the practitioner can see herself against the mirror of guides and peers to receive feedback that may be affirming or disconfirming. Either way she takes this positively, given the explicit non-judgemental nature of the guidance. Boyd and Fales (1983: 12–13) write,

> The need to test one's self-changes [insights] against the mirror of others is an essential component of all growth. It is our belief that the changes experienced in the resolution stage are never completely lost, whether or not they are shared. However, they are bolstered and reinforced by the commitment to test them publicly. Negative evaluation by others may force the individual back into a new cycle of reflection, may be discounted in the service of the self's certainty, or may be experienced as disastrously disconfirming of self. It appears, however, that the individual is intuitively cautious at this stage, and evaluates the probable effectiveness of the action before deciding to go public with the change.

I take my reflection about Peggy to guided reflection.

Peggy

The guided reflection group meets for 75 minutes once a month. We take it in turns to facilitate the group so we can all develop guidance skills. Initially we bought in a guide for six months to teach us to self-manage. It is a voluntary group open to all staff within the hospice, although few attend. I've discussed this with some of the nurses and therapists. A number of excuses were offered:

'I'm too busy!'
'I don't believe it will help my practice.'
'I don't like sharing myself within groups.'
'I talk with others if I have any problems.'
'I never liked reflective practice as a student nurse.'
'Navel gazing!'

Those that do attend seem more committed and more caring than others, as if they take their practice seriously and welcome the learning opportunity. I asked staff who do attend why they attend. Some responses were:

'It's good to talk over issues with colleagues. It creates a sense of community that spills over into practice itself.'
'I realise that what bothers me is shared by others.'
'It helps me deal with any conflicts I have.'
'I have learnt a lot about ethics and ways of talking with patients.'
'It's good professional practice.'

'Rotating the group's guide facilitates guidance skills. That's useful because it actually teaches me to listen and weigh up options that I can transfer to my clinical practice.'
In the group we take it in turns to share experiences. We have contracted[1] to reflect on these experiences before each session using the Model for Structured Reflection.[2] In this way we work through issues before presenting them. Five other staff arrive: three nurses, a new young doctor and the senior physiotherapist. There are no other therapists and no senior nurses. Why do they never attend? Perhaps they are anxious of exposing themselves as lacking in some way?

Today, Connie, the senior physiotherapist, is the group's guide.
She asks, 'Does anyone have anything particular to share today?'
'Yes,' I say.
'Anyone else?'
Marie, the young doctor, has something to share but is happy for me to go first.

The group listen to my story with respect. Connie opens my story to the group. It seems a common story. Group confession! Everyone recognises 'passing people by' and how such self-management becomes embodied and hence invisible.

Someone asks, 'Have you considered the ethical dimension? Did you act for the best?'[3]
'No, not directly. What do you think?'
'Well, consider Peggy's autonomy.'

'I know I should always respect her autonomy. To do so I need to put Peggy in a position of taking responsibility and making a decision. Umm, that's interesting.' As such, a fourth response might have been – 'Would you like a therapy now, Peggy? I have time.' Saying 'I have time' frees Peggy to accept. I can see this response would be better. It acknowledges and respects her autonomy.'

The group like this response. Someone says, 'You can really see the utilitarian ethic at work in your experience – the demand on time and its influence on the way we set priorities.'

Perhaps I should not have offered any of my own alternatives but asked them to generate alternatives before sharing my own; for example, *'if you were in my shoes how might you have responded?'* I sense it would have been a better learning curve. Learning how best to share stories and work within the group is an ongoing developmental process.

Connie feeds in some theory concerning defence against anxiety stemming from the work of Menzies-Lyth, in particular, the assertion of the need for practitioners to develop a necessary professional detachment as a protection from not being overwhelmed by the other's suffering. I argue that if concern for Peggy is vital in opening a healing space then I must rewrite Menzies-Lyth (1988) as 'the need to develop a necessary professional involvement' if I am to realize my vision of easing suffering. As I wrote, *'I was touched by her sense of being alone.'* And saying that I feel emotional, as if I am back in that moment. But then involvement is not easy. Being detached, we can surf through the day, not oblivious to suffering, but keeping it at a distance. Such an approach is governed and sanctioned by the medical model with its primary gaze on the person as symptom management whereby social, psychological and spiritual issues become problems to solve rather than being seen from a holistic perspective.

Marie emphasizes, 'We need to have poise or emotional intelligence – the ability to be fully available to the other within the moment by managing our vulnerability to the other's suffering.'

I say, 'My experience with Peggy suggests poise is not simply a technical knowhow that can be applied. It is much deeper than that.'

I had expected Marie, the doctor, to be defensive, but she surprises me by agreeing that 'easing suffering', as enshrined within the WHO definition of palliative care, should be emphasised as the Hospice's primary value.[4]

I feed in my thoughts about whether I was suffering from 'situational blindness' or lack of compassion influenced by a current controversy within the nursing literature. I offer to circulate these papers for others to consider and perhaps pick up in our next session if desired. Connie says, 'I will share this story at the next senior clinical team meeting. Wake them up a bit!'

I say, 'Like throwing a stone into a still pond, creating disturbing ripples.'

Marie then shares her story. As she does she relates it to my story, her anxiety about relating to a male patient who won't talk to her. Do men need men to talk to, especially older men fearful of death? How can she, a young woman, help? It is a question I had reflected on in my journal when one of the female consultants asked me if I would talk with a male patient.

Connie summarises the session, skilfully drawing the assumptions that govern our practice and how these assumptions have been challenged, even transformed.

I never got to share my ideas about rescheduling.

Jennifer offers to write up the session and post it on the staff noticeboard to illustrate the significance of guided reflection. Perhaps it will influence others to attend, or if not, at least to dialogue about care. Her idea reminds us of the value of both individual and group-guided reflection, to get underneath the stories to reveal and challenge core values. We are all more mindful, more energised. From a group perspective the practitioner joins peers and guides within a community of learning. In my extensive experience of guiding both individuals and groups, group guidance has many advantages over individual guidance.

Guidance

As the guide, Connie's role is to facilitate the deepening of insights. The practitioner has a partial view and guidance helps her expand this view from wider perspectives, pulling away any masks that distort seeing self and reality for what they really are, cleaning smudges from the reflective mirror. We cannot learn if the basis of understanding is built on distortion. Lather (1986a, 1986b) terms this self-distortion 'false consciousness'. Brookfield (1996: 33) writes,

> An intrinsic problem with private self-reflection is that when we use them, we can never completely avoid the risks of denial and distortion. We can never know just how much we're cooking the data of our memories and experience to produce images and renditions that show us off to good effect.

In a similar vein, Cox, Hickson and Taylor (1991: 285) write,

> Reflection in isolation is difficult to sustain because of the difficulty in surfacing and transcending our own distorted self-understandings, asking ourselves difficult, often self-exposing questions, facing difficult answers to such questions, and, perhaps most particularly, keeping our vision directed toward new possibilities for understanding and action.

Perhaps one reason why practitioners *smudge the mirror* is to distort the image of self being reflected back in order to give a better impression. This is a defence mechanism protecting the threatened ego. It may not be easy for the practitioner to recognise distortion without guidance.

Co-creation of Insights

The practitioner and guide shape meaning, craft insight, and fuse horizons whereby their partial perspectives are transcended in reaching a new shared perspective (Gadamer

1975). Horizon is a metaphor for our understanding. Horizons constantly shift as we move towards them. As such, horizon suggests the limits of our vision to understand things. Gadamer (1975: 183) writes, 'Our own horizon is constantly in the process of formation, not least through our encounters with the past.' Both the guide and practitioner are mindful of the limitations of their own understanding, and so through dialogue work to expand their understandings, hence the *co-creation of insights*, insights for both the practitioner and the guide.

Dialogue

The intended pattern of 'guidance talk' is dialogue. Dialogue comes from the Greek word *dia-logos*, which can be taken to mean 'meaning flowing among and through us, out of which may emerge some new understanding' (Bohm 1996: 6).
Isaacs (1993: 25) describes dialogue as

> a discipline of collective thinking and inquiry, a process for transforming the quality of conversation and, in particular, the thinking that lies beneath it … a movement towards creating a field of genuine meeting and inquiry where people can allow a *free flow of meaning* and vigorous exploration of the collective background of their thought, their personal predispositions, the nature of their shared attention, and the rigid features of their individual and collective assumptions. As people learn to perceive, inquire into, and allow transformation of the nature and shape of these fields, and the patterns of individual thinking and acting that inform them, they may discover entirely new levels of insight and forge substantive and, at times, dramatic changes in behaviour. As this happens, whole new possibilities for coordinated action develop.

Issacs (1993: 24) contrasts dialogue with debate:

> in debate one side wins and the another loses; both parties maintain their certainties, and both suppress deeper inquiry. Unfortunate, most forms of organizational conversation, particularly around tough, complex, or challenging issues lapse into debate (the root of which means 'to beat down'). In debate one side wins and another loses; both parties maintain their certainties, and both suppress deeper inquiry. Debate reflects patterns of power relationships and rivalry, where people jostle for control typified by people lining up to get their point across and win the argument. Very little genuine listening takes place. People partially listen to what they want to hear, seeking feedback to reinforce their position rather than be open to new possibility through dialogue.

Bohm (1996) discerned six *rules* of dialogue that provide a basis for exploring and contracting dialogue within the guided reflection group:

1 commitment to work with others towards consensus for a better world
2 awareness and suspension of one's own assumptions and prejudices
3 pro-prioception of thinking
4 openness to possibility and freedom from attachment to ideas
5 listening with engagement and respect
6 having a mutual appreciation of dialogue.

Dialogue can be with oneself or within groups of people. It always *moves towards* consensus for a better world. The emphasis on *moving towards* acknowledges a *letting go of attachment* to old ideas. The idea of a better world suggests that all action is moral social action towards this end. To dialogue people must not only know and suspend their assumptions and opinions, but also be aware of the thinking that gave rise to these assumptions in the first place. Where do they arise from, how tenacious do we cling to them? Why do we cling to them? This requires a *proprioception of thinking*, an awareness of where the mind is at the moment. Within the dialogical process there is a shift from problem solving towards acknowledging and resolving a paradox that requires thinking about the way people think about things. If we use the same thinking that caused the problem to try and solve the problem, we fail. Hence we need to change the way we think to view the problem differently.

Bohm (1996: 25) writes,

> We could say that practically all the problems of the human race are due to the fact that thought is not proprioceptive. Thought is constantly creating problems that way and then trying to solve them. But as it tries to solve them it makes it worse because it doesn't notice that it's creating them, and the more it thinks, the more problems it creates – because it's not proprioceptive of what it's doing.

Only then can people transform their perspectives to see things differently. Dialogue is *listening*. Only when people *really* listen can they hear what is being said or not being said. Yet listening seems a rare quality in the patterns of talk that dominate practice and education. Do we listen to what we want to hear, or distort what we hear in order to fit into our own scheme, to confirm our own assumptions?

Talking Stick

Using a talking stick might aid develop dialogue until people 'get it'. The person holding the stick is the only person allowed to speak and must summarise what has been spoken before and move on from that point. As you might expect, some people just like talking and dominating talk. It is interesting to see how people in a guided reflection group who use the 'talking stick' confront those who don't get it or revert to old ways, especially if the dialogue becomes heated and people's emotions run high.

Air Time

There is only so much 'air' time within a session for practitioners to share their experiences. However, practitioners can benefit more by listening and relating to others' experiences than by sharing their own. This may benefit less vocal or reticent practitioners who feel threatened by individual guided reflection. In groups, there are more diverse views and more support for practitioners. However, people can feel more vulnerable sharing their experiences in groups. As such groups may take longer to create a safe environment, moving through forming norms.[5]

Finding Voice

As I suggested above, writing a journal enables practitioners to find their 'voice'. In guided reflection the practitioner now 'voices' her voice. The group is a sound box reverberating her voice back to her so she can hear herself clearly. Expressing voice at this level is what Belenky et al. (1986) describe as the 'subjective' voice – giving vent to opinions, ideas and so on (see Table 5.1). The practitioner refines this subjective voice with dialogue with literature and now with guides and peers to develop her 'constructed' voice. Belenky et al.

(1986) note that to learn to speak in this unique and authentic voice, women must jump outside the frames and systems authorities provide and create their own frame. *It is the voice of the reflective practitioner.*

Finding voice develops from critical yet non-judgemental voices of others, both peers and guides, within the guided reflection group. Indeed, sharing clinical experiences where it has been difficult to voice self becomes a significant focus within the development of guided reflection groups, especially where not voicing self for whatever reason compromises patient health (Bradbury Jones, Sambrook and Irvine 2011). Indeed, dialogue around student perceptions of each other's experiences or simply a work of art are visual thinking strategies that have the potential 'to improve observational and communication skills, teaching students to speak out in safe ways which may mitigate errors in patient care' (Moorman 2015: 754).

The Reality Wall

In a rational world it is easy to see how performance could be improved. However, the world is not rational. It is governed by norms and assumptions grounded in issues of authority, tradition and embodiment – *the reality wall*. These norms that govern everyday practice are not easy to appreciate simply because they are normal. The guide helps the practitioner understand these norms and ways in which they might be shifted towards a more desirable state of affairs. However, such is the constraining power of these forces, the practitioner may choose to rationalise the contradiction or tension and decide to let matters lie, particularly if the practitioner is fearful of consequences. She may fear disapproval and sanction.

Smyth (1987: 40) notes, 'Most of us, unless we feel uncomfortable, shaken, or forced to look at ourselves, are unlikely to change. It is far easier to accept our current conditions and adopt the least line of resistance.' Lieberman (1989: 88 – cited by Day 1993) writes, 'Working in bureaucratic settings has taught everyone to be compliant, to be rule governed, not to ask questions, seek alternatives or deal with competing values.'

In this respect the guide enables the practitioner's empowerment to take action or reassures the practitioner when this is not possible for whatever reason.

In Kieffer's (1984) study of empowerment of grassroots community leaders in the United States, participants referred with great emotional intensity to the importance of the *external enabler* to support their struggle against more powerful others who were motivated to maintain the status quo. The practitioner connects with her guide as a representative of the wider community, the gatekeeper and guide to this new world. In order to do this, the guide must connect with the practitioner in terms of her existing reality and simultaneously in terms of a potential new reality. I meet few practitioners who are happy with 'their lot'. The guide may struggle with the trauma stories the practitioner reveals and it becomes an ethical issue to urge the practitioner to take action and then watch them stumble and fall against the hard edge of reality. The key is not to fix the problem for the practitioner but guide them to see ways they can fix it for themselves.

The guide disturbs the surface of normal practice, planting seeds of doubt in tune with the practitioner's notion of desirable practice. The guide waters these seeds to grow and blossom, weeding away old ideas that are no longer tenable. The guide disturbs the idea of desirable practice, challenging the practitioner to find meaning in these words beyond the cliché.[6] Through continuity of guidance, new ideas can quickly be put into practice and subsequently reflected on. If the seeds don't take because the soil is stony, then the stone is chipped away slowly, until the moment when the new seed takes hold. Then the practitioner can emerge transformed into a new horizon.

Margolis (1993) considers that new ideas compete with existing ideas. The success of adopting new ideas depends on the robustness of existing ones and the force of argument available to support the new idea. Practitioners are likely to feel anxious when their 'old ways' are challenged. They are caught between defending self from this anxiety and opening self to new possibilities. However, in exploring new, more congruent ways, the practitioner may experience a crisis of isolation or separateness (Isaacs 1993) whereby group norms and ways of relating must shift. This may overflow into personal lives as practitioners find their voices and speak out. Isaacs (1993: 38) writes, 'Such loosening of rigid thought patterns frees energy that now permits new levels of intelligence and creativity.'

Power

Issues of power underline every experience and can be revealed if the practitioner goes deep enough to bring them to the surface. Yet power relationships are difficult to shift, rooted as they are deep within the organizational and professional culture.

For dialogue to work, it requires the development of trust within the guided reflection group. Dialogue will take time to flow freely until trust is established. This requires an active realignment of power. However, authority is in the room. Power norms must be surfaced and suspended. Dialogue gets stuck when the power issue is not addressed. But people are authority. People have different roles and status that are a reality. Hence the guide actively works at deconstructing power so that authority is left at the door, so 'the elephant is not in the room'.[7] It is part of the developmental process to shed fear of authority and realise your own power.

Power is embodied through socialization processes and reinforced through everyday patterns of relating. Hence it is normal and largely unchallenged. From an authoritative perspective, power is invested in position, for example in management roles. Hence subordinates get told what to do. Play the game, do as you are told, keep your head down to avoid sanction, and then one day you too will become a manager and have power! Power is also invested in professional roles – so doctors often perceive themselves as superior to nurses, coining the expression that 'nurses are the doctor's handmaiden'. Nurses are taught 'to know their place' within the order of things. It is natural for dominant professions such as medicine to reinforce subordinate behaviour in other healthcare professions, such as nursing (Oakley 1984). In other words, doctors are always motivated to maintain the status quo and resist rivalry for power. Nurses rationalise their compliance with medical domination because of the need to be valued. Chapman (1983) suggested that doctors reinforce nurses' subordination through humiliation techniques that become a normative pattern of relating. Hence it becomes difficult for nurses to claim autonomy to move into the right place to nurse desirably, kept in place by both managers and doctors. It is also the same with students and teachers. Even in universities, teachers traditionally set the agenda and control the classroom. Students learn to be 'good', otherwise sanctions will ensue.

The guide checks herself not to fall back into a dominant teacher mode of being or not being mindful of being contradictory, especially if she feels anxious about the way the group is performing. To help her, she can use student feedback to check out her own assumptions and enable students to express their voice.[8]

As a guide, I usually wait for peers within the group to respond to another student practitioner's sharing of experience before myself, not because I am unduly humble or courteous, but because I know that my voice is acknowledged as the expert voice. Practitioners know this, so let's not play at collaborative games. They want to hear my voice and learn from it. As a guide, knowing how to assert one's own voice is like tuning into the community's wavelength – not easy with large groups, and yet groups settle and create norms. The astute guide is always checking out the control of the community through practitioner feedback, and yet the practitioner must feel able to voice true feedback if the community is to achieve optimum performance.

Finding Your Own Way

Pirsig (1974: 191) writes about climbing mountains that resonates strongly with the practitioner finding her own way:

> some practitioners travel into the mountains accompanied by experienced guides who know the best and least dangerous routes by which they arrive at their destination. Still others, inexperienced and untrusting, attempt to make their own routes. Few of these are successful, but occasionally some, by sheer will and luck and grace, do make it. Once there, they become more aware than any of the others that there's no single or fixed number of routes. There are as many routes as there are individuals.

Even though I am an experienced guide, I sometimes get caught out by assuming I know the best way rather than helping the practitioner find their own way. Recently, I kept saying to one student: 'Just practise, and it will come.' And of course it doesn't just come. I recognized my frustration that she could not get it, a blind spot that emerged when another student recognised her own difficulty in getting it. Sometimes people do need to be shown the path and stick to it, and that's OK! It is a creative tension between prescription and finding your own way.

The Guidance Process

The guide invites the practitioner to share her experience. The group listens carefully, with respect. Perhaps, in the early sessions, the guide reminds the group to pay attention to and suspend their opinions. At some point the practitioner will pause, offering the guide a cue for clarifying issues, guiding the practitioner towards formulating insights. The guide invites other group members to clarify, perhaps using the MSR cues, to ensure breadth and depth of reflection. By this time, the practitioner is usually able to focus on what was significant in this experience. Other group members are also able to relate to this experience from the perspective of their own experiences. This deepens and enriches the dialogue.

The guide then asks the group to consider how each of them might respond if they were in the practitioner's shoes and for the practitioner to consider alternative, more effective ways of responding given the situation again. This is often difficult for the practitioner locked into normal and habitual patterns of responding. The group generates a range of options and offer these to the practitioner to consider alongside her own options and the potential consequences. The guide inputs theory to inform the debate to which she directs the group to pursue before the next session.

The practitioner determines her preferred choice and whether she could actually respond in this way. Is she skilled or empowered enough? What factors might constrain her from taking action and working towards understanding and shifting these factors? This can involve role modelling and rehearsal. The guide then 'wraps up' by asking each practitioner to summarise their learning and ensures that emotional issues have been worked through.

Of course, all sorts of distractions take place as in the nature of such groups. At no time is the guide judgemental, but rather confronts by asking questions: 'Do you think that was the best way?' or 'What other options could you have?' At all times the guide invites practitioner self-assessment and responsibility for actions.

Inputting Theory

As explored above, the practitioner is challenged by the MSR cue 'How does extant theory/ideas inform and deepen my insights?' However, the guide may help by inputting theory, as illustrated by Connie in my experience with Peggy (see above).

As a guide I was famous for having a stack of 'theory' papers in my briefcase to pull out at appropriate moments to inform the practitioner's experience. I knew from experience that certain topics always emerge from shared experiences, topics such as conflict management and therapeutic relationships. This suggests that the guide requires an eclectic knowledge base. Inputting theory leads practitioners into critical conversations with others – 'I have been reading this …' – noting its challenge, inspiration or even rejection of the ideas offered. I encourage students to research relevant theory and share these texts with the community for critique and assimilation into personal knowing. Inputting theory links with the MSR influencing factor (What knowledge informed my practice'? – see Chapter 3).

Balance of Challenge and Support

Guidance is the *intense* balance of challenge and support. Inevitably, revealing and exploring self creates anxiety, as deeper parts of self become exposed. The guide *holds* the practitioner to face up to anxiety rather than to defend against it. In this respect the guide becomes part of the practitioner's defence system; a safety harness. The guide is comfortable being with the practitioner in this way. In my experience, this is not a big deal, a big psychotherapeutic drama. It is a mindful, caring way of being in dialogue whereby the guide is non-attached to the other, connected to them yet separate from them. The guide is skilled at not absorbing the practitioner's emotions and mindful of his own assumptions and suspending these assumptions in order to listen and respond dialogically to the learner's reflections. Lisa noted,

> *I felt that being challenged is an essential element of guidance, providing you feel comfortable in your environment and at ease with your guide. The challenge element encouraged me to think further than I had been and to deal with issues in a way I would not have considered before.*
> (unpublished journal notes)

The balance of challenge and support can be visualized using the challenge/support grid (Table 5.2). Ideally, the practitioner would score their guide ten out of ten for both

Table 5.2 Challenge–support axis

		10	**High challenge / Low support**	**The optimum learning milieu**
		9	creates high anxiety for the	The guide can challenge without
	High	**8**	practitioner.	the practitioner feeling threatened.
		7	People do not learn well under	Indeed the practitioner thrives on
Challenge		**6**	situations of high anxiety.	this challenge.
		5	**Low support / Low challenge**	**High support / Low challenge**
		4	Leads to apathy-what's the	Comfort work. This may be
		3	point?	appropriate for periods when
		2		practitioners disclose experiences
	Low	**1**		of stress.

				Support					
Low	◄─────────────────────────────────►								High
1	2	3	4	5	6	7	8	9	10

challenge and support – perfect balance; the optimum learning environment that should be explored when guided reflection is contracted.

Perhaps the easiest mode to fall naturally into is low challenge/high support, as if people have a natural reluctance to be critical of each other. As Bohm (1996: 13/18) writes,

> If five or six people get together, they can usually adjust to each other so they don't say things that upset each other – they get a 'cozy adjustment'. When a dialogue group is new, in general people tend to talk around the point for a while. In all human relations nowadays, people talk around things, avoiding the difficulties.

Skill Box

- *If you are in either individual or group supervision, where would you score your guide? Ask your guide to score her/himself. Do these scores match? Discuss.*
- *In your next guided reflection group, pay attention to the balance of challenge and support – actively move towards more challenge and more support.*

Six Category Intervention Analysis

Specific communicative techniques such as the 'Six Category Intervention Analysis' (Heron 1975, Sloan and Watson 2001) may be helpful to structure dialogue. Heron proposes six basic therapeutic interventions that can be either authoritative or facilitative.

Authorative interventions are:

- *Giving information* – enabling the other to make a rational decision based on information
- *Giving advice* – helping the other see other, better ways of seeing and doing things
- *Confrontation* – challenging the other's restrictive attitudes, beliefs or behavior.

Facilitative interventions are:

- *Being cathartic* – enabling the other to express a difficult emotion so it can be resolved
- *Being catalytic* – enabling the other to talk through an issue
- *Being supportive* – communicating a sense of 'being there' for the other (balancing the impact of challenge).

Heron further categorizes these interventions as manipulative or perverse, where the practitioner abuses the responses to meet their own agendas.

Think of confrontation. From a perverse perspective, confrontation is used to challenge someone's behavior, rather like a critical parent with a naughty child: 'Don't do that.' From a therapeutic perspective, confrontation is more subtle – 'Do you think that was the best way to act?' – suggesting that the way the person did respond was not the most effective.

As with clinical practice, the guide chooses the most appropriate interventions to suit the situation, moving easily between each response as appropriate.

For example:

1 When an underlying emotion is sensed, the guide will use a cathartic response; 'You seem angry at your manager?' The intention is to release and bring to the surface the underlying emotion so it can be dealt with. At this level practitioners may fear releasing the emotion because they do not know how to respond to it.
2 Having released the emotion, the guide uses a catalytic response to help the person talk through the issue with the intention of helping them find meaning in their feelings, and through talking through it, to understand deeper underlying reasons and assumptions for these feelings. In this way the supervisee is helped to convert the released negative energy into positive energy for taking action.
3 Confrontation can then be used to challenge, yet always within a supportive framework. Confrontation is a subtle rather than direct intervention – for example, 'Can you see other ways of responding?', implicitly suggesting that the practitioner's response was not effective, yet without direct judgement. Confrontation is easier within a trusting relationship because the practitioner is naturally more open to challenge, especially when challenge is balanced with support.
4 Information can be given, but I am always wary of giving advice because it is taking responsibility for the other person. Much better to say, 'What options do you have', rather than 'I would do this', even for novice practitioners who seek direction. When I do think it is appropriate to give advice I say, 'I am going to give you advice' and imagine I have a neon warning sign over my head that says 'Giving advice' –to remind me that this is a power intervention and to remind the supervisee to take it with caution.

In using these interventions the guide is mindful of making them available to group members to use in both guidance and clinical practice. Burnard and Morrison (1991) note that practitioners are generally not skilled at cathartic, catalytic and confrontational responses, and yet these are the very essence of therapeutic work, not just with patients but also with guidance.[9]

Skill Box

> • *Reflect on your use of each of Heron's six interventions within an experience.*
> • *Play with each of them and consider how you could use these interventions more skilfully.*
> • *Be mindful when next in practice about using Heron's communication skills, notably catharsis, catalytic and confrontation. Reflect on a new experience and review your use of these skills.*

Energy Work

Being able to tell a trauma story is healing. Being heard, the practitioner is remoralised (Frank 2002); their self often becomes demoralised through loss of care, both the care they give and the care they receive. Without doubt, low morale and stress are endemic within healthcare. As a guide working with students it is vital to prepare the students to be 'fit for practice' through self-care to become poised or emotionally intelligent – having the ability to know and manage self within relationships. Stress accumulates within the body and creates stiffness and fatigue. It is not healthy and requires energy to balance it, often leaving the practitioner drained, with little in reserve to give to patient care.

As explored in Chapter 3, one strategy is for the guide to help the practitioner visualise a water butt or stress butt – and help the practitioner open the drainage tap, using the stress as positive energy for taking action (Hall 1964).

In Figure 5.1, the single curly line represents the practitioner's unproblematic practice until it she hits a crisis where her normal thinking and responses fail her, resulting in anxiety or negative energy. Being open systems, practitioners can convert this energy with the environment to create positive energy for taking future action to resolve the crisis and emerge at a higher level of consciousness. The guide is a catalyst converter.

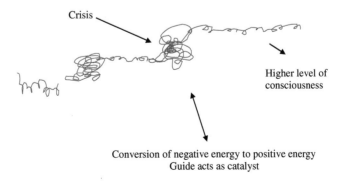

Figure 5.1   The guide as catalyst. Inspired by Newman (1994, 38) based on Prigogine and Stenger's theory of dissipative structures (1980).

Pulling Free

When energy gets really stuck, I might ask the practitioner to imagine a rope extending into her body connected to her feelings. I ask her to imagine I am pulling out the negative energy from her body. Hand over hand, I pull the imaginary rope until it pulls free, and stamp on it. It works!

Contracting

A contract forms a formal yet dynamic background to guided reflection (clinical supervision). Proctor (1988, cited by Hawkins and Shohet 1989: 29) note,

> if supervision is to become and remain a co-operative experience which allows for real rather than token accountability, a clear, even tough, working agreement needs to be negotiated. The agreement needs to provide sufficient safety and clarity for the student/worker to know where she stands; and it needs sufficient teeth for the supervisor to feel free and responsible for making the challenges.

What Issues Need to be Contracted?

In establishing a guided reflection relationship, the supervisor and practitioner(s) agree to collaborate within a set of mutual expectations, responsibilities and boundaries.

Key points:

- *The practitioner accepts responsibility for using the learning space in the most appropriate and effective way.* I contract with practitioners to bring at least one experience they have reflected and are willing to share to each session even though time may not permit its actual sharing.
- *Practitioners will keep a record within a portfolio.* This can be an extension of the practitioner's reflective journal or a summarised formal record used for professional registration or required educational submission. Guided reflection is a continuous developmental process. As such, the guide is mindful to 'pick up' issues from the previous sessions. Between sessions practitioners will have reflected deeper on issues and drawn on an informing literature. They may have used ideas generated within the previous group. Other similar experiences may have arisen.
- Notes can be structured as follows:
  - 'pick up' from last session; what was talked about in the guided reflection session in response to shared experiences both my own and others (if in group guided reflection)
  - what was significant about what was talked about – linking to my own insights
  - what actions taken as a consequence in future practice (as revealed through subsequent experiences)I do not ask to see the portfolio because I do not want the practitioner to feel inhibited (although a summary of learning may form assignment work if linked to a formal learning programme). Session notes build the practitioner's CPD file that are useful for any CPD requirement. Keeping a portfolio will also enable practitioners to accumulate reflections necessary for maintaining professional registration, just as time spent in 'guided reflection' will substantially contribute to the 'professional development' hours requirement.[10] What stronger motive can you ask for?

- *Distinguish guided reflection work from therapy.* The guide is mindful of transgressing into therapy by keeping a focus on the practitioner's practice. Guided reflection is not psychotherapy or counselling.
- *Maintain confidentiality.* The maxim is that whatever is discussed within guided reflection should stay in guided reflection. This is the basis for safety and trust. Trust may take some time to establish because of the vulnerability in self-revelation, but can be quickly shattered if talk is taken out of the session and gets back to the practitioner. There may be times when confidentiality must be breached in terms of patient safety, although in my experience this is a very rare and should always be negotiated.
- *Monitoring the effectiveness of guided reflection.* The effectiveness of the guidance process should never be taken for granted and should be constantly scrutinised. Evaluation is itself a significant developmental exercise for the practitioner to analyse the guidance process and to give critical feedback, for example using the 'Guided reflection evaluation' and 'Classroom critical incident' questionnaires (see Appendices 4 and 5).

Skill Box

- *If you are involved in guided reflection (clinical supervision), prompt a review of your contract for its suitability (either as guide or participant).*
- *Consider how guided reflection can be evaluated for its effectiveness.*

The Learning Environment

Guided reflection within clinical practice (as opposed to something done at home in the practitioner's own time) requires time out from practice itself. In the fast pace of clinical practice, time is a premium and costs money. Yet what value does the organisation give to guided reflection? It must be seen as a part of legitimate staff development and support rather than a sticking plaster papering over a failing system, dealing with the consequence of stress rather than the causes of stress. Indeed, guided reflection may become a stressor in itself by demanding more from the practitioner. How long is a piece of string?

A Quiet Eddy

Imagine clinical practice as a fast-moving river. In the busyness of the day, many practitioners feel they are being swept along in the current, reacting to events as they unfold about them. Guided reflection is like an eddy within the fast-moving water that enables the practitioner to pause in relative stillness, and reflect on what goes on in the fast-moving water. In this way, the practitioner prepares herself to practise more effectively and be more able to negotiate the fast current. The eddy must be seen as a legitimate place to pause because the current will not let you go easily.

Returning to my guided reflection group where I shared my experience with Peggy – it was voluntary, open to all disciplines, and peer-led. From this, we can discern four key variables for guided reflection:

- Who should the guide be?
- Individual vs. group-guided reflection;

- Single or multi-disciplinary?
- Voluntary or mandatory?

Who Should the Guide Be?

From an educational perspective, the 'teacher' is inevitably the guide. There is really no escape from this perspective and nor should there be, although it does require a radical shift in assumptions about the nature of the teacher–student relationship, and indeed about the culture of teaching and learning. Perhaps third-year students could be involved with guiding first-year students alongside teacher guides. This would enable them to develop guidance skills ready for guidance and mentoring roles as qualified practitioners.

Who the guide should be in clinical practice is more complex

A number of positions are possible:

- line-managed
- non line-managed within the organisation
- non line-managed from outside the organisation
- peer-led

Establishing professional supervision[11] at Burford Hospital as clinical leader and manager, I naturally took the role of supervisor/guide, justified as an experiential approach to clinical leadership. However, analysing patterns of recorded dialogue,[12] practitioners did not share experiences concerning myself, illuminating that even with collaborative intent and collaborative role-modelling, and viewing me with caution. Why was that? I suggest it reflects an essentially oppressive transactional culture whereby practitioners have been socialised into subordinate-type relationships that are not easily overthrown. It reminds me of supervision as someone looking over your shoulder ensuring you do your work competently. If so, supervision is threatening, asking the practitioner to reveal their practice for scrutiny, no matter how good the supervisor's intention. Through guiding other line-manager supervisors, I discovered this was normal (Johns 1998). It wasn't until I guided practitioners as a non-line manager that I came to realise that the most common shared topic was conflict with the organisation. Ipso facto – line manager guidance inhibits the practitioner.

Analysing patterns of guidance dialogue, a number of potential advantages and disadvantages with line management guidance emerged (Table 5.3). The potential disadvantages are set against a background of the transactional nature of healthcare organisations, and was essentially concerned with targets and its own smooth running. The transactional attitude dampens professional accountability in the demand for organisational accountability.

The non-line manager as guide, especially if imported from outside the organisation, is likely to be more objective, to see things more broadly when outside the situation, and is less likely to have their own practice agenda than a line manager guide. Hence guided reflection is likely to be less outcome-focused and less judgemental. As a consequence, the practitioner may have a greater sense of control and feel less threatened.

I wonder, in my Burford leadership role, if I would have allowed an *outsider* to guide Burford practitioners? Could I have 'let go' my need to control the practice environment? Would I have felt my leadership role usurped?

The availability and potential resource cost of non-line managers is another factor to consider, especially when it is unlikely that guidance will have an organisational budget.

Table 5.3 Advantages and disadvantages of line managed guidance within the organisation. (Adapted from Johns & McCormack 1998.)

Potential advantages

- The guide knows the practitioner's practice and therefore has a better understanding of issues the practitioner reveals, so they can tackle issues together.
- Guidance talk spills over into everyday practice, facilitating more professional and collaborative ways of relating within practice. It breaks development out of the guidance bubble into everyday practice.
- Enables managers to acknowledge and value practitioners [in a culture that generally has not done that].
- Facilitates mutual reflection and learning because the manager/ guide shares practice with supervisees.
- Facilitates the manager developing and fulfilling leadership role.

Potential disadvantages

- The guide, wrapped up in her own perspective, lacks vision to see other ways of doing things and hence moulds the practitioner to conform to guide's image of how she should be.
- The guide takes action on behalf of the practitioner [i.e. it becomes the guide's issue].
- The manager manipulates agenda to suit the manager's own needs/ anxiety [Line managers know
  that they, rather than individual practitioners, are held to account for what takes place within their units. In the attempt to control this anxiety, they act to control their environments. The effect is to impose conformity and stifle practitioner responsibility].
- Guides act as managers by imposing authority over the practitioner and being overly judgemental.
- Practitioner may only share certain types of experiences to avoid censure and create a 'good impression'.

Perhaps the bottom line is that practitioners can choose their guides. Yet the organisational complexity of enabling that would be difficult, and the reasons for choice questionable. Put another way, if guides were skilled, it wouldn't matter who the guide was. Every guided reflection relationship must inevitably work through teething issues to develop genuine collaborative relationships. Indeed, this work is itself developmental.

Emancipatory vs. Technical Supervision

Depending on the intent and emphasis of the guide (Johns 2001), guided reflection can be a very different experience. I describe this as a tension between an *emancipatory* and *technical* approach. The terms emancipatory and technical are two specific types of knowledge-constituted interests (Habermas 1984). The *emancipatory* is knowledge that seeks to liberate people to fulfil their best interests, whereas the *technical* is knowledge that seeks to shape people towards performing competently. The emancipatory approach focuses on process, using facilitative-power ways of relating. The technical approach focuses on outcomes using authoritative-power ways of relating[13] (Figure 5.2). Ideally, guided reflection is negotiated where the guide and learner surface their agendas and agree a mutual path that serves the interests of both parties. Habermas terms this as *communicative* knowledge that mediates between the emancipatory and technical knowledge interests. The tension between the emancipatory and technical is lived within each practitioner – on one hand seeking liberation to practise as desired, and on the other hand, a compelling need to conform to transactional pressure. The supervisor too lives this tension, and in doing so, may emphasise either the emancipatory or technical.

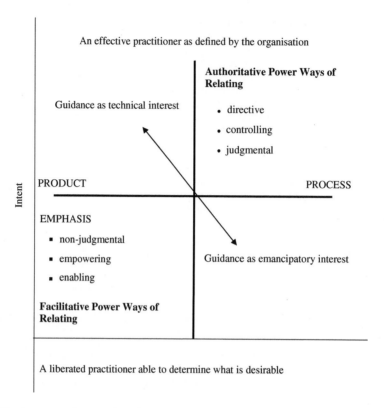

An effective practitioner as defined by the organisation

Authoritative Power Ways of Relating

Guidance as technical interest

- directive
- controlling
- judgmental

Intent

PRODUCT   PROCESS

EMPHASIS

■ non-judgmental
■ empowering
■ enabling

Guidance as emancipatory interest

Facilitative Power Ways of Relating

A liberated practitioner able to determine what is desirable

Figure 5.2   The intent–emphasis scale (Johns 2001a).

Skill Box

- *If you are in guided reflection, where do you experience yourself within the intent–emphasis scale?*
- *Next time you are in guided reflection, reflect on this position and mindfully move to a more emancipatory position. What is the impact of this move on yourself and the others involved?*

Peer Guidance

My group at the hospice was peer led. The guide's role is rotated within the group. This enables a more overt realignment of authority within the group, even though people with different positions within the hierarchy may constitute the group. As such, it cannot be assumed that collaboration will exist from the outset. An advantage of this arrangement is that this collaboration will spill into everyday practice where the group also work with each other.

Peer guidance will also enable the development of group guidance skills. Each member of the group takes responsibility for their own performance and for the group's performance as a whole – what I term *a community of inquiry*. Practitioners new to guided reflection will require a period of time to 'learn' this role and would benefit from specific guidance training.[14] Such groups embody the values of the learning organisation.

Group Versus Individual Supervision

When I established supervision at Burford Hospital I contracted individual guidance arrangements with staff. I had no rationale for this approach, even though I used group-guided reflection with nursing students as a curriculum model.

When I teach guided reflection as a group it is fascinating to watch the group learn to work together, breaking down their own vulnerability to self-revelation, even for the more reserved practitioners. Without doubt, the synergy of peer learning is powerful and, in my view, its effectiveness far outweighs individual guidance.

In a research project with ward sisters to develop leadership (Johns 2003) I used individual supervision. My reflections on this project led me to the conclusion that group-guided reflection would have been more enabling because the ward sisters were isolated within their clinical and organisational practice. They would have benefited from developing strong peer relationships and learning from each other, especially as they shared similar experiences. This would have enabled them, in my view, to become politically stronger as a group. As it was, individual guided reflection reinforced their isolation.

Establishing groups can be fraught with pragmatic difficulty, for example, who should be in the group and managing time for the group to meet. This might make group *norming* more difficult, especially if the group takes place within normal hours of clinical practice when supervision time, no matter if allocated, becomes a victim of the exigencies of the clinical moment. One contentious solution would be to suggest that clinical supervision takes place outside clinical hours. I do not think this unreasonable in terms of professional responsibility to be 'fit for practice' and CPD fulfilment. Resistance to this idea may stem from a traditional 'shift culture' of doing work. Despite the forming difficulties of group supervision, it fosters collaborative teamwork, shared vision, team learning, mutual support, role responsibility and quality; all advantages over individual supervision.

Skill Box

- *Do you think you should take responsibility for keeping 'fit for practice'?*
- *Would you participate in peer-led supervision outside work hours with like-minded people? If so, what are you waiting for?*

Single or Multi-professional

My guided reflection group at the hospice was multi-professional. I felt it worked well without any obvious power plays between professionals involved. I think this was due to shared values and personal responsibility to collaborate. Certainly, working within multi-professional healthcare teams, it is logical to promote multi-professional group-guided reflection. Unfortunately existing power relationships, for example between nurses and doctors, get played out within guided reflection, undermining the group's impact. Or doctors won't participate, as if they are above such indulgence.

Voluntary or Mandatory?

Clinical supervision is not mandatory for nursing, with the exception of safeguarding and midwifery. It was promoted as a professional activity rather than a managerial activity

(UKCC 1996) in response to increasing nursing's accountability to offset public concern. Yet clinical supervision is implemented most often as a top-down organisational approach with very little resource attached to it. From this perspective, it is inevitable that the implementation of supervision becomes the responsibility of unit leaders, leading to a managerial approach despite its 'professional' rhetoric. A mandatory approach would require significant resourcing in terms of development and sustainment. It is likely that practitioners would be reluctant to use their 'own time' where supervision is viewed as yet another task to be undertaken by staff already under workload pressure. Practitioners are likely to view mandatory guided reflection as a form of social control and surveillance (Gilbert 2001) and therefore to be resisted rather than as a developmental opportunity.

A voluntary arrangement may only attract practitioners already committed to their professional development. However, NMC registration demand from 2016 may shift this perspective, whereby practitioners come to view guided reflection as an opportunity to meet NMC requirement and therefore will be more likely to respond to opportunities such as guided reflection, although I imagine such people will see reflection as a necessary evil and merely conform by doing the least amount of work required. In other words, it becomes a task.

My view may seem unduly pessimistic. So view my pessimism as a challenge to any complacency to existing clinical supervision/guided reflection arrangements. My hospice group was open to all, yet few attended. A survey revealed their reasons as indicated above. I sense this as a failure of leadership. An attribute of effective leadership is to create a dynamic learning community where the growth of practitioner responsibility and learning opportunity is built into the fabric of practice (Johns 2015). Perhaps this suggests that formal guided reflection sessions become more flexible through creating dialogical communication. Voluntary arrangements may exist outside normal work hours as a reflection of professional commitment and professional patterns of working, especially when such arrangements are peer-led, breaking out of a 'shift-bound' transactional and subordinate culture.

Karen, an associate nurse at Burford, reflects on her supervision 'breakthrough',

> *Sessions 1–6 were very much led by my supervisor, but in session 7 we had a sudden break-through and I took control. From then on I felt I was growing through supervision – I remember telling my supervisor that I felt like a seedling in spring which has felt the sun and is now growing big and strong into a tree. I knew how much I benefited, but I also knew how much energy it took and I often felt drained afterwards. (Johns 1998, unpublished PhD notes)*

Karen's words reflect that it takes effort. Her learning patterns had not prepared her for such a learning experience.[15] She also felt threatened that her lack of competence would be exposed and that she would be judged as a poor nurse. She was anxious to demonstrate her competence after qualifying with a nursing degree. As such, at the time when she most needed support, she resisted it because she wanted to show she was competent. An ironic twist, yet seemingly a common response from newly qualified practitioners (Cherniss 1980).

If reflection was accommodated within pre-registration curriculum, then it would become second nature for the newly qualified professional. It is no good saying 'Reflection is good for you'. The practitioner must experience this value for herself. It takes time to sense the point.

Game Playing

Practitioners may be reluctant to be critical of peers due to a collusive strategy to make the dialogue space safe so they can avoid criticism when telling their own stories. Kadushin (1968) notes that practitioners (supervisees) may initiate games as a defence against the anxiety that revealing self might create. In a similar vein Hawthorne (1975) reveals games supervisors (guides) might play concerning authority in order to construct 'a comfortable and effective guide identity' (179).

Kadushin (1968: 30) writes,

> Supervisors play games out of felt threats to their position in the hierarchy, uncertainty about their authority, reluctance to use their authority. A desire to be liked, a need for the supervisees' approbation and out of some hostility to supervisees that is inevitable in such a complex intimate relationship.

Working within transactional organisations does not prepare either the guide or practitioner for their respective roles within guided reflection or clinical supervision. Indeed, some guided reflection relationships may be built on existing authoritative roles to ensure practitioner conformity designed to meet organisational objectives. Perhaps this is one reason why I avoid using the term 'clinical supervision' because of this legacy whereby one person (the supervisor) stands over another person (the practitioner) to ensure the practitioner is competent (competence being defined by the supervisor). I take the position that all guided reflection relationships are constructed as collaborative relationships and that this inevitably requires a realignment of transactional authority relationships, no matter the setting, as contracted. Of course, this is more easily said than done because of embodied ways of being learnt over time. People simply cannot just become different. It needs to be actively worked towards. Indeed, stripping away learnt ways can leave people vulnerable, anxious and uncertain of how to respond and subsequently prone to game playing to minimize threat.

Games are defensive postures played to reduce threat, taking responsibility and anxiety. They disrupt learning, with its emphasis on playing the game. Hence both guides and practitioners are alert to this possibility. Games are minimised when the guidance process is constantly monitored for threat. As such, a part of every session should involve this. In this way all concerned become mindful of process and actively work towards ensuring the learning process is not compromised. If not, then guided reflection will inevitably degenerate into power plays that reflect dominant transactional authoritative patterns of relationships.

Summary

Dialogue with literature, guides and peers enhances the learning potential of reflection. Indeed, without guidance, novice reflective practitioners would struggle to learn from this approach. It is likely that exposure to reflection will take place within formal settings facilitated by supervisors or teachers. The quality of this guidance is vital. Guidance is not unproblematic. It is contextual and strongly influenced by the relationship between the guide and practitioner, notably in situations where embodied patterns of relationship have led to traditional subordinate-type relationships. For example, the guide may view herself as an authority and demand compliance, impose the practitioner's agenda, and even determine what insights the practitioner has gained.

In Chapter 6 I explore writing narrative to communicate insights gained through the first four dialogical movements and the potential of performance narrative as a more expressive narrative form that opens exciting potential for teaching and learning.

Chapters 14 and 15 have been written from the perspective of guiding students. Chapter 24 gives an exemplar of guidance and a critique of guidance contract.

Endnotes

1 Endnotes See Chapter 5 for details of contracting.
2 See Chapter 3 for a review of the Model for Structured Reflection.
3 See Chapter 3 to review the Model for Structured Reflection.
4 The WHO definition of palliative care: 'Palliative care is an approach that improves the quality of life of patients and their families facing the problems associated with life-threatening illness, through the prevention and relief of *suffering* by means of early identification and impeccable assessment and treatment of pain and other problems, physical, psychosocial and spiritual' (http://www.who.int/cancer/palliative/definition/en/).
5 The forming – storming – norming – performing model of group development was first proposed by Bruce Tuckman in 1965, who maintained that these phases are all necessary and inevitable in order for the team to grow, to face up to challenges, to tackle problems, to find solutions, to plan work, and to deliver results (https://en.wikipedia.org/wiki/Tuckman′s_stages_of_group_development).
6 A cliché is an expression, idea or element of an artistic work which has become overused to the point of losing its original meaning or effect, even to the point of being trite or irritating, especially when at some earlier time it was considered meaningful or novel (https://en.wikipedia.org/wiki/Cliché).
7 'The elephant in the room' or 'Elephant in the living room' is an English metaphorical idiom for an obvious truth that is either being ignored or going unaddressed. The idiomatic expression also applies to an obvious problem or risk no one wants to discuss (https://en.wikipedia.org/wiki/Elephant_in_the_room).
8 See Appendix 5 for an example of how student feedback can be utilised.
9 See my narrative with Tony (Chapter 20) for an example of using these skills in practice.
10 I refer here to the Nursing and Midwifery Council's new registration requirements introduced in 2016. [http://www.nmc.org.uk/standards/revalidation/]
11 In clinical practice guided reflection is most often termed clinical supervision.
12 Implementing guided reflection/supervision was established as a research project (Johns 1998).
13 The terms facilitative and authoritative ways of relating are from French and Raven's leadership power styles (1968) (see figure 15.2).
14 At the University of Bedfordshire I led a supervision development programme that consisted of 12 three- hour sessions spread over 30 weeks (contact me for further details).
15 See exemplar of guided reflection involving Karen in C. Johns (2004), *Becoming a reflective practitioner* (2nd edition), 131–144.

References

Belenky, M. F., Clinchy, B. M., Goldberger, N. R. and Tarule, J. M. (1986) *Women's ways of knowing: the development of self, voice, and mind.* Basic Books, New York.
Bohm, D, (1996, ed. Lee Nichol) *On dialogue.* Routledge, London.

Boud, D., Keogh, R. and Walker, D. (1985) Promoting reflection in learning: a model. In D. Boud, R. Keogh and D. Walker (eds.) *Reflection: turning experience into learning.* Kogan Page, London.

Boyd, E. and Fales, A. (1983) Reflective learning: key to learning from experience. *Journal of Humanistic Psychology* 23.2, 99–117.

Bradbury-Jones, C., Sambrook, S. and Irvine, F. (2011) Nursing students and the issue of voice: a qualitative study. *Nurse Education Today* 31, 628–632.

Brookfield, S. (1996) *Becoming a critically reflective teacher.* Jossey-Bass, San Francisco.

Burnard, P. and Morrison, P. (1991) Nurses' interpersonal skills: a study of nurses' perceptions. *Nurse Education Today* 1, 24–29.

Chapman, G. (1983) Ritual and rational action in hospitals. *Journal of Advanced Nursing* 8, 13–20.

Cherniss, G. (1980) *Professional burn-out in human service organisations.* Praeger, New York.

Cox, H., Hickson, P. and Taylor, B. (1991) Exploring reflection: knowing and constructing practice. In G. Gray and R. Pratt (eds.) *Towards a discipline of nursing* Churchill Livingstone, Melbourne, pp. 373–390.

Day, C. (1993) Reflection; a necessary but not sufficient condition for professional development. *British Educational Research Journal* 19.1, 83–93.

Dewey, J. (1933) *How we think.* D. C. Heath, Boston.

Dworkin, R. (1993) *Life's dominion: an argument about abortion, euthanasia and individual freedom.* Alfred Knopf, New York.

Frank, A. (2002) Relations of caring: demoralization and remoralization in the clinic. *International Journal of Human Caring* 6.2, 13–19.

French, J. and Raven, B. (1968) The bases of social power. In D. Cartwright and A. Zander (eds.) *Group dynamics.* Row Peterson, Evanston, IL, pp. 150–167.

Gadamer, H-G. (1975) *Truth & method.* Seabury Press, New York.

Gilbert, T. (2001) Reflective practice and clinical supervision: meticulous rituals of the confessional. *Journal of Advanced Nursing* 36.2, 199–205.

Habermas, J. (1984) *Theory of communicative action. Vol. 1: Reason and the rationalisation of society.* Beacon Press, Boston, and Basil Blackwell, Oxford, in association with Polity Press, Cambridge.

Hall, L. (1964) Nursing – what is it? *Canadian Nurse* 60.2, 150–154.

Hawkins, P. and Shohet, R. (1989) *Supervision for the helping professions.* Open University Press, Buckingham.

Hawthorne, L. (1975) Games supervisors play. *Social Work* May, pp. 179–183.

Heron, J. (1975) *Six-category intervention analysis.* Human Potential Resource Group, University of Surrey, Guildford.

Isaacs, W. (1993) Taking flight: dialogue, collective thinking, and organizational learning. *Centre for Organizational Learning's Dialogue Project.* MIT, Boston, MA.

Johns, C. (1998) *Becoming a reflective practitioner through guided reflection.* PhD thesis. The Open University.

Johns, C. (2001) Depending on the intent and emphasis of the supervisor, clinical supervision can be a different experience. *Journal of Nursing Management* 9, 139–145.

Johns, C. (2003) Clinical supervision as a model for clinical leadership. *Journal of Nursing Management* 11, 25–34.

Johns, C. (2015) *Mindful leadership: a guide for health professions.* Palgrave Macmillan, Basingstoke.

Johns, C. and McCormack, B. (1998) Unfolding the conditions where the transformative potential of guided reflection (clinical supervision) might flourish or flounder. In C. Johns and D. Freshwater (eds.) *Transforming nursing through reflective practice.* Blackwell, Oxford.

Kadushin, A. (1968) Games people play in supervision. *Social Work* July: 23–32.

Kieffer, C. (1984) Citizen empowerment: a developmental perspective. *Prevention in Human Services* 84.3, 9–36.

Lather, P. (1986a) Research as praxis. *Harvard Educational Review* 56.3, 257–277.

Lather, P. (1986b) Issues of validity in open ideological research: between a rock and a hard place. *Interchange* 17.4, 63–84.

Lieberman, A. (1989) *Staff development in culture building, curriculum and teaching: the next 50 years.* Teachers' College Press, Columbia University, New York.

Logstrup, K. E. (1997) *The ethical demand.* University of Notre Dame Press, Notre Dame, IN.

Lorde, A. (1980) *The cancer journals.* Spinsters Ink, New York.

Margolis, H. (1993) *Paradigm and barriers: how habits of mind govern scientific beliefs.* University of Chicago Press, Chicago.

Menzies-Lyth, I. (1988) A case study in the functioning of social systems as a defence against anxiety. In *Containing anxiety in institutions: Selected essays.* Free Association Books, London.

Moorman, M. (2015) The meaning of visual thinking strategies for nursing students. *Humanities* 4, 748–759.

Newman, M. (1994) *Health as expanded consciousness* (2nd edn). National League for Nursing Press, New York. (esp. p. 38).

Oakley, A. (1984) The importance of being a nurse. *Nursing Times* 83.50, 24–27.

Pirsig, R. (1974) *Zen and the art of motorcycle maintenance.* Vintage, London.

Prigonine, L. and Stengers, L. (1988) *Order out of chaos.* Bantam, New York.

Proctor, B. (1988) *Supervision: a working alliance* (videotape training manual). Alexa Publications, St Leonards-on-Sea.

Schön, D. (1987) *Educating the reflective practitioner.* Jossey-Bass, San Francisco.

Sloan, G. and Watson, H. (2001) John Heron's six-category intervention analysis: towards understanding interpersonal relations and progressing the delivery of clinical supervision for mental health nursing in the United Kingdom. *Journal of Advanced Nursing* 36.2, 206–214.

Smyth, W. J. (1987) *A rationale for teachers' critical pedagogy.* Deakin University Press, Melbourne.

Steinbeck, J. (1937/2000) *Of mice and men.* Penguin, London.

Tann, S. (1993) Eliciting student teachers' personal theories. In J. Calderwood and P. Gates (eds.) *Conceptualizing reflection in teacher development.* Falmer Press, London.

Tuckman, B. W. (1965) Developmental sequence in small groups. *Psychological Bulletin* 63.6, 384–399.

UKCC (1996) *Positional statement on clinical supervision.* UKCC, London.

Woods, S. (2007) *Death's dominion.* Open University Press, Buckingham.

Chapter 6

Weaving and Performing Narrative: The Fifth and Sixth Dialogical Movements

Christopher Johns

Performance spirals narrative into social action

Introduction

In the previous chapters I explored dialogical movements 1–4 towards constructing reflexive narrative. In this chapter I explore the fifth dialogical movement in weaving narrative and the sixth dialogical movement in performing narrative as social action.

To commence, I set out my experience with Peggy as a performance narrative entitled 'Passing people by', which includes sharing the narrative with my guided reflection group.

Passing People By

In the blink of the eye I pass people by;
in passing you by
what message do I give you?
That I do not care?
That I am blind?
That I am not mindful enough of your despair?

Another Monday. I arrive at the hospice day-care centre and look about the sitting room. Some people have already present, sitting in their usual chairs. People become territorial.

Becoming a Reflective Practitioner, Fifth Edition. Edited by Christopher Johns.
© 2017 John Wiley & Sons Ltd. Published 2017 by John Wiley & Sons Ltd.
Companion Website: www.wiley.com/go/johns/reflectivepractitioner

On the surface a normal day, judging by other Mondays during the six weeks I have been working here as the 'Monday therapist'.

Can any day be described as normal without immediately deflating it?

The morning briefing. The room filling. 20 patients attending. As has become my practice, I go round and say hello to each person and take requests for therapy. I am surprised when Peggy smiles and calls out, 'I'm first on the list.' I had not previously given Peggy a treatment. In fact, I have rarely spoken to her beyond the usual social pleasantries. She had not requested a therapy and other patients claimed my time. Caught off guard, the pang of guilt hits! I struggle to frame her demand and my emotional response.

I say, 'What treatment would you like, Peggy?'

'Some reflexology, please.'

Reactively I say, 'OK, let's do it.'

She walks with her stick to the treatment room. As she walks she talks about her grief for her partner who died of cancer in March. This grief lies thick on the surface, a grief made more poignant with the death of her dog a few months later.

She cries. 'I'm sorry for the tears', she says, as if her tears might burden me.

I respond in a somewhat facile manner, 'The tears are better out than in.'

She is gracious. 'I know. Many people tell me that.'

And perhaps it is true. Opening the floodgates for the grieving heart. Opening a healing space for her raw wound of grief.

'Tell me about your partner, Peggy.'

She tells the story of his cancer diagnosis and death just a few weeks later, such a contrast to her own prolonged treatment from breast cancer and bone metastases in her pelvis. Her story is limited to his cancer. I do not push her to tell me more about him. I sense she is caught between the world of the living and world of the dead (Walter 1994), the vitality for her to talk about him so she can put him to rest in her heart as a loving memory. The continuing bonds theory of grief helps me frame her grief but risks closing down an interpretative space (Klass, Silverman and Nickman 1996).

'How do you feel about coming to the day-centre, Peggy?'

'I have mixed feelings. It's not easy sitting with other people but on the other hand I do like the company. Does that make sense?'

'I think so … as if part of you wants to come and another part doesn't. Do you feel alone?'

'Yes, I do, even though I'm surrounded by well-meaning friends and neighbours. I miss him so much, and my dog."

'What was your dog's name?'

'Alfie.'

'I'm sorry about him. I don't have a dog but I imagine he must have been great company.'

Silence between us. I feel her aloneness. I sense she has lost her significant connections to life. I notice she says surrounded by well-meaning friends and neighbours, but not family. But I do not pursue this. The idea of aloneness and loneliness are complex elements to suffering that are not easily understood and perhaps not easy to explore with someone (Elias 1985).

For a conversation filler I ask, 'Are you religious, Peggy?'

'I do believe in God, but have no strong religion. I mean I don't go to church. Believing in God doesn't comfort me.'

'I can see you limp and grimace when walking. Do you have any pain?'

'Oh yes. My pain is managed well enough with paracetamol and diclofenac. I also take some tummy protection tablets.'

We reach the therapy room. She sits on the edge of the therapy couch. She surprises me by easily removing her boots and getting herself onto the couch.

'I bought these boots recently for the winter,' she says, as if reading my mind.

I place a blanket over her and ask, 'What smells do you like, Peggy?'

'Um, I'm not fussy.'

'How about I mix lavender, frankincense and grapefruit essential oils into my reflexology cream. Grapefruit is described as a sunny oil bringing sunshine into grief's darkness. Lavender lifts the veil of sadness, while frankincense helps to slow the breath and instil calm.'

'Sounds good. Mmm, the aroma is lovely. I've always loved grapefruit and lavender. Frankincense was one of the gifts of the Three Kings.'

I know aromas hold memories. Or at least I assume that they do, based on one particular experience with the daughter of a woman who died in the hospice. The mother was agitated and the family became agitated in response. They begged me to help. I used a cream mixed with oils to massage her hands. She became calm and lucid, enabling the family to have a positive death experience. The daughter asked if she could have a small pot of the cream I had used to remember her mother by. When I met her again she said how much the cream had helped her deal with her grief (Johns 2006). This is anecdotal evidence, but there is support for my experience within the literature. For example, Worwood (1995: 95) writes, 'Is it any wonder that smell has such a profound effect on us, or that extended memory can be triggered by certain aromas? Aroma is one of the means by which memory is laid down by its yet mysterious recording mechanism.' Telling Peggy about the oils also intends a placebo effect.

I hold Peggy's feet. She closes her eyes as I guide her to relax. She falls asleep. Halfway through the treatment she cries out. When she wakens she says, 'I feel a weight has been lifted from me.'

I respond, 'Grief is a heavy burden.' (Am I really so clichéd?)

But Peggy again responds graciously, 'Yes. It feels like that.'

It makes me think how much health talk is grounded in platitudes or clichés that fill empty spaces or are spoken to ease the health giver's anxiety over not using negative talk.

Peggy on my arm. We walk back to the sitting room in silence. Faces turn to stare, the room heavy with expectant people, no doubt wondering about their turn. Mrs Perkins shouts out, 'Ah, there you are.' I feel the pressure but I now see a bigger picture, my gaze no longer so focused on those with the loudest voice. I wonder if there is anybody else in the room I have 'passed by'.

As I write I again feel a twinge of guilt at passing Peggy by. How I had seen her but not seen her in terms of her suffering? It is unwitting, for I would never intentionally pass her by. Have I avoided patients in the past who make no demands? Or when I'm busy, avoided eye contact? If so, what message does that give the patient or relative eagerly searching out my eyes? I suspect this is a common phenomenon as practitioners struggle to control their workload or avoid demanding patients.

Did I pass Peggy by to manage my anxiety? The clamour of demand for my services each week – those who ask get and those who don't ask don't get. I can see that, in the crowded room, I only paid attention to those with the loudest voices. Is that my modus operandi? It is certainly the route of least resistance. Perhaps meeting so many new people in my new role, it is easier for me to be approached. But that is just a lame excuse! I imagine Peggy seeing me each week, waiting for me to offer her a therapy and her growing discomfort watching others have a therapy week after week. She may have not wanted a treatment but then I should have known that rather than assume it because she didn't ask.

Looking at the bigger picture, I can see my practice of letting people ask rather than me enquiring is problematic. That I hadn't seen Peggy is a powerful confession. To see everyone in the crowded room, I must be more mindful of the crowded room, stand back, and see each individual within the crowd rather than just the crowd – not to let my mind be crowded out. Caught up in my self-concern, I hadn't looked deeply enough into Peggy's eyes. I can see that my attempt to impose order through my schedule is not sensitive enough. One thing springs from another. I wonder if I pass people by as a defence from the vulnerability of emotional work and entanglement? This idea takes me deeper within myself. Do I keep myself separate from the other so as not to be overwhelmed by their suffering? Ramos (1992) notes the emotional and power impasses that face the nurse in establishing therapeutic relationships. This experience teaches me to listen on an emotional level – to myself and to the other. How Peggy is feeling is a vital cue. I wonder if I should have pursued her aloneness. It bothers me.

Could I have responded more effectively to her demand, 'I'm first on the list'? Just saying these words to myself confirms my suspicion that she would have liked a therapy on previous Mondays or at least to have been asked.

Perhaps I could have responded, '*You should have asked, Peggy.*' But would that have put the onus on her when her natural inclination is not to ask, not to be a burden? I know from experience that women who care deeply for others, as she has for her partner, do not find it easy to ask for their own care. It would have increased the burden on her, to make it seem as if it was her responsibility to ask rather than mine to offer. Responding like this would be me projecting my anxiety at having been caught out, as if a naughty boy anxious to shift the blame.

Another option might be to say something like, '*OK, I'll fit you into the schedule.*' At first glance this response seems reasonable. It acknowledges that I plan a schedule of therapies for the day. Yet such a formulaic response might seem insensitive. It would not have acknowledged her desperate cry. It might have put her in her place, reminding her of her status and my authority.

Another possible response might be an act of apology, '*I'm sorry, Peggy, I hadn't realised.*' In doing so I acknowledge my responsibility and that I can get it wrong. Humility. But by apologising, would I have burdened her with my guilt and made her feel she needed to care for me? The repentant child seeking forgiveness?

These alternative responses all seem feasible but in considering their potential consequences I reject them. Even so, exploring them is insightful, especially the child-mode perspective as a response to guilt. Using Transactional Analysis (TA) as a framework (Stewart and Joines 1987), I need to be in adult mode and enable the other to respond likewise unless it is therapeutically necessary to be otherwise. TA offers an excellent reflective framework for seeing patterns of communication and relationships.

My actual response to Peggy – '*Let's do it now*' – still feels the most appropriate because it acknowledged her desperate cry. It was intuitive, a response in the moment. I did not figure it out. You might argue that it was a reaction to my guilt, of having been caught out. Perhaps sharing this experience in the group will throw more light. It usually does.

I share my experience with my multi-profession-guided reflection group[1] that meets every six weeks. We take it in turns to facilitate the group.[2] Connie, a physiotherapist, is the group facilitator today. It seems a common story. Everyone recognises 'passing people by' and how such self-management becomes embodied and hence invisible. Everyone feels the tension between involvement and detachment with patients. It becomes uncomfortable when we pay attention to this tension as if somehow we are lacking. But then involvement is not easy. Being detached, we can surf through the day, not oblivious to suffering but keeping it at a distance. Such approach is governed and sanctioned by the medical model with its primary gaze on the person as symptom management whereby social, psychological and spiritual issues become problems to solve rather than being seen from a holistic perspective reflected in suffering.

I had expected Marie, a doctor, to be defensive but she surprises me by agreeing that 'easing suffering', as enshrined within the WHO definition of palliative care, should be emphasised as a hospice's primary value.[3]

Someone challenges me with the MSR cue, 'Did you act for the best?'

'No, not directly. I always think this cue is implicit. What do you think?'

'Well, consider Peggy's autonomy?'

'I know I should always respect her autonomy. To do so I need to put Peggy in a position of making a decision. Um, that's interesting. As such, a fourth response might be, '*Would you like a therapy now, Peggy? I have time*.' Saying 'I have time' frees Peggy to accept. I can see this response would be better. It acknowledges and respects her autonomy.'

The group concur. Perhaps I should not have offered any of my own alternatives but asked them to generate alternatives before sharing my own, for example, 'If you were in my shoes, how might you have responded?' I sense it would have been a better learning curve.

Someone says, 'You can really see the utilitarian ethic at work in your experience – the demand on time and its influence on the way we set priorities.'

Connie feeds in some theory concerning defences against anxiety stemming from the work of Menzies-Lyth (1988), in particular, the assertion of the need for practitioners to develop a necessary professional detachment as a protection from not being overwhelmed by the other's suffering. If compassion is vital in opening a healing space then I must rewrite Menzies-Lyth as 'the need to develop a necessary professional involvement' to realize my vision of easing suffering.

Marie emphasises, 'We need to be emotionally intelligent or poised in order to be fully available to the other within the moment by managing one's vulnerability to the other's suffering.'[4]

The group concur and share experiences of emotional disturbance with both patients and colleagues. I share my reading of articles by Paley (2014) and Rolfe and Gardner (2014). Paley's article in particular challenged me as to whether I had a case of 'situational blindness', which led me to pass Peggy by. I find his argument compelling, although his perspective is challenged by Rolfe and Gardner. I can see that my need for order was a reaction to my anxiety faced with a daunting caseload. Anxiety, when it becomes overwhelming, can create situational blindness. It narrows the focus. But does it diminish my compassion? If I am wrapped up in concern for myself, does it diminish my concern of the other? Yes, if I am not mindful enough. But then I have become doubtful about compassion as a desirable attribute simply because the word is bandied about without due appreciation of what it implies. I give copies of the papers to the group to consider.

Connie, in summarising the group's work today, says, 'I will share this story at the next senior clinical team meeting. Wake them up a bit!' Like throwing a stone into a still pond, creating disturbing ripples.

What insights have I gained? Peggy taught me a lesson about paying attention, to take nothing for granted and to listen more carefully. There is no such thing as a normal day when you pierce it rather than slide along its surface. I can see that 'poise' is not simply a technical knowhow that can be applied. It is much deeper than that. To be present to

Peggy is to be present to myself. I can better appreciate that suffering is a disruption of the spirit. If I absorb it as my own it will disrupt me. Caring *is* mindful, *is* intentional. It can never be routine, scheduled, taken for granted, unexamined. Then it becomes careless, and adds to suffering, just as my passing Peggy by added to her suffering last week. Every moment is the opportunity to learn if we are mindful enough.

Reflecting on the session, I wonder if perhaps I should not have offered any of my own alternatives but asked them to generate alternatives before sharing my own, for example, '*If you were in my shoes how might you have responded?*' I sense it would have been a better learning curve. Learning how best to share stories and work within the group is an ongoing developmental process.

Next Monday. My gaze takes in the whole room. I am more mindful of the bigger picture. Peggy smiles at me from across the room. I sit with her awhile and ask how she's been. Not so bad. 'A therapy today, Peggy?'

'No, not this week. Maybe next week.'

A new lady sits alone. I focus my breath. I go and sit with her. I introduce myself and invite her story. I feel no demand on my time. More stillness. Listening, I am better able to plan my schedule rather than simply react to the loudest voices, even as they pull at me. Suddenly it hits me. That the way I plan my day is flawed. I need a schedule that is not at the beck and call of the loudest voices. What are my options?

1 Get people to put their name down for a therapy on arrival. I can then review and plan a schedule based on fairness, recognising I cannot give a therapy to everyone who wants one in one day.
2 We have two therapy rooms. If demand is greater than supply, then perhaps seek a second volunteer therapist – explore this at the team meeting.
3 Shorten time span of each therapy, to enable more patients to have a therapy.

I think option (1) will work. I go and speak to the hospice manager to get her viewpoint. I can also discuss option (2) with her. Perhaps option (3) might work, but would the therapy benefit be compromised with shorter treatments? I sense my integrity as a therapist would be compromised.

The hospice manager is enthusiastic about my schedule options. She agrees that getting people to sign up for a therapy is a good idea. She will think about recruiting a second therapist, but that goes against the grain as the other days of the week are serviced by one therapist – so what makes me special? She respects the fact I do spend longer with each patient than other therapists, but the feedback from patients is very positive. We will commence next week with the 'sign in' – she says she will organise it.

Fifth dialogical movement

The narrative 'passing people by' is woven around my insights within the broader plot of 'easing suffering'. Reflexive narratives always have a major plot. My narrative does not stand alone. It is part of an evolving narrative that stems back to 1998 when I began writing reflexive narratives. As such, my experience with Peggy is informed by past experiences – the deepening of understanding within the hermeneutic circle. As I suggest 'next Monday', the narrative continues.

I do not *tell* the reader what my insights are. These are *shown* within the narrative for readers to discern from their own experience. To tell would be to close down an interpretative space.

Skill Box

- *What significance do you draw from the narrative?*
- *How do you relate to these significances in terms of your own practice?*

Methodology and Plot

Reflexive narrative is a *reflexive journey of self-inquiry and transformation towards developing professional artistry and identity.* My development of reflexive narrative methodology has been reflexive and a constant focus of my inquiry in much the same way as my teaching and clinical practice (Johns 2004, 2006, 2010).

Narrative has a significant theoretical basis through diverse intellectual traditions such as anthropology, psychoanalysis, literary criticism and performance (Mattingly 1998). My own approach to narrative has been influenced by a bricolage[5] of influences: autoethnography, reflective and narrative theory, hermeneutics, critical social science, feminism, chaos theory and ancient traditions (Table 6.1). However, for purposes of this text, such theoretical background can be put aside unless, of course, you wish to pursue reflexive narrative as formal research, as indeed many practitioners have chosen to do.[6] The process of self-inquiry through reflection on one experience is a first step along a research path. Reflexive narrative is constructed through layers of reflected-on experience. The insights gained from one experience are picked up in subsequent experiences, creating the reflexive movement (Dewey 1933).

Dewey (1933: 4–5) writes,

> The successive portions of reflective thought grow out of one another and support one another; they do not come and go in medley. Each phase is a step from something to something. Technically speaking, it is a term of thought. Each term leaves a deposit that is utilised in the next term. The stream or flow becomes a train or chain. There are in any reflective thought definite units that are linked together so that there is sustained movement to a common end.

Over time, themes or threads can be discerned within the major plot, however you choose to express that, for example, 'becoming a patient-centred practitioner' or 'to ease suffering', or more broadly 'professional artistry'.

Mattingley (1998: 813) writes,

> It is the plot that makes individual events understandable as part of a coherent whole, one which leads compellingly towards a particular ending. Any particular event gains its meanings

Table 6.1 Reflexive narrative theoretical and philosophical influences (Johns 2010)

Critical social science and empowerment theory	Auto-ethnography and performance studies	Ancient wisdom [Buddhism and Native American lore]
Hermeneutics and dialogue	Reflexive narrative as a process of self-inquiry to develop professional artistry and identity	Reflection and reflexivity
Feminism	Chaos theory	Narrative theory

by place within this narrative configuration, as a contribution to the plot. This configuration makes a whole such that we can speak of the point of the story. Yet this is an always shifting configuration for we live in the midst of unfolding stories over which we have a very partial control.

Skill Box

- *Ask yourself: What do I value about my practice? Consider 'being compassionate' – what does being compassionate mean as something lived? What are its consequences? How would you know if you were truly compassionate? Try this with any caring concept. Reflect on two experiences; one where you felt you were compassionate and one where did not feel compassionate. What insights do you gain? How does your experience link with my experience with Peggy? How does compassion fit into a broader vision of practice? What does the literature say about compassion? As a consequence you will never be complacent about compassion in the future.*

Narrative Form

Constructing narrative is an art–form that can only really be appreciated and developed through practice. I cannot prescribe how it should be written, although I can give broad guidelines and examples such as 'passing people by'. Narrative creates drama around insights or what Carson (2008) describes as transitional moments or *turning points* that are pivotal in the journey of becoming or moments of significant resistance to becoming.

Inserting questions demands attention, as if the writer is inviting the reader to consider and answer them, especially around insights. Asking questions begs answers that sometimes I answer and at other times leave open.

Narrative is being open to the words, letting the words flow through me, as if they pattern themselves below the threshold of conscious thought. It is intuitive, a kind of poetic prose. It is tuning down the left brain and letting the creative juices run free. It is chaos theory, letting go of control as if the writing is self-organising, 'penetrating beyond what is superficial or obvious' (Carson 2008: 205).

Wheatley (1999: 126) writes,

> to see patterns, we have to step back from the problem [text] and gain perspective. Shapes are not discerned from close range. They require distance and time to show themselves. Pattern recognition requires that we sit together reflectively and patiently. I say patiently not just because patterns take time to form, but because we are trying to see the world differently and there are many years of blindness to overcome.

In other words, the mind is not trained to see reflexive patterns. Yet there is always connection between experiences, however random they may appear. As the practitioner becomes more mindful, she learns to pay attention to specific experiences that pursue and deepen insights. Practice becomes an unfolding narrative. I find writing in the present tense and using dialogue also helps create a sense of drama, of pulling the reader into the text. Given the complexity of the whole, it is not possible to capture the wholeness of everything. Narrative is always fragmentary.

As Fay (1997: 168) writes,

> No narrative of actual human lives can ever be characterised as the 'genuine one'; the results of human activities are forever occurring, so that any narrative about them must be inherently fragmentary and tentative.

Often I repeat myself, as I am sure readers have noticed. This is deliberate, to get messages across. Often when we read, we read something and it slips by. Hence, if it is important enough I repeat it, perhaps many times, so it registers.

When Eva Hesse was asked, 'Repetition is very prevalent in your work. Why do you repeat a form over and over?', she replied, 'Because it exaggerates. If something is meaningful, maybe it's more meaningful said ten times. It's not just an aesthetic choice. If something is absurd, it's more greatly exaggerated, absurd, if it's repeated' (2002: 11).

Creativity

Narrative is creative art, shaping words into images to enchant and disturb the reader. Symbols, images and metaphors are significant forms for holding meaning.

Tuffnell and Crickmay (2004: 41) write,

> An image evokes a world, a solar system of connections and meanings, of associations, qualities, textures and memories … an image forms a bridge between what's inside us and what is outside … it brings us more fully into a felt relationship with the world.

A variety of media can be utilised — metaphor, poetry, art, dramatic prose, storyboards, photographs, nature, music, installation, movement, film, dance — to represent meaning, often with a commentary that links the whole. The idea is of *show not tell*, where the narrative pattern reveals meaning to the discerning reader. However, narrative that is subject to academic scrutiny might demand an explanation of events. In other words, *show and tell*. Or even, don't bother showing, just tell! Such is the nature of academic writing, demanding adherence to the left brain!

Different media forms give texture to the narrative. They engage the reader's imagination more than the dry words of prosaic intellectual language. Parker (2002: 104) writes, 'Art and aesthetic expression unite us and contribute to our wholeness. They are essential means of communication and move us all toward increased wellbeing.'

The potential of narrative for wellbeing reflects the cathartic impact of writing and reflection. It is a way of working through emotion and trauma. Fordham (2010) used the ideas of 'the net' and 'the spider's web' as a metaphor and image to represent organisational services through which the homeless fell through. She envisaged her role as a specialist nurse working with the homeless as a 'net weaver'. In an earlier article, Fordham (2008) uses the metaphor of a 'bridge' to span the homelessness void. In a similar vein, Jarrett (2008, 2009) used the idea of 'opening space' in her work with disabled people, literally opening space for their physical disability and opening space metaphorically for giving them more satisfying lives, inspired by the sculptures of Barbara Hepworth. At times I expand reality or write fiction if I consider it will help to dramatise my insights to engage the reader or audience. The reader will know if the narrative 'rings true' in terms of her own experiences.

Empathic Poems

Despite dialogue with an informing literature and guides, narrative can only present a partial view of the particular experience. Tools such as ethical mapping[7] encourage the practitioner to reflect on the perspectives of others involved in the experience. For example, how would Peggy see my experience with her? Would she view it very differently? Putting myself in the shoes of others facilitates empathic connection and challenges my own perspectives. Indeed the guide may facilitate this by asking the practitioner to do just that – 'put yourself in the others' shoes', just as she might ask other members of the guided reflection group to 'put themselves in my shoes' to consider how they might respond in the particular situation.

The use of empathic poems can bring involved others into focus by imagining their perspective. Besides giving a broader perspective, empathic poems help to deepen the empathic connection with others — what were they really thinking and feeling? Why did they feel or think that way? Could I have helped shift their thoughts and feelings into a better frame of being? They also add to the drama.

One example of an empathic poem is in 'Smoking Kills' (Chapter 24) when I reflect on Max's perspective. In 'Anthea' I write empathic poems to represent the different Anthea, her family and staff (Chapter 25). In 'Through a glass darkly' (Johns 2013) I wrote similar poems to represent patients and family framed within nursery rhymes. Murphy is the husband of Jeannie, who is unresponsive and close to death. He is in despair. As I left the hospice one evening, Murphy was walking alone in the garden.

> ### Murphy's Lament
>
> Round and round the garden
> Like a teddy bear
> One step, two step,
> Yet I stumble alone into the gathering darkness.
> My children's noise deafens me
> Fine words fade like dew
> I am beyond words now
> Stumbling on
> No 'tickly under there'. (Johns 2013: 284)

Writing such poems deepened my appreciation of Murphy's experience. He wasn't an easy man to speak to and yet I felt my words spoke for him. Of course, I might be wrong but there is an uncanny realness to empathic poems as if the poems capture something embodied.

Another approach is to ask someone to put themselves in the shoes of others – someone not involved in the situation but who might be sensitive to the issues. The poems written by Colleen Marlin in 'Jane's Rap' to represent attempted suicide and self-harm patients in a hospital Accident and Emergency department are brilliant examples of this art (Johns and Marlin 2010).

> Walls tighten
> The press of your diagnostic gaze
> My head in a vice
>
> You, in nurse fashion, ask
> "What upset you so much today?"'
> Today …
> Not only today …every day.
>
> You want me to talk,
> I can't, can't breathe

Can't risk wasting precious air on stupid words
They won't be enough for you anyway

You send my family away
Thinking now I'll talk

To you?
In your peach polyester uniform?
So you can do, what,
Feel better about your own sweet life
Tell my woes at your dinner table and tsk tsk
At the hardship that doesn't touch you
All safe, smug, employed … loved.

You press again
I turn away, conflicted
Don't want to answer and
Satisfy your curiosity
As you crane your neck
At me, poor victim of an awful accident

And yet
To answer, to dislodge this stone blocking my airway
Inch it in your direction,
What it would unleash,
A geyser of bile would land on your hospital frock
And never wash out
With all the chemical laundering
It's just not safe …

I turn to the wall
So you can't see
I want to cry

"I'm here if …" you say, before leaving
As if …

Coherence

Using empathic poems as a type of fiction, or indeed fiction, raises the question of narrative coherence: 'When something has *coherence*, all of its parts fit together well. An argument with *coherence* is logical and complete — with plenty of supporting facts. *Coherence* comes from a Latin word meaning 'to stick together'. When you say policies, arguments and strategies are *coherent*, you're praising them for making sense.'

Wilber (1998) argues that different research paradigms have different rules of injunction to determine what counts as proper research. Reflexive narrative is, by its very nature, subjective, in contrast to empirical research that demands objectivity to counter bias and ensure reliability and validity. Narrative is your experience! Reflection guides you to step back and move into a subjective–objective stance with the story text in order to see yourself more clearly. At all times, the practitioner challenges herself: 'Am I being authentic? Are my partial views correct?'

As with self-inquiry, the narrative must firstly be coherent to oneself. Wheatley and Kellner-Rogers (1996: 890) write,

> Every self makes sense. It creates a world and an identity that feels coherent to itself. From infinite possibilities, it chooses what to notice and how to respond. As we look at any living being, we are observing its particular coherence, the logic it has used to create itself.

The idea of *coherent to itself* challenges any idea of imposing criteria for coherence on narrative. By this I mean the narrative has to fit certain criteria or rules of injunction (Wilber 1998) to be coherent. That it might be expected to fit into specific criteria is usual within research methodologies. However, the nature of reflexive narrative does not lend itself to judgement against external criteria. Reflexive narrative is chaotic simply because life is. This is not to advocate 'anything goes'. Reflexive narrative must 'ring true'. It must be compellingly crafted to engage and draw the reader into its plot. It should be authentic to enable the reader to dwell within it (Okri 1997).

Okri notes that narrative should:

- Be enchanting and disturbing, where beauty and horror lie side by side; whilst much of suffering might be described as 'horror' there is also a 'beauty' in caring.
- Be transgressive, *disturbing* the taken for granted, the complacent, the oppressive state of affairs. Such transgression can be something quite normal or something dramatic. It does not matter. I emphasise '*disturbing*' as a practical word – the idea of disturbing the apparent normal surface of practice. Hence narrative should always have this edginess. It is not merely descriptive of a situation but shakes it out.
- Reveal and critique the hidden bullies [misplaced assumptions, hegemonic structures, authority, tradition, embodiment] that constrain our self-realisation. This is very much the *critical reflection* agenda inspired by critical social science whereby narrative goes deep into the background of practice to reveal the assumptions, norms and relationships that govern existing practice and are necessary to shift if a better, more satisfactory state of affairs is to be established.
- Be transformational. Of course, by now, I hope the reader will appreciate this word – that as a consequence of reflection things change through gaining insight. Hence narrative reveals such transformation, however slight or subtle it may be.
- Plant seeds in the reader's mind that will germinate at a later date when ready. Where this is not possible it poses questions to inform subsequent reflections, building layer on layer of experience through which transformation is revealed.

Auto-ethnography has a natural fit with its emphasis on self-inquiry, if less so with reflexivity. I dialogue with Ellis (2004):

E: Does the narrative have the possibility for changing the world?

CJ: I view narrative as reflexive in enabling practitioners to become who they desire to be. In realising self, they change themselves. In changing themselves they change the world.

E: Good auto-ethnographic writing should motivate cultural criticism.

CJ: I view narrative as 'critical' — that in order to change self, then the nature of reality and the assumptions that govern this reality are exposed, understood and worked towards shifting to support a more desirable state of affairs.

E: Narratives must be hopeful, well-written and well-plotted stories that show memorable characters and unforgettable scenes.

CJ: Narrative must be compelling and engaging to draw the reader into the text, as if they were present within the scenario, feeling it as well as thinking it; leaving indelible marks and planted seeds to explode at later moments in terms of their own experiences and social action.

Using the six dialogical movements gives reflexive narrative structure that strengthens claims for rigour. Self-inquiry is systematic, through using a well-tested model for reflection to cover the breath and depth of experience. Using such a model counters any claim that reflection is haphazard. Dialogue with literature places insights within the existing field of knowledge. Dialogue with guides challenges partial views. Reflexivity reveals transformation in a meaningful way, with evidence of experience to support it. At the end of the day I urge the practitioner to simply write what they want without anxiety about criteria that might validate it as 'narrative'. Virginia Woolf (1945: 105) writes,

So long as you write what you wish to write that is all that matters; and whether it matters for ages or only for a few hours, nobody can say. But to sacrifice a hair of the head of your vision, a shade of its colour, in deference to some professor with a measuring rod up his sleeve is the most abject treachery.

Constructing narrative is like following a stream and seeing where it flows. It seeks to capture the drama of the unfolding journey of becoming within the broad plot of understanding and realising professional artistry and identity, however that might best be expressed. Like experience itself, narrative is not formulaic, even though we seek to impose order on the world. However, the demand for coherence does impose some structure to the banks of the stream.

> Be soft in your practice
> Think of the method as a fine silvery stream, not a raging waterfall.
> Follow the stream
> Have faith in its course.
> It will go its own way,
> Meandering here, trickling there.
> It will find grooves, the cracks, the crevices.
> Just follow it.
> Never let it out of your sight.
> It will take you.

Sheng-yen (Levering 2000)

The Sixth Dialogical Movement

Narrative is constructed primarily for self, a reflexive expression and feedback of the practitioner's learning, answering the question, 'What insights have I gleaned through reflection?' However, because of narrative's value in informing others and opening dialogical space, I construct it with an audience in mind as potential social action towards creating a better world. This takes us into the sixth dialogical movement as a dialogue between the text and its audience. Okri (1997: 41) writes,

> The writer does one half of the work, but the reader does the other. The reader's mind becomes the screen, the place, the era. To a large extent, readers create the world from words, they invent the reality they read. Reading, therefore, is a co-production between writer and reader.

This extends to the audience where the narrative is performed. Meaning is not something the author creates within the text for the reader to simply pull out. Such a view is naïve. The reader interprets meaning for themselves.

Mattingly (1998: 8) writes,

> It [narrative] casts events in a particular light that allow the audience to infer something about what it is really like to be in that story … Narrative offers meaning through evocation, image, mystery of the unsaid. It persuades by seducing the listener or reader into the world it portrays, unfolding events in a suspense-laden time in which one wonders what will happen next.

Gadamer (1975) asks the reader not take offence at the text. This is quite likely if the text says something the reader or listener does not agree with. It is as if people project meaning into the text, expecting it to say things they will agree with. Readers or listeners should read or listen with a sceptical mind, simply because the text may be provocative or even a devil's advocate, and particularly sceptical if the narrator spells out what the text means. As Louise Bourgeois (2008:) writes,

> An artist's words are always to be taken cautiously … the artist who discusses the so-called meaning of his work is usually describing a literary side-issue. The core of his original impulse is to found, if at all, in the work itself. Just the same the artist must say what he feels …

I sense the truth in these words, that I may have implanted many ideas I am not even aware of in my text, such has been my partial gaze. Any text is a microcosm of the whole and hence the whole of practice can be discerned within any text.

This is the posture of the reflective practitioner — open, curious, sceptical as to what the text has to say in dialogue with her own experiences.

Performance Narrative

To reiterate, I construct narratives such as Peggy with a view to performing them. By performance I mean standing in front of an audience and reading the narrative with visual, musical and installation aids ,as appropriate. Other players may be involved, such as in Anthea (see Chapter 25). As such, I imagine the impact of my words upon an audience.

Langellier (1999:) writes,

> Performance is the term I used to describe a certain type of particularly involved and dramatized oral narrative. Of special importance is how performance contributes to the evaluative function of personal narrative – the 'so what? How is this interesting? Who's interested in this/who interest is this?'

Performance narrative is opening a dialogue with an audience whereby insights within the narrative can be teased or shouted out, enticing the audience towards social action.

Perhaps I have to shout out to be heard to disturb the complacent din that characterises much of healthcare. I need to prod the audience and disturb with my words and voice and voices of others. Perhaps I need to say shocking things. Otherwise it makes no difference; water off a duck's back. This may sound intense but I sense the way reflective practice rubs along the surface of smooth running with barely a scratch, let alone reconstructs a more satisfactory surface and the supports that hold it up.

I risk performance because I am uncertain about how to do it well. And it must be done well. With my partner Otter, we construct performance, considering visual images, movement, light, voice, music, installation, props and such like. A multimedia extravaganza to showcase the insights gained, yet without imposing these insights on the audience. D. Soyini Madison (1999: 106) writes, 'Performance helps me see. It illuminates like good theory. It orders the world and it lets the world loose.'

The audience may ask, 'What was all that about?' And I answer, 'What do you think it is about'? In other words, performing narrative does not intend to be a passive experience. If so, I have failed, although some people are so passive that no amount of enticing will stir them. Performance is creative. It is exciting and it gets to the core of practice discipline. It enables both performers and audience to feel and see what is going on, moving beyond cognitive to bodily understanding. It is living or acting out theory. Dry, lifeless theory comes to life.

Soyini Madison (1999: 109) writes,

> Performance helps me live a truth while theory helps me name it – or maybe it is the other way around. My mind and body are locked together in a nice little divine kind of unity: the theory knows and feels, and the performance feels and unlearns. I know I am un/learning body in the process of feeling. You too.

I know that audience can struggle to dialogue, as if overwhelmed by what they have experienced. Perhaps they feel intimidated by the demand to dialogue. Perhaps they need time to process. Sensing this, I can ask the audience before the performance commences to write down just one thing that seems significant about what they have witnessed. I recently did this with a performance of 'Smoking kills'[8] with an audience at the University of Minnesota. Many of the audience wrote a number of things and were invited to share and dialogue with these ideas. Knowing a task to be done may also encourage attention that they are part of the performance.

Some of my performance narratives are about personal experiences. These include 'My mother's death' and 'The angiogram'[9]. These experiences have proved valuable to inform my understanding of suffering from the perspective of a relative rather than a health professional.

Skill Box

- *Rewrite any reflexive narrative as a performance narrative. Imagine performing it. Create the practice or learning situation where you can perform it. Think about multimedia enhancement. Use your peers to help you. You might want to review Chapters 23, 24 and 25 (all examples of performance narrative that have been performed in public) before doing this.*

Performing narrative engages students in meaningful learning. This is proven time and time again as I share my stories in the classroom, in workshops, in conferences. In developing performance I consider ways to engage the audience more actively in the performance. For example, in 'Jane's Rap' (Groom and Johns 2010, Johns and Marlin 2010), I recruited drama and psychiatric students to read the empathic poems that represented the voice of eight self-harm patients. I read the voice of Jane — a staff nurse working in a hospital Accident and Emergency department. The topic was her attitude towards self-harm patients. Feedback from the participating drama and psychiatric students was very positive, offering real insight into self-harm. The students dialogued with the audience and between themselves following each performance. Some of the psychiatric and drama students had a history of self-harm and reading their poems was cathartic. It led to a deeper understanding of themselves and was intensely moving. In one performance a student nurse in the audience commented, 'I've learnt more about self-harm and A&E in one hour than in any previous theory class.'

In 'Anthea'[10] I built in pauses whereby an artist performing with me intuitively painted in dialogue with the words. We extended this by supplying art materials to the audience for them to engage in the same way.

Skill Box

- *Review any reflexive narrative you have written. Consider the different people you have mentioned in your narrative. Now write empathic poems to reflect deeper on their perspectives of the experience.*
- *Ask someone else to write empathic poems for people in your experience.*
- *What insight do you gain from this exercise?*

Curriculum Potential

One of the most exciting things about performance narrative is the way it can transform the curriculum in ways to enable students and practitioners to take responsibility for their learning in a very active and dynamic way. By this I mean that students construct performance narratives and perform these to their peers as a way of exploring particular curriculum aspects. I develop this idea in Chapters 8 and 15.

Summary

Weaving narrative enables the practitioner to put the pieces together, to bring learning to a coherent whole. It is of course the stuff of assignments and portfolios, and hence significant for those who are constructing such stuff. It is also the stuff for teachers who wish to teach through story and performance. It is also the stuff of researchers who want to research self through reflexive narrative. All this stuff is picked up in later chapters, so hang on in there! However, before I do that I develop the idea of poetic expression with my narrative of being with Veronica in Chapter 7.

Endnotes

1   The hospice describes this as clinical supervision, although I prefer the term guided reflection.
2   Different approaches to facilitating group-guided reflection are explored in Chapter 5.

3 'Palliative care is an approach that improves the quality of life of patients and their families facing the problem associated with life-threatening illness, through the prevention and *relief of suffering* by means of early identification and impeccable assessment and treatment of pain and other problems, physical, psychosocial, and spiritual' (www.who.int/cancer/palliative/ definition/en/).

4 See the Being Available template (Table 4.3).

5 Bricolage is '(in art or literature) construction or creation from a diverse range of available things' (https://www.google.co.uk/?gfe_rd=cr&ei=afSPVr2PDKq8wesnZWwBQ&gws_ rd=ssl#q=bricolage+definition).

6 Within my school of reflective practice, narrative and performance at the University of Bedfordshire.

7 See Figure 3.2.

8 See Chapter 24, where I also explore its multimedia construction.

9 'The angiogram' was developed and retitled 'People are Not Numbers to Crunch' (see Chapter 23).

10 See Chapter 25.

References

Bourgeois, L. (2008) *Destruction of the father, Reconstruction of the father: Writings and interviews 1923–1997*. Edited and with texts by M-L. Berbadac and H-U. Obrist. MIT Press, Cambridge, MA in association with Violette Editions, London.

Carson, J. (2008) *Spider Speculations: a physics and biophysics of storytelling*. New York Theatre Communications Group.

Dewey, J. (1933) *How we think*. D. C. Heath, Boston.

Elias, N. (1985) *The loneliness of the dying*. Basil Blackwell, Oxford.

Fay, B. (1987) *Critical social science*. Polity Press, London.

Fordham, M. (2008) Building bridges in homelessness, mindful of phronesis in nursing practice. In C. Delmar and C. Johns (eds.), *The good, the wise, and the right clinical nursing practice*. Aalborg Hospital, Arhus University Hospital, Denmark, pp. 73–92.

Fordham, M. (2010) Falling through the net and the spider's web: two metaphoric moments along my journey. In C. Johns (ed.), *Guided reflection: a narrative approach to advancing practice* (2nd ed). Wiley-Blackwell, Oxford, pp. 145–163.

Gadamer, H-G. (1975) *Truth & method*. Seabury Press, New York.

Groom, J. and Johns, C. (2010) Working with deliberate self-harm patients in A&E. In C. Johns (ed.), *Guided reflection: a narrative approach to advancing practice*. Blackwell, Oxford, pp. 169–185.

Hesse, E. (2002) *Eva Hesse* (ed. M. Nixon). MIT Press, Cambridge, MA.

Jarrett, L. (2008) From significance to insights. In C. Delmar and C. Johns (eds.), *The good, the wise, and the right clinical nursing practice*. Aalborg Hospital, Arhus University Hospital, Denmark, pp. 59–72.

Jarrett, L. (2009) *Being and becoming a reflective practitioner, through guided reflection, in the role of a spasticity management nurse specialist*. Unpublished PhD thesis, London City University.

Johns, C. (2004) *Being mindful, easing suffering: reflections on palliative care*. Jessica Kingsley, London.

Johns, C. (2006) *Engaging reflection in practice: a narrative approach*. Blackwell, Oxford, esp. pp. 158–160.

Johns, C. (2010) Constructing the reflexive narrative. In C. Johns (ed.), *Guided reflection: a narrative approach to advancing practice* (2nd ed.). Wiley-Blackwell, Oxford, pp. 27–50.

Johns, C. (2013) Through a glass darkly. In C. Johns, *Becoming a reflective practitioner* (4th ed.). Blackwell, Oxford, pp. 280–292.

Johns, C. and Marlin, C. (2010) Jane's Rap: guided reflection as a pathway to self as sacred space. In C. Johns (ed.), *Guided reflection: a narrative approach to advancing practice* (2nd ed.). Wiley-Blackwell, Oxford, pp. 236–255.

Klass, D., Silverman, P. and Nickman, S. (1996) *Continuing bonds: new understandings of grief*. Taylor and Francis, Washington, DC.

Langellier, K.M. (1999) Personal narrative, performance, performativity: two or three things I know for sure. *Text and Performance Quarterly* 19, 125–144.

Levering, M. (2000) *Zen*. Duncan Baird, London.

Madison, D. Soyini. (1999) Performing theory/embodied writing. *Text and Performance Quarterly* 19, 107–124.

Mattingly, C. (1998) *Healing dramas and clinical ploys: the narrative structure of experience*. Cambridge University Press, Cambridge.

Menzies- Lyth, I. (1988) A case study in the functioning of social systems as a defence against anxiety. *In Containing anxiety in institutions: Selected essays*. Free Association Books, London.

Okri, B. (1997) *A way of being free*. Phoenix House, London.

Paley, J. (2014) Cognition and the compassion deficit: the social psychology of helping behaviours in nursing. *Nursing Philosophy* 15, 274–287.

Parker, M. (2002) Aesthetic ways in day to day nursing. In D. Freshwater (ed.), *Therapeutic nursing*. Sage, London.

Ramos, M. (1992) The nurse–patient relationship: themes and variations. *Journal of Advanced Nursing* 17, 496–506.

Rolfe, G. and Gardner, L. (2014) The compassion deficit and what to do about it: a response to Paley. *Nursing Philosophy* 15, 288–297.

Stewart, I. and Joines, V. (1987) *TA today: a new introduction to Transactional Analysis*. Russell Press, Nottingham.

Tuffnell, M. and Crickmay, C. (2004) *A widening field*. Dance Books, Alton.

Walter, T. (1994) *The revival of death*. Routledge, London.

Wheatley, M.J. (1999) *Leadership and the new science: discovering order in a chaotic world*. Berrett-Koehler, San Francisco.

Wheatley, M.J. and Kellner-Rogers, M. (1996) *The simple way*. Berrett-Koehler, San Francisco.

Wilber, K. (1998) *The eye of spirit: an integral vision for a world gone slightly mad*. Shambhala, Boston.

Worwood, V. (1999) *The fragrant heavens*. Doubleday, London.

Chapter 7

Moving Towards a More Poetic Form of Expression

Christopher Johns

Poetic expression opens the mind beyond reason

Introduction

In Chapter 6 I briefly explored using empathic poems as a way to include other voices, different perspectives within narrative. In this chapter I consider writing narrative as a prose poem. In doing so, I endeavour to open the reader's mind to possibility.

Veronica[1]

I rewrite the narrative as a prose poem. Prose poetry transcends the mind. It opens up the imagination in free flow, freeing me from cognitive constraint to flow more with the experience in an embodied way. Poetry is parsimonious. It cuts to the quick. Reading poetry facilitates reading between the lines, where insights are often revealed. It is more evocative of mood than prosaic language and hence more engaging.

Poetry is a narrative form that for some reflective writers may offer a more creative form of expression.

> Dawn peels back the night.
> Fallen leaves damp from the rain litter the verges.
> Headlights dipped
> Another shift at the hospice.

Becoming a Reflective Practitioner, Fifth Edition. Edited by Christopher Johns.
© 2017 John Wiley & Sons Ltd. Published 2017 by John Wiley & Sons Ltd.
Companion Website: www.wiley.com/go/johns/reflectivepractitioner

Veronica is curled up in the corner of the four-bed ward.
No visitors again this afternoon.
Her sight taken by the brain tumour.
blind, yet what does she sense as she approaches death?
What does she see in the darkness?
Perhaps childhood memories?
Or bright lights of spent romance?
Or perhaps regret?
Perhaps I should ask or would I intrude?
I sit with her.
A touch of pity stirs within
That she is alone
Sadness quickly smiled away in the moment.
'Shall I massage your hands,
Play you some music?'
She turns her head towards me
A faint smile
As she folds her hand over mine
'Only if you aren't too busy.'
She makes no demand for herself,
So easy to pass her by
Or merely superficial presence;
Her spirit glows
And lifts me beyond the throws of any pity
As my hands respond to ease her.
Other women watch me.
One woman furtively says to her visitors
'He's a complementary therapist.'
The relatives look at me as if I am a curio.
Am I a curio?

But I wonder – who is alone?
Is it she or I?
Why might I think she is alone?
True, no one sits by her side
Yet … perhaps inside
She brims with memories of relationships
Perhaps she dwells in rich company
Perhaps that is why
She can smile and gently fold her hand
Over mine;
A hand gnarled with age
Caresses mine like silk
So I am no longer alone
In the quiet afternoon where we dwell.
Do I ease her suffering
Or does she ease mine as I seek to be useful?
Perhaps a bit of both
Suffering is not easy to assuage deep within us.
Elias (1985) guides – *for some of the dying it might be right to be alone.*
Perhaps they are able to dream and not want to be disturbed.
'One must sense what they need'.
The link between dying with loneliness cannot be assumed.

Linda

People are careless
Caught up in their minds or task
They lose sight of the bigger picture.
Linda suffers from multiple sclerosis.
Here for pain management.
I gave her a reflexology last week.
Reading her notes
She has a 17-year-old daughter called Zoë.
Sexual relations with her husband have ceased
Such comment disturbs me.
Intrusive
Putting her on public display.
And yet, it acknowledges her as a sexual being.
She threw me a cue last week
Discussing *ylang ylang* as being an aphrodisiac
She said, '*That won't be of much use to me now.*'
I hadn't pursued it, feeling uncomfortable with the topic.
Do other staff explore sexuality with her?
This afternoon, she lies on her bed
Tired and uncomfortable but looking forward to reflexology.
The aroma stone is dry.
'*I didn't want to make a fuss,*' she says
Frustration
Aroma-stones are outside the nurses' gaze
A recurrent story
I say '*I'll wag my finger at the staff later.*'
My frustration leaking out.
But I do not want to draw Linda into warfare.
Shift the topic
'*I've plotted the pattern of your pain management.*'
She laughs,
Tells me about big boxes of methadone arriving from the chemist.
'*You're not on any neuropathic pain analgesia?*'
'*I was on gabapentin but it didn't suit me but I may have to go
back on it. The shooting pain down my leg is sciatic on top of my
normal pain.*'
My perception confirmed.
'*How do you feel about having multiple sclerosis?*'
'*It hangs heavily over an uncertain and disabling future.*'
Perhaps it would have been better not to ask
For it hangs heavily over us
Loud noise drifts through the pulled curtains that separate us from
the outside world.
Two women are with Veronica.
Routinely turning Veronica who is unable shift her own position.
Surely they might quieten their talk?
Gossip about personal stuff
They consider with uncertainty how best to use the sliding sheets.
One calls Veronica 'darling', then 'sweetheart', then 'darling' again.
My brow frowns.

Veronica has lost her name.
She is quiet and makes no demand.
They move across the ward and call Andrea 'Andrea'.
She has a name.
Is Veronica aware of the distinction?
If so, does it bother her?
Frustration, but must I refocus on Linda.

Later, I attend the shift report.
Tentatively I say, '*I suspect Linda has neuropathic pain.*'
Bridget [the nurse in charge] replies, '*Her pain management is being reviewed later.*'
Not daunted, I enquire, '*Do you explore sexuality with Linda?*'
Bridget looks at me askew, '*No, it's not relevant to her care. She's admitted for pain management.*' Linda framed by her presenting symptoms
I note the reference in her notes.
News to them.
Notes are then not so carefully read
Is sex is a taboo topic?
'*She might appreciate talking about sexuality? I avoided it myself because I'm not comfortable with the topic.*'
A nerve hit.
The nurses do not respond.
I want to say something more but I hold my tongue.
At least I've made my point.
I can write my concerns in Linda's notes
But what is my concern?
And, would anyone read them?
I must write facts not concerns.
I wonder at my discomfort to talking with women about sexuality.
Am I anxious about boundaries?
Especially being a man?
Could I be more open?
Maybe say, '*Would you like to explore that?*'
To open a potential space.
After all, it was she who mentioned it.
At least I mentioned it at the shift report.
Explore the literature

I resonate with Charmaz (1983): '*Sexuality is integral to the person's identity and is a major factor in their perceived sense of loss of self.*' These words resonate. I know Linda has an impaired body image and diminished view of herself as a [sexual] woman.
Lemieux et al. (2004) feed my insight:

For patients in this study, sexuality was an important aspect of their lives, even in the last weeks and days of life. Sexuality encompassed many things but was centred on emotional connectedness. Their experience of sexuality changed over time, from expressions that usually included sexual intercourse prior to the disease, to one of intimacy through close body contact, hugging, touching of hands, kissing, 'meaningful' eye contact and other non-physical expressions of closeness and companionship. These expressions were a key component of their quality of life.

Words that resonate with my experience.

Lemieux et al. further note that the therapeutic impact of their study to create a space in which the participants could talk about sexuality.

Nurses are generally not good at 'intimacy'.

But if so, do we fail our patients?

I find Erica, a nursing student.

'*I overheard your loud conversation with Marion when you turned Veronica earlier.*

I was behind the curtain with Linda. It disturbed us. I noticed Marion called Veronica by endearments.'

Erica, apologetic, '*I'm sorry. I hadn't realised. I got caught up in Marion's conversation. I know it's wrong to call people by endearments but everyone seems to do it especially if the patient is dependent, like Veronica.*'

'*Yes, I noticed Andrea was called by her name. How would you feel if I called you "darling"?*'

'*Not good. We need to treat everyone with respect and dignity. Veronica didn't seem to mind, though.*'

'*Is that because she likes it or simply because she's passive?*'

'*Um … passive, I would guess.*'

'*Why not offer her a hand massage? It is one way to communicate with her.*'

'*Actually, I am a trained holistic therapist but I lack confidence because I haven't practised for two years since becoming a student nurse.*'

'*Come, let's go and see Veronica.*'

Erica inquires, '*Veronica, would you like a hand massage?*'

Veronica's eyes are alive and she eagerly accepts.

Afterwards, Erica, '*It was good to massage Veronica, she appreciated it.*'

'*Does she have dry feet?*'

Erica exclaims, '*She does. I am on tomorrow afternoon, maybe I could how much do her feet then?*'

I open up possibility for both Erica and Veronica.

But I have doubt
Erica responded positively.
How would Marion respond if I took her aside?
Confronted her less than caring behaviour?
Ethically, I should confront uncaring wherever I meet it.
But was it uncaring?
Perhaps endearments are fine?
Do they reflect a lack of dignity?
Do I avoid conflict with her?
She has been working at the hospice for years and can be abrasive.
Perhaps I can inform Marion of my response to Erica?
She might make the association with her own behaviour?
Perhaps just feign outrage at her,
give it to her straight?
Perhaps that's the only way she would 'hear'.
But then, would I just impose my own values?
Do I act as Veronica's advocate because of her diminished
autonomy?

Absorb her imagined suffering
I know she wouldn't complain.
But Marion should have been more respectful of my therapy with
Linda. Perhaps a word with Chloë, the unit sister?
Pass my concern up the hierarchy.
Make it someone else's responsibility.
Without doubt practice is complex loaded with potential conflict
Writing releases frustration
yet fuels frustration reliving
I don't give Marion feedback
I don't confront the aroma stone management
I am a conflict avoider
It bothers me
My integrity aches with such failure.
I am alone.

Skill Box

- *Rework your narrative as a prose poem. Does it open up meaning for you?*
- *Note how much you rewrite as a consequence*

Summary

Poetic prose and poems offer a creative approach to narrative that feeds the imagination and evokes insight by breaking open text where insights are hidden. In moving away from technical rational language it helps balance the whole mind. In Chapter 8 the idea of using storyboard as story and narrative is explored.

Endnote

1   'Veronica' was originally published in Johns (2006: 221–225).

References

Charmaz, K. (1983) Loss of self: a fundamental form of suffering in the chronically ill. *Sociology of Health & Illness* 5.2, 168–195.
Elias, N. (1985) *The loneliness of the dying*. Basil Blackwell, Oxford.
Johns, C. (2006) *Engaging reflection in practice*. Blackwell, Oxford, esp. pp. 221–225.
Lemieux, L., Kaiser, S., Pereira, J. and Meadows, L. (2004) Sexuality in spiritual care: patient perspectives. *Palliative Medicine* 18, 630–637.

Chapter 8

Reflection Through Art and Storyboard

Otter Rose-Johns and Christopher Johns

A picture paints a thousand words

In the previous chapter I explored the significance of prose poetry to access the right brain and nurture the creative mind. Remember, the right brain is the centre for perception, imagination, intuition, curiosity and creativity; all significant reflective and clinical skills (see Table 2.1). In this chapter we explore reflection through art as a more embodied way to stimulate and nurture the creative mind.

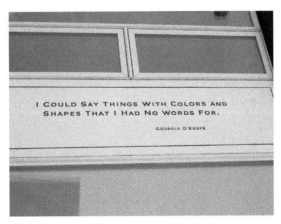

These words, photographed from a building in Boulder, Colorado, suggest that words can limit our ability to express our experience. How we present our stories in a journal is a creative act. Explore Perrella (2004) to inspire your potential and imagination. My own journal is littered with sketches and doodles alongside words.

I am sure many readers have experienced the value of art therapy in enabling patients to explore their experiences around death and dying, especially when experiences seem too traumatic to write about. It seems art offers a gateway to deeper thoughts and feelings. The work by Cameron et al. (2008) and Gaydos (2008) illuminate the potential of reflection through art.

Becoming a Reflective Practitioner, Fifth Edition. Edited by Christopher Johns.
© 2017 John Wiley & Sons Ltd. Published 2017 by John Wiley & Sons Ltd.
Companion Website: www.wiley.com/go/johns/reflectivepractitioner

Cameron et al. worked with Canadian pre-registration students. They note (2008: 115),

> the purpose of the aesthetic assignment is to invite students to participate in a journey that stretches and challenges self in the paradoxes of life experiences. The student begins to engage in a form of 'academic play' which gives them permission to 'think outside the box' and leads them to ponder, analyze and develop their own perspectives. They apply the theoretical underpinnings of a critical social theory, which includes the values of justice and equity, inclusion, empowerment and respect as related to 'lived experience' of their clients. Expression through art brings to life suppressed and repressed feelings, attitudes and beliefs and increases insights and self-awareness.

The results of this project are beautifully illustrated with colour plates. Gaydos (2008) used collage with midwives on a maternity unit in the United States to help them reconnect with their values after a severe period of disruption. The results are deeply symbolic. Gaydos (2008: 168) cites Eliade (1991: 12): 'the symbol reveals certain aspects of reality – the deepest aspects – which defy other means of knowledge'.

Moorman (2015)[1] used art appreciation as a visual thinking strategy with nursing students. Her results indicated that students developed the ability to see the 'whole clinical picture', to pay more attention to detail, and to explore surface signs for deeper meanings. Sharing their perceptions with peers and guides enabled them to appreciate ambiguity and to speak out, especially in a clinical climate where they had felt silenced through fear of being judged by senior nurses. As such, it is not just the art that is important but the safe sharing of it.

However, an approach to reflection through art requires careful preparation. In Otter's practitioner workshops there are usually not more than 12 practitioners (the workshop outline is shown in Table 8.1). First, Otter sets out the aim of the session: to explore reflection through art. She shares some of her own images and the techniques she used to give the participants some scope of possibility, either portraying experience through a

Table 8.1 An example of a workshop timetable.

Exercise		Time frame
1	**Introduction** ● Aim of session ● introduction to art and storyboard and techniques ● VTS	15 minutes
2	**Warm-up exercises** 1 Draw a Zen circle [quieten the mind] 2 Draw a series of circles using the left hand with eyes closed 3 Draw a self portrait using the left hand blind with eyes closed [tune into the body] 4 Draw a red ball of wall unravelling with threads hanging down left-handed with eyes closed [tune into the imagination] 5 Draw – 'the moon is what I've been telling you about'.	30 minutes
3	Construct an image/ storyboard of six images that reflects on and tells the story of an experience.	60–90 minutes
4	Share image/ storyboard within your small group [no more than four]. Write caption notes. Lay out images as an exhibition for others to view.	75–105 minutes
5	Plenary – how was the session useful, if at all? [feed-in left–right brain theory]	90–120 minutes

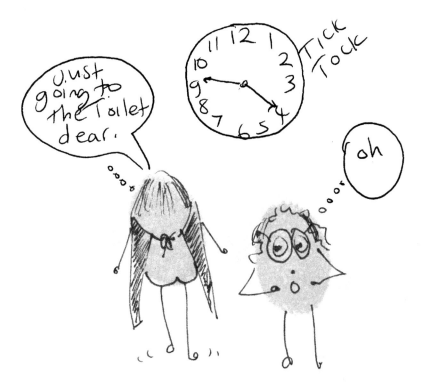

Figure 8.1   Thumb print impact.

single image or as storyboard. Practitioners are often anxious that they lack artistic skill. However, people can easily be represented as stick people or thumbprints. Thumb doodles books (Klutz 2008) offer an introduction to using thumbprints. Google 'draw with stick people' and you will find several sites offering guidance.[2] Both are easy and fun to use. Figure 8.1 shows a scene from 'People are not numbers to crunch' using thumbprints.[3]

Otter then outlines any appropriate research to support reflection through art, as noted in Chapter 2, for example Moorman (2015). Otter then uses a series of 'tuning' exercises.

'Tuning' Exercises

1 To draw a Zen circle with one breath and one stroke of the hand. This exercise aims to tune the practitioner into quieting her mind or to 'bring the mind home' (as set out in the MSR – see Tables 3.1, 3.2 and 3.3, as explored in Chapter 2).
2 This leads into a second exercise to let go of the concentration and free-flow a series of circles, as if releasing the quietened mind into play, using the left hand with the eyes closed.
3 To invite the practitioner to draw a self-portrait using the left hand, with her eyes closed. This exercise aims to tune the practitioner into her body. Using the left hand opens a pathway into the right brain where imagination and creativity are located. Closing the eyes focuses the task.[4]

4 To draw an image of a red ball of wool unravelling with threads hanging down,[5] again left-handed, with the eyes closed. This exercise is playful and develops the practitioner's ability to tune into her imagination.

5 To draw an image of the 'the moon is what I've been telling you about'. This is a more abstract idea that demands greater imagination.

Practitioners are urged to do the 'tuning' exercises quickly without too much thought. A brief discussion can take place between exercises and afterwards. Following the tuning exercises practitioners are guided to reflect on a recent personal or clinical experience that seems significant in some way. This can either be drawn or painted. The practitioners then share and explore these images in small groups followed by a plenary with the whole workshop to explore the insights gained and significance of the workshop. An exhibition of the collected images gives other workshop practitioners the opportunity to view all the work and exchange views.

Otter reinforces the significance of making the connection between the left (or less dominant) hand and the right brain function[6] and how the imagination has become trimmed in the demand to 'grow up', reinforcing the idea that our imaginations have been trimmed in the demand to grow up (Paramananda 2001).

Storyboard

Storyboard takes the idea of drawing or painting images into narrative form. As such, it offers the practitioner an engaging approach to constructing narrative that is creative and effective. It is a technique developed in the 1930s from the Walt Disney Studio (Canemaker 2010) and forms the basis for filmmaking.

Storyboard literally draws or paints the narrative. The scenes chosen capture the drama of the experience, each scene significant as a *turning point* (Carson 2008), evident to the discerning reader yet without distracting the reader from drawing their own insights in relation to their own experiences. One scene prompts the next. A brief commentary usually accompanies each scene enough to reinforce the visual message. Storyboard might also be termed narrative visualisation.[7]

To illustrate, we set out a storyboard of Otter's experience of visiting her father in hospital and witnessing a nurse attempting to put on TED stockings (Figure 8.2). It is entitled 'Can care be so careless?' The title doesn't mince with words. Getting to the point graphically is characteristic of storyboard.

Otter reveals her experience through nine scenes. Of course, more or fewer could be used. Condensing the situation to nine scenes concentrates the mind and sharpens its impact, as does the dramatic expression of the commentary. The significance of Otter's experience is obvious. She uses such words and phrases as 'robot nurse', 'no *stop*', 'she's dangerous', 'poor communication', 'defensively' and 'porky pies'. Otter's insight is that hospitals are potentially dangerous places because routine practice is unreflective and careless. Practitioners need to be reflective about every situation. Nothing can be taken for granted. Practitioners should always introduce themselves,[8] welcome relatives and inquire into their wellbeing. Within a reflective culture nurses would always be open to dialogue, rather than being defensive and lying to cover up poor practice, and welcome feedback and complaint as a learning opportunity. We wonder what retribution, if any, the ITU nurse experienced as a consequence?

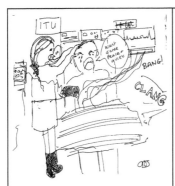

I arrive in ITU. Dad's just had a triple by-pass. The noise is deafening!' Dad cries 'I want some peace and quiet!'.

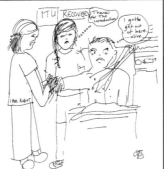

A nurse is doing observations. No introduction from her. I muse 'Robot nurse.' My anxiety increasing.

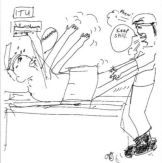

The nurse then attempts to put TED stockings on Dad's swollen legs. No explanation to dad. 'That hurts!' he moans.

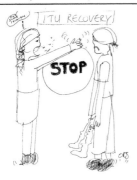

"STOP" I shout '"You're doing it wrong! She confesses she doesn't know how to put them on correctly. Am I really hearing this?!

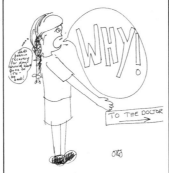

I ask 'Why are you putting them on?' She says 'We put them on every person.' I retort 'But hang on, he's got arterial problems. Where's the doctor?!'

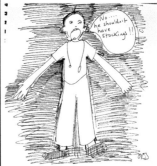

The doctor is shocked. He confirms Dad shouldn't have TED stockings. Talk about the danger of routine practice and poor communication!

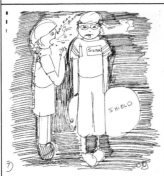

I challenge the sister. Defensively she responds 'All our nurses are trained to apply TED stockings.'

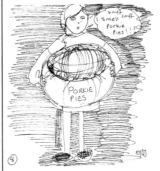

'Really?' I say. **Porky pies.** Why can't she be honest! Dad was put at risk by such mindless action.

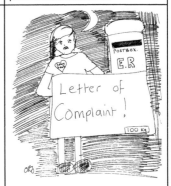

I reflect that such care and response is unacceptable. I decide to complain via PALS. Writing helps dispel my anxiety.

Figure 8.2   Otter's storyboard.

Otter could also construct a complementary storyboard to respond to the MSR cue, 'Given the situation again, what are my options for responding more effectively?'[9] Visualising such options plants the seeds of resistance and possibility. It enables the reflective practitioner to *see* herself in a new situation as opposed to thinking about herself in a new situation. Visualisation is more embodied and cathartic and better prepares the person for actually taking the envisaged action. For example, see 'Nurse bully and the timid sheep' (Johns 2013: Ch. 20), where Otter visualises how she could respond more effectively to confront being bullied.

In the workshop, practitioners are guided to reflect on an experience through storyboard using six transitional frames. As with Otter's storyboard, writing a commentary helps tell the story and minimises writing text on the image. The images are then shared within the group. The sharing is often emotional, reflecting the cathartic nature of reflection through art. We suggest no more than four people in each small group for two reasons. First, it is difficult to pay attention and absorb too much of other peoples' images. Secondly, sharing takes time. We then ask the participants to set out their storyboards as if in an exhibition for everyone to review each other's images. This draws everyone together for a plenary to dialogue the value of the workshop. Caption notes can be added after dialogue when insights or transitional moments have become clearer.

The workshops, including *tuning exercises*, take approximately 90 to 120 minutes, depending on whether one image or a storyboard is being developed. The talking phases of the workshop are vital for helping practitioners draw insight. Often the artist has a limited focus, whereas others can help her see the 'bigger picture'.

As I noted, people are often anxious about artistic skill, just as people unaccustomed to writing poetry worry about writing poetry. This type of response reminds us that people's imagination has been trimmed. They are uncomfortable with play, sensing that they will be publicly exposed and judged as not very good. In our storyboard workshops, people learn to play again and recover their imagination that has been trimmed in the demand to 'grow up' and be rational (Paramananda 2001). It seems that perception is sharpened through a more intuitive response to experience, leading to a more embodied learning. However, these workshops are very cathartic and require very sensitive guidance. Otter is good at that, at infusing this sense of play with her wild enthusiasm and conviction that everyone can succeed – yet in a secure way.

Skill Box

- *So, play time! Draw a recent experience and see where it takes you. Open up your box of crayons and recover the imagination that has been trimmed and suffocated by the technical, rational mind.*
- *Imagine yourself in Otter's shoes. How might you like Otter to respond differently given the situation again? Use storyboard to envisage this response.*
- *How do you think the nurse and sister felt being confronted by Otter? Again, use storyboard to imagine this.*
- *Reflect on a recent clinical experience that seems significant somehow, using storyboard. Use just six scenes, although more can be used (Figure 8.3 offers a template based on using six scenes]. Write caption notes. If possible share with others and note how the dialogical process reveals deeper insights.*

Summary

Storyboard offers a visual and creative approach to constructing narrative through a sequence of scenes that depict the essential *turning points* of the narrative that point towards insights. In a similar way to writing prose poetry, drawing and painting storyboard opens up the text, enabling the practitioner to draw insight.

1	2	3
Image	Image	Image
Caption	Caption	Caption

4	5	6
Image	Image	Image
Caption	Caption	Caption

Figure 8.3   Typical storyboard template

In Chapter 9 I imagine the reflective curriculum whereby art-based workshops are significant to nurture right brain creativity.

Endnotes

1   Google 'Visual thinking strategies'.
2   For example, http://www.thedrawingwebsite.com/2012/10/10/stick-figures-with-style-basic-design/.
3   See Chapter 23.
4   We are grateful to Kate Walters for introducing Otter to this approach.
5   This image is taken from 'People are not numbers to crunch' (see Chapter 23).

6   See Table 2.1.

7   For example, see Edward Segel and Jeffrey Heer, Narrative Visualization: Telling Stories with Data (posted online 2010; http://vis.stanford.edu/files/2010-Narrative-InfoVis.pdf, accessed 17 December 2016).

8   The failure of nurses to introduce themselves is a significant theme within 'People are not Numbers to Crunch' – Chapter 23.

9   See Table 3.2.

References

Cameron, D. et al. (2008) Expressing voice and developing practical wisdom on social justice through art. In C. Delmar and C. Johns (eds.), *The good, the wise, and the right clinical nursing practice*. Aalborg Hospital, Arhus University Hospital, Denmark, pp. 59–72).

Canemaker, J. (2010) *Paper dreams, the art and artists of Disney storyboards*. Hyperion Press, London.

Carson, J. (2008) *Spider Speculations: a physics and biophysics of storytelling*. Theatre Communications Group, New York.

Eliade, M. (1991) *Images and symbols: studies in religious symbolism* (trans. P. Mairet). Princeton University Press, Princeton, NJ.

Gaydos, H. (2008) Collage: an aesthetic process for creating phronesis in nursing. In C. Delmar and C. Johns (eds.), *The good, the wise, and the right clinical nursing practice*. Aalborg Hospital, Arhus University Hospital, Denmark, pp. 163–178.

Johns, C. (2013) *Becoming a reflective practitioner* (4th ed.). Wiley-Blackwell, Oxford, esp. pp. 260–269.

Klutz (2008) *Thumb doodles book*. Klutz, Palo Alto, CA.

Moorman, M. (2015) The meaning of visual thinking strategies for nursing students. *Humanities* 4, 748–759.

Paramananda (2001) *A deeper beauty: Buddhist reflections on everyday life*. Windhorse, Birmingham.

Perrell, L. (2004) *Artists' journals and sketchbooks: exploring and creating personal pages*. Quarry Books, Gloucester, MA.

Chapter 9

The Reflective Curriculum

Christopher Johns

Pick the lock and open the door

Introduction

Educational institutions are locked into technical rational approaches to a curriculum that accommodates reflective practice as a technical rational approach. As such, the impact of reflective practice is diminished and education is impoverished. Reflection picks the lock and opens the door to self-inquiry and understanding whereas a technical rational approach closes this door, with its focus on obtaining competence in a particular field and conformity to set ideas. Put another way, the technical rational approach breeds a fear of failure (Krishnamurti 1996). A professional artistry-envisioned curriculum is necessary to enable reflective practice to flourish and its learning potential to be fully realised. However, the difference between a technical rational and professional artistry-driven curriculum is like chalk and cheese. You might argue, 'Never the twain shall meet.' And so teachers live out illusions that they know and teach reflective practice. I know. I worked in a university nursing department for over twenty years gnashing my teeth.

In this chapter I imagine the potential structure and ensuing issues associated with implementing a truly reflective curriculum. Such a curriculum, as far as I am aware, does not exist.

Taking nursing as an example, the Nursing and Midwifery Council (NMC) advocate reflection in the curriculum. What is their rationale for doing so? There are studies on teaching reflective practice that any curriculum group would naturally investigate to support the need for a reflective curriculum and its delivery, for example, O'Connor, Hyde and Treacey (2003), McGrath and Higgins (2006), O'Donovan (2007), Mann, Gordon and Macleod (2009), McCarthy, Cassidy and Tuohy (2013) and Clarke (2014). However, these studies offer little the empirical support to justify the NMC's decision. But then we might argue, what is the empirical support for using lectures?

Becoming a Reflective Practitioner, Fifth Edition. Edited by Christopher Johns.
© 2017 John Wiley & Sons Ltd. Published 2017 by John Wiley & Sons Ltd.
Companion Website: www.wiley.com/go/johns/reflectivepractitioner

Journal Entry

A group of second-year nursing students invite me to talk about reflection. They are frustrated with reflection. It is a chore with little value except to answer reflective-type assignments that make them anxious. Can I help? We have two hours.

I ask about the way they have been taught reflection. As I suspect, they are given a model of reflection with little commentary and told to apply it to an experience.

I share my story concerning my experience with Violet (Johns 2014). It takes about 20 minutes to narrate. When I teach reflection, I generally begin with a story, especially if I expect students to write and tell their own stories. This role-models what a story might look like and my risk in sharing it. Within the story, I question my practice. I pose the MSR reflective cue, 'How might I respond differently given the situation again?' and consider alternative responses. I finish by summarising my tentative insights and a potential informing literature.

The students say the story was engaging. Some reported that they actually experienced the situation, as if they were there. Two students, bold enough, relate to my story with their own similar stories. There's a buzz about the place.

I then invite the students to write a story. I give them 15 minutes. After an initial flurry of comment between them, the room is very quiet as pens race across pages.

I then illuminate how the MSR cues (Table 3.1[1]) enable me to explore the experience towards drawing tentative insight. I emphasise my experience as a contextual moment situated in history – a personal, social, cultural, professional, political, environmental, professional, gendered history. I say, 'It's like peeling back an onion skin to reveal deeper contextual layers.' A bit deep for them, but I want them to think about that, that reflection has critical depth.

I prompt the students to apply the cues to their own stories and draw out tentative insight. I then invite them to share their stories, guiding them to reveal insight by asking, 'What do you learn from this?' The two hours pass quickly. However, some students stay on, wanting to talk more about reflective practice. Some say that they had no idea that reflection could be so creative and exciting. Some exclaim, 'Why haven't we been taught reflection like this?'

I suggest it is a problem with accommodating reflection within a programme grounded in a dominant technical rational approach to knowing. Reflection is bolted on and taught from a technical rational perspective rather than from a professional artistry perspective. The students understand but are frustrated. I further explain that their reflective assignments are designed to measure their application of a reflective model supported by references (a pseudo-intellectual game) with no credit for aesthetic expression. I suggest that reflective assignments should be constructed around insights gained. The students say they play the game. 'What game is that?' I enquire. 'Guess what is in teacher's head – that way at least you pass.' What kind of education is that? 'If I had submitted my story as an assignment would I pass?' 'No,' is the general consensus, 'it doesn't tick the boxes.' Is education no more than ticking the boxes? If so, what a parlous approach to learning, and yet this story is normal throughout nurse education.

Some days later, their course teacher, who is also head of curriculum development for pre-registration nursing, approaches me and feeds back the students' enthusiastic response. The power of students' voices could not be easily discounted. She is convinced of a need for a new approach to reflection within the curriculum. She asks if I would lead a specialist sub-group for the curriculum revalidation for the degree course in nurse training. I agree, but that's another story – not a good one. Perhaps I went about it the wrong way, suggesting our existing curriculum wasn't good enough and needed to be grounded in reflective practice. Resistance was overwhelming, although not unanimous. Perhaps now, five years on, the reflective tide has gathered momentum to seriously challenge the dominance and validity of a technical rational curriculum.

Imagine

Imagine the curriculum development team, led by Laura, settling down around the table. Their mandate is to develop a truly reflective curriculum. Imagine the team listening to my journal entry above. I argue that the existing curriculum is inadequate to accommodate a truly reflective curriculum for a number of reasons:

1 Reflection is bolted on to the curriculum in a very limited way rather than integrated within the curriculum. Clarke (2014) writes,

> Reflection and reflective practice has become a key issue for curriculum development within nurse education. The Nursing and Midwifery Council has linked the demonstration of reflective skills to clinical competence to gain entrance onto the professional register. However, despite a significant volume of literature on reflection there is a paucity of research evidence regarding how nurse educators teach mental health nursing students to reflect and become effective reflective practitioners and, little research exploring experiences of staff and students engaged in reflection for teaching and learning purposes.

Clarke emphasises the need for reflection to be an integral part of teaching, and should not be perceived as something to add on.

2 The sessions we give students on reflective practice are no more than introducing a reflective model of nursing and setting some case-study assignments where the student is asked to reflect on an experience. This approach is buried within the college's dominant technical rational approach. In fact, reflection is delivered as a technical rational approach, reflecting a fundamental dominant technical rational approach to nurse education in contrast with a professional artistry perspective that, in my view, would offer a more meaningful and effective approach to nurse education.

3 The majority of nurse teachers do not practise nursing (at least in any meaningful way to be a credible nurse). Nor do they practise reflection. Or, put another way, they are not reflective practitioners and thus not credible to teach reflective practice. Indeed, many of nurse teachers resist reflection because it is threatens their credibility and control. As a consequence, both nursing and reflection are generally taught from a technical rational perspective.

Imagine a small working party led by Ken who have been given the remit to come up with a reflective curriculum plan. They have one month to report back.

Ken: Well, we met weekly over the past month. We are aware of strong diverse views within Faculty. As such, there was a lot of resistance to work through but we came up with a proposed plan. Without doubt, a truly reflective curriculum is a radical idea that evokes strong feelings for and against. From what we have gathered, voices against outweigh the voices who favour a truly reflective curriculum.

Our existing curriculum is based on a theory driven or, in Schön's (1983) terms, a technical rational approach that intends to be predictable. It is very teacher-centric. Teachers are comfortable with this approach. A reflective curriculum would be much less predictable and more student-centric. It offers the opportunity for more flexibility, to wander off the beaten paths and explore the surrounding areas. We believe that learning through reflection is deeply meaningful because it focuses on the individual's and collective journey of becoming a nurse. As such, each step along the journey becomes significant rather than looking at the outcomes. Each step is an event in itself not merely a means towards the end. This paying attention to experience creates the reflexive momentum. As Pirsig (1974: 208) writes, 'to live only for some future goal is shallow. It's the sides of the mountain which sustains life, no the top. Here's where things grow.'

We acknowledge that the curriculum has to respond to the demand of governing bodies, for example the Nursing and Midwifery Council, for approval of the nursing programme where specific regulations and outcomes must be met. In addition approval of programmes is determined by university validation events and the demand of NHS Trusts within the vagaries of tendering. NHS nurse education contracts are big money! As such, the reflective curriculum is not a blank canvas. It is a contested political canvas.

We have constructed a potential model, explored the advantages of a reflective curriculum and identified the staff development we feel is vital to make it work as a reality. We had to admit, or confess might be a better word, that we, as a school, had sunk into a normalised technical rational approach to teaching reflective practice. I think we have 'forced' reflection into the curriculum because we didn't understand it enough or felt we had to conform to it as a teaching technology. These are concerns highlighted in the literature. Beauchamp (2015: 126) quotes Russell (2013): 'Has reflective practice done more harm than good in teacher education?' Beauchamp (2015: 127) notes that Russell identified that 'teacher educators have failed to provide adequate clarity on the meaning of reflection, have not necessarily modelled its practice themselves and have maintained their focus on it outside the realm of real action and experience.' We all felt the truism in these words.

We sketched the potential curriculum model (see Figure 9.1). It is straightforward as it stands. We recommend Schön's (1983) terminology of 'professional artistry and identity' as the goal of practitioner training – *the knowing* that practitioners need to practise. This is in stark contrast with our current technical rational approach to reflection and also what we believe to be our greatest challenge – how can we view our curriculum from a professional artistry perspective when we are so rooted in technical rationality? How do our assumptions need to change?

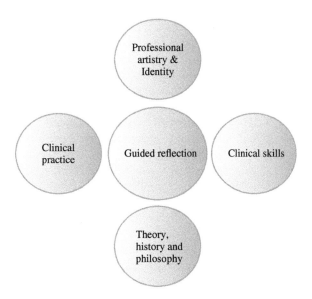

Figure 9.1 The basic structure of the reflective curriculum.

'Professional identity' sets 'professional artistry' against a professional background of values – 'what it means to be a nurse'. In essence, it is about being a certain sort of person besides doing certain sorts of practice.

We recognise that there are two stems to reflective practice – reflection-on-action and reflection-in-action, or what Johns (2013) terms mindful practice. Following Johns, we consider that one leads to the other – that through reflection-on-action practitioners learn to become increasingly more mindful of their experience in action, and able to note and respond to contradictions between their desired practice and their actual way of going about the situation. It becomes a way of doing practice (Rolfe 2014).

As befits any practice discipline, practice must be at the core of the curriculum. So we put guided reflection as the core learning mode informed by reflection on practice, theory and other forms of knowledge deemed necessary, and clinical skills learnt in the school. The model seems obvious but the consequences are phenomenal.

Ken pauses to let the model sink in.

Mary continues: The relationship between theory and practice is redefined. In a practice discipline, such as nursing, it is self-evident that we learn through doing. We may have theories of how to do it but that doesn't mean we know what it is to nurse. As such, our existing curriculum has blocks of theory and blocks of practice but that doesn't mean the twain shall meet. It is legend that nurses learn one thing in the classroom and another thing in clinical practice – what is historically described as the theory–practice gap.

The problem with theory prior to practice is that the student has *nothing to hang the theory upon*. As such, it is difficult to assimilate theory into personal knowing. It remains 'out there' as an abstract idea. The problem with theory after practice is to let students loose in practice with little idea about what they might be trying to achieve with patients. So, clearly, students need to be informed before going into practice. However, within guided reflection, significant aspects of practice become a focus for attention, yet always set against the experience's context and wider theoretical, philosophical background. In other words, theory is introduced at a time when it is most meaningful and can be assimilated into personal knowing. The student *has a hook to hang it on* (Ausubel 1967)! Of course, teachers will need to know a broad range of theory in order to feed it in. We consider at least a two year lead-in period to prepare.

Someone asks: 'How do you envisage the guided reflection core working?'

Glynis takes over: We want to be both realistic and within current budget. We envisage that all practitioner students would spend 4 hours each week in guided reflection groups guided by a teacher for the whole training duration. We see reflective practice as a reflexive development unfolding, a process of student's reflexive self-inquiry – what Ryan (2013: 145) describes as 'treating self as a subject in relation to others and the contextual conditions of study or work'. The emphasis on 'contextual conditions' stains self-enquiry as overtly political, which of course, may not be popular with NHS Trust who may linger for a docile rather than political practitioner. In other words, wanting a docile reflective practitioner, if that's not a contradiction in terms. Research (Ramsey 2010, Beauchamp 2015) indicates that if students are permitted to make decisions about the focus of reflection and the process of reflection, more meaningful reflections are generated.

In practical terms, we suggest groups of about 12 students. The teacher would be the practitioners' personal mentor for the first year. After the first year it might be beneficial to have different guides/mentors. We aren't sure about the relative merits of that. We would need to 'suck it and see'. We also advocate that teachers spend one day a week in clinical practice to support both students and mentors in practice, to be more credible teachers and collect story material for teaching. We need to become highly visible. At the moment very few of us get into practice. There is nothing like the real stuff to develop person-centred learning. One obvious risk with our simulation teaching is that if you talk to a doll object long enough, that's the way you will be with patients and families.

Leslie continues: Supporting students in clinical practice is a growing headache. Feedback suggests that mentoring has become more problematic with the pressure on clinical staff in a stressed clinical environment due to fewer staff and a greater workload. Perhaps even more so, with the government funding more nurse training places.[2] Fewer qualified staff means less mentors. As such, our presence, at least once a week, will be vital to sustain and develop the clinical learning environment.

Mentors need to be reflective practitioners, role-modelling reflection as a way of being in practice, offering a running commentary of their narrative practice. We need to look at the professional practice part of our existing programme to develop our third-year students' ability to provide this role. Equally we need to offer a guided reflection programme for existing staff. We can link that to the NMC requirement for revalidation with its reflective practice requirement. It plays a bit into our hands![3] It is noticeable when I teach clinical supervision to experienced healthcare professionals that professions that have seriously incorporated reflection into curriculum are better equipped for supervisory roles than those professions, such as nursing, that have not. Of course, this is a generalisation.

Ken: What Leslie says is vital and a major focus for our attention. We must get the clinical environment right. The curriculum space/time to accommodate guided reflection is not an issue. We consider that the groups will teach much of the required theory by feeding it in as appropriate and setting students literature searches.

Betty adds: Space within the curriculum for guided reflection is created with a reduction in traditional classroom teaching on topics that we consider are better learnt within guided reflection. Short lectures on topics can be picked up and applied to practice within guided reflection.

Clare: Yes, topics such as caring, relationships, ethics, knowing self and poise, communication skills, and professional issues such as conflict management and assertiveness, would naturally be taught within the group. Of course that necessitates we widen our own theory base.

Glynis: Yes, the relationship between students and teachers radically shifts. It is a model that depends on students taking responsibility and teachers *serving* them to succeed. This is possible if we commence guided reflection from the beginning of training. It cuts across the maternal approach we take at the moment.

Some unrest in
the audience: 'We don't like the aspersion we treat students as children.'

Ken: One thing that is important is that we move forward positively in dialogue. I know for some teachers it will be kind of 'future shock'[4] – that's why we propose a developmental period over two years. It is exciting and creative. In fact it is liberating for us teachers.

Rupert quips, 'Oh Ken, you could sell coal to a coalman!'

Laura, the curriculum leads, asks, 'Can you summarise the benefits of such a reflective curriculum over our existing traditional curriculum, which is essentially theory-driven despite the 'bolt-on' reflective bits?'

Ken: Teaching and learning through reflective practice can claim a number of benefits that are generally lacking in the non-reflective curriculum. We've split this into two parts; benefits of reflection as a process and outcome.

Table 9.1 Potential benefits of a reflective curriculum

Outcome

Practitioners emerge from the programme with a strong sense of professional identity and professional artistry.

- They are adept reflective practitioners.
- They are clinically poised and competent in person-centred practice.
- They are responsible for ensuring that their ongoing clinical performance is effective.
- They speak with an informed, politically astute and assertive voice.
- They are leaders; adept at conflict management and collaborative ways of working.
- They can articulate a strong professional vision and identity.

Process

- It is grounded in a philosophy of genuine student-led practice, grounded in the students' own practice – thus ensuring learning is both practical and meaningful.
- It is contextual through stories where theory and ideas can be seen in context of the particular moment, and the relationship between things can be seen as a whole.
- It is 'whole brain' teaching enabling the development of right brain attributes; intuition, perception, imagination, and creativity, notably through art.
- It juxtaposes theory in relation to emerging issues from practice – hence the student will find theory more relevant and meaningful and hence assimilate it within personal knowing.
- It accesses the swampy lowlands where real issues lie rather than focusing on hard high ground of abstract concepts. Many students may struggle in practice because of its complexity – reflection gives direct focus to their experience and enables them to make sense of contradictions, develop problem-solving and survival skills. It also acknowledges and accepts their difficulties.
- It is values based – constantly challenging and clarifying vision and purpose - balancing 'being a nurse' with 'doing nursing', addressing such issues as ethics, relationships, compassion, therapeutic use of self, and poise that are essential to effective practice but which we do not teach well within a theory-led curriculum.
- It is experiential, leading to creative modes of learning such as performance.
- It fosters students' responsibility for their learning, and as a consequence, it radically shifts the power relationships with teachers.
- It is political – focusing on areas of contradiction, ethics, politics, tradition, power and change – enabling practitioners to become political, empowered and assertive.
- It makes a difference to practice through its reflexive focus of gaining and applying insights to new experiences. In this way we get 'joined-up learning'.
- It prepares practitioners for lifelong learning and ongoing guidance roles.
- It is supportive, dynamic and engaging, and … hopefully fun!

Tania talks through the benefits as perceived by the working group (Table 9.1): We emphasise the idea of competence but armed with the knowhow towards developing expertise. On the other hand, we see it as the potential resistance to the reflective curriculum. I've summarised this (Table 9.2). I would say that these resistors based on applying Lewin's (1951) force field analysis.[5] We've split them into students and teachers.

As we have noted, the resistors are very powerful to protect the status quo and reflect how a rational approach to curriculum change won't work, especially when the change is so radical. To reiterate, as Ken mentioned earlier, the biggest resistor is our own embodied selves, reinforced by working within a technical rational-dominated university that has always and always will value technical rational

Table 9.2 Potential constraints to the reflective curriculum

Students
- They may feel threatened by the intense gaze particularly if they lack commitment to practice or study. It is less prescriptive and therefore more 'adult' and requires more responsibility and self-direction. It is not what they have been used to in schools.

Teachers
- We've been socialised into a set of assumptions that support a traditional teacher-led technical rational curriculum. We are so rooted in a technical rational approach to learning/ reflective practice – How can we view the curriculum from a professional artistry perspective? The technical rational is so embodied within us as individuals and within the university system that we naturally resist a shift. This approach has not privileged students' voices. As such, the truly reflective curriculum is possibly beyond our scope.
- We feel threatened due to democratising the classroom and shift of power leading to issues of control. As hooks [1994] writes – 'Focusing on experience allows students to claim a knowledge base from which they can speak.' [p. 148]. '[However] many professors are critical of the inclusion of confessional narrative in the classroom, where students are doing a lot of the talking because they lack the skill needed to facilitate dialogue' [p151].
- We are generally not reflective on our practice. We lack both reflective and facilitative skills.
- As much as I hate saying this, we have become comfortable and complacent in our teaching roles within a non-reflective culture that has made virtually no demand for us to demonstrate teaching development and excellence.
- Returning to clinical practice is threatening. The neglect of any clinical role may leave reluctant and resistant nurse teachers scratching their heads as to how best to fulfil this role.
- The bottom line is that we like the 'status quo' and resist any attempt to disturb this when we might be disadvantaged in some way. In other words, our 'comfort' as teachers is more important than effective teaching and learning.

knowledge, as indeed does healthcare generally, with its neon sign buzzing 'evidence-based practice rules OK'. We can bring to the surface the assumptions that support the technical rational and highlight a new set of assumptions to support professional artistry. The logic of professional artistry is compelling, it's just our embodied selves resisting. It means we have to unlearn, which can be uncomfortable when we are so comfortable doing what we've always done, especially when the technical rational evidence to support the shift is weak.

Laura: Is there evidence to support these benefits?

Glynis: We've threaded in comment from a number of papers. However, it's like a catch-22 situation. We need professional artistry research, not technical rational research.

Laura: Like narrative studies?

Tania: Yes. Studies grounded the lived experience of doing or being reflective.

Ken: We have talked to NHS Trusts. They would support this shift as long as students emerged as competent practitioners against a set of competence criteria. However, these criteria would inform the reflective process. The link between reflective practice and competency is being made by professional bodies. One example, the International Federation of Sports Physical Therapists (IFSPT), to quote Paterson and Chapman (2013: 133), 'requires physiotherapists applying for their accreditation process to demonstrate a variety of reflective pieces relating to their devised sports physiotherapy competencies' (Bulley et al. 2005). This need to evidence professional development and its impact on an individual's practice increases pressure for physiotherapists to become competent reflective practitioners. Paterson and Chapman (2013: 133) note Mann et al.'s (2009) observation that there is little direct evidence in the literature associating reflective practice and competency.

Perhaps a reflective curriculum would naturally lead to a return to an apprenticeship-type education. Now, there's a thought. Perhaps the NMC would be willing to pilot such a scheme?

Laura: It seems you have painted a broad canvas around the concept of a 'reflective curriculum' that is very challenging in the sense of making it a reality, not least amongst ourselves. However, we are committed to this approach and hence must see resistance as a stimulus for dialogue between us. If that's the way we want to work with students then we must work that way between ourselves. I emphasise 'dialogue' as our method of communication so we can be positive and move towards consensus. In this way we become a learning organisation or community of enquiry. I would like to quote from Wheatley and Kellner-Rogers (1996: 70). They state,

A system [such as the curriculum] is fluid relationships that we observe as a rigid structure. If we look past these structures, we see that systems spring to life from agreements among individuals [us] on how best to live [and work] together. From this multitude of individual explorations, a system may suddenly appear [that] individuals didn't know they were creating.

Ken: I would like to add that within the broad idea of the Community of Inquiry, student practitioners and teachers *collaborate* to ensure the optimum learning environment towards enabling students to successfully register and be effective in their practitioner roles. Each individual, both students and teachers, must take responsibility for her own performance and for the group as a whole. This is the bottom line. Without responsibility the group will fail.

As hooks (1994: 152) writes,

'That's the difference education as the practice of freedom makes. The bottom-line assumption has to be that everyone in the classroom has to act responsibly. That has to be the starting point – that we are able to act responsibly together to create a learning environment. All too often we have been trained as professors to assume students are not capable of acting responsibly, that is we don't exert control over them, then there's just going to be mayhem.

Collaboration extends to peers. Peers can offer an invaluable resource to each other as they relate to each others' experiences. Wheatley and Keller-Rogers (1996: 53) write,

When we link up with others, we open ourselves to yet another paradox. While surrendering some of our freedom, we open ourselves to even more creative forms of expression. This stage of being has been described as communion, because we are preserved as our selves but are shorn of our separateness or aloneness. What we bring to others remains our self-expression. Yet the meaning of who we are changes through our communion with them. We are identifiable as our selves. But we have discovered new meaning and different contributions, and we are no longer the same.

Learning becomes co-creative. However, the shift from passivity to agency can seem threatening, if not frankly overwhelming. Again, quoting hooks (1994: 143),

> The difficulty getting students to take responsibility is that they have already learnt that they are not the ones with legitimate authority. Students have learnt the left brain approach and expect to be taught in the manner they are accustomed to.

However, the teacher/guide is mindful of this transitional period and sensitive to power relations between self and other(s). She acknowledges the ideological basis of her teaching, mindful not to impose collaboration in any hegemonic or contradictory way. How are we doing?

Laura: Thanks, Ken. Adding this pedagogical slant is helpful. It both informs and strengthens our dialogue. As I said, we have a broad canvas. It would be useful to consider staff development for our next large meeting.

One Month Later

Staff Development

Ken: With regard to staff development. We plan to establish teacher-guided reflection groups for all staff to mirror the proposed student groups. Same numbers, same contract,[6] expertly guided but less frequent! In fact we suggest monthly. After six sessions the groups will revert to being peer-led with an expert guide shadowing. After 12 sessions we are on our own.

Art and Performance Workshops

Candice: We know that learners are either verbal or visual. I am verbal, although I live with an artist. I have been inspired and encouraged to engage art more overtly in some of my own narratives. Just look at the work by Cameron et al. (2008) and Gaydos (2008). Such powerful stuff! *We envisage* engaging students in art and drama workshops, perhaps sharing curriculum with other practice disciplines, art and drama faculties. Take a topic like stroke. The traditional approach would be to set learning objectives and then sequentially move through anatomy and physiology, aetiology, signs and symptoms, medical treatment and patient care. No different than with a host of other medical conditions.

Imagine – taking a class of 50 students and dividing the class into five groups of ten. Imagine a one-day workshop collaborating with drama and dance teachers, perhaps a shared class with drama students that introduces the group to drama technique. Imagine setting out five projects around medical disorders, for example – stroke, depression, myocardial infarction, receiving chemotherapy, dementia. Imagine prepping the group to talk to patients, relatives, nurses, doctors and other healthcare workers, to gain their perspectives of living with and treating these health disorders. Imagine the student practitioners reading the literature and then putting together a performance around caring for a patient to perform to their colleagues. The students take responsibility. The performance is stunning. They say, 'We have learnt so much.' The other projects are equally brilliant. The buzz about the place is great. Learning is both profound and fun. What odds are there that the students learn more through performance than lecture?[7]

Laura: Indeed, what odds? Why not set up a project to test the viability and impact of this. Perhaps with one of your student groups, Candice?

Journal Entry 2

A first-year student nurse suggests that students always focus on negative experiences for two reasons; first, that's what teachers expect, and secondly, how can you reflect on a positive experience? He gave an example of a male patient thanking him for giving him a bath – 'What is there to reflect upon?'

I say, 'Tell me, how do you feel if patients don't thank you? Does it make you feel differently towards them than those who do thank you?'
The student looks at me. 'I don't know, I've never thought about that.'
'Well, think about it.'
'I suppose I do expect to be thanked. Some patients are very grumpy whatever you do to help them.'
'Do you know the literature on the unpopular patient?'
'It's been mentioned in class, but I haven't read it specifically.'
'I suggest you do, and consider the idea of the "grumpy patient". Do male patients like being bathed/touched by male nurses?'
'Again, I've never considered that. The gender thing. It's never come up in the class. Sounds like more homework!'

These questions (and perhaps many more) seem obvious, yet it was not the student's natural way to think. What is normal on the surface becomes potentially problematic when the surface of the experience is scratched to expose deeper significance. The student's experience suggests the need for guidance perceptive enough to pose these types of questions. Such a rich teaching opportunity stemming from one line – '*A male patient thanked me for helping him bathe.*'

Journal Entry 3

The first-year MSc Leadership in Healthcare programme. It is our fifth session. Rick (yet again) raises concern with what is expected of the second assignment. Patiently, I explain it requires a reflection on a specific experience that explores the creative tension between realising your vision of leadership and an understanding of your current reality. I sense his anxiety – his need to know exactly what is required. I ask (perhaps slightly less patiently), 'What is your problem?' It stems from his uncertainty with reflective writing – his ability to 'get it'.

When we explore this difficulty it emerges that many of the students have no meaningful learning experience with reflection. So, even though it is a master's programme I must respond to them as reflective novices. I cannot assume a prior knowledge. Many of the students do not keep a reflective journal. Between sessions they get caught up in their everyday work-worlds.

Lucy asserts she does reflect, but does this in her head. I make the point that she needs to write it down – that something deeper happens when we write it down and move into disciplined reflection. She agrees that in writing she is more attentive to the experience. The students agree they must be more disciplined to set aside time to write and reflect. I state my frustration that they are not writing their journals. I know it is early days and this is a familiar pattern but, slipping into an unhelpful parental mode, I nag them to take responsibility for their learning. Not good dialogue! I assert that the connection between this activity, at this early stage of the programme, and becoming a mindful leader is vital. Yet I know from experience, that the more they invest in systematic serious reflection at this stage the more they will benefit from the programme and succeed at assignments. We agree to spend the next 30 minutes of the session writing and reflecting to get into a reflective groove. We agree that the students will bring two experiences, one self-affirming and one problematic, to the next session.

Journal Entry 4

Lucy shares an experience. It is very descriptive. I challenge her with the MSR cues – notably, 'How did she and others feel within the situation'? She laughs nervously. Her feelings are not easily expressed.

'Perhaps anger?' I suggest
'Yes, I did feel angry at my colleague,' she reluctantly confesses.
'So why is it difficult to admit?'
'I don't know.'
'Well?'
'Well, anger isn't easy to admit. I need to be more poised.'
'What do the group think?' I ask expansively
Someone says, 'Could you not be angry, given the situation again?'
'I don't know. This woman gets under my skin.'
I say, 'Anger is an embodied response. Lucy – consider the "influences grid".[8] Better still, the whole group consider this and put yourself in Lucy's shoes.'

In the ensuing dialogue a culture of conflict and conflict avoidance emerges.
Someone asks, 'Why does so much conflict exist?'
Someone responds, 'So why does it?'
Lucy responds, 'Perhaps because we are frustrated in trying to realise our visions of practice as a reality. That's a problem with vision – it makes you think, and when you

think you get frustrated and see all these people blocking you. Perhaps it's better not to have a vision and put your head down. Turn a blind eye to injustice and rationalise it's not my responsibility.'

I say, 'Behaviours are governed by socialised patterns of authority, tradition and embodiment. As such, it's not an easy culture to shift, certainly from any rational perspective. Note Fay (1987).'

Lucy is in the groove, 'Yeah, Fay is a great book, although not that easy to appreciate on first reading. A new language. Issues of control and unspoken hostility weave a toxic mix to demoralise staff. I feel confronted as a leader to shift this, at least within my scope of responsibility.'

Someone adds, 'It becomes a moral quest but do you have the courage to achieve this?'

I say, 'We can pick it up next session.'

The group buzzes. I sense their subversive hackles rise towards action. The tension between the transactional organisation and a transformational type leadership becomes clearer.

Journal Entry 5

Platzer et al. (2000) note that students may resist revealing self. Cotton (2001) makes the same point. Cotton also suggests that reflection is a type of surveillance, assessment and control. Yet education is always a socialisation process. If teachers use reflection from a teacher-centred perspective, then it is likely be resisted. Plazer et al. (2000) must be more specific about context. They further noted that the nurses' previous educational experience made the self-directed approach associated with the adult-learning process difficult, as nurses had not been encouraged to think for themselves. Of course, this is not the fault of reflection. It is the dominance of a received type of knowledge. Resistance can only be expected and played with. Reflection has been shown to be beneficial in enabling students to develop self-awareness and caring potential (Novelestsky-Rosenthal and Solomon 2001).

Journal Entry 6

A study, involving 50 students from one cohort in their final-year degree course in community healthcare nursing, sought to ascertain whether the students found reflection to be a meaningful activity, whether there are perceived benefits associated with reflective practice, and whether it is a valid process on which to access the outcomes of the course relating to the competencies of specialist practice (Smith and Jack 2005). The data were collected via a web-based discussion board and focus-group interview. The findings neither fully support or refute the usefulness of reflective practice. It became apparent that the student's learning style was pertinent to his or her perception of the usefulness of reflection. However, it is not possible to draw any insight from this study because it paid no attention to the quality and exposure of the student's reflective experience. Clearly such variables are paramount to appreciate in judging the efficacy of reflective learning.

Journal Entry 7

Email from Marcia Ring, University of Vermont, August 2008:

I can't believe this is the first time I am writing to you since June when you graced us with your presence and wisdom. Some of the Masters in Expanded Psychiatric Nursing (MEPN) students found your work and conference life altering. I even changed the final assignment for the MEPN students in psych to allow them to do their final Interpersonal Process Recording utilizing your method. Only one took advantage of that but it was truly stunning. If you like, I can find out if I can send it to you. You'd love it. I think she should publish it'.

Skill Box

- *If you are a teacher, take action towards creating a reflective environment in your teaching practice. To start with, replace a theory-led session with a practice-led session through sharing a story that encapsulates the theory. Open a dialogical space so students can relate to your story with their experiences. Evaluate the experience.*
- *Question what a reflective curriculum should be like at meetings and conversations. Share your evaluations.*
- *Students – challenge the way your curriculum is delivered from a reflective practice perspective. Remember – it's your learning and your learning is vital!*

Summary

The shift from a technical rational to a professional identity and artistry curriculum is a revolution in terms of pedagogy. However, if we are ever to have reflective practitioners we require compatible educational and clinical environments. If not, then we will always be scratching at the surface of what being a reflective practitioner might mean. Scratching that becomes painful to the point whereby even bothering is just a waste of effort. A reflective curriculum necessarily turns on its head the traditional relationship between teachers and students, and between theory and practice. Reflective learning cannot simply be bolted on to an existing technical rational curriculum without it being perceived as itself a technical rational perspective. It requires committed and courageous reflective teachers and teacher programmes that promote reflective practice.[9]

In Chapter 10 Margaret Graham explores the value of story in creating a reflective learning environment.

Endnotes

1 This was prior to the development of the 17th edition (Table 3.2).
2 NHS Forward Review 2015 (https://www.england.nhs.uk/wp-content/uploads/2014/10/5yfv-web.pdf, accessed 16 December 2016).
3 http://www.nmc.org.uk/standards/revalidation/provisional-revalidation-requirements/ (accessed 16 December 2016).
4 *Future Shock* is a book written by the futurist Alvin Toffler in 1970. In the book, Toffler defines the term 'future shock' as a certain psychological state of individuals and entire societies. His shortest definition for the term is a personal perception of 'too much change in too short a period of time' (https://en.wikipedia.org/wiki/Future_Shock).

5 Force field analysis offers an effective reflective framework in change management for looking at forces for driving or resisting change in relation to the status quo. The theory suggests that change agents should focus primarily on minimising resisting forces, as strengthening driving forces would lead to strengthening resistance.

6 I explore guidance and contracting in Chapter 5.

7 This idea is explored further in Chapter 16.

8 See Table 3.4.

9 See Chapters 17 and 18 where Adenike Akinbode reflects on becoming a reflective teacher of teachers and its impact in teaching teachers.

References

Ausubel, D. (1967) *Learning theory and classroom practice*. Ontario Institute for Studies in education, Toronto.

Beauchamp, C. (2015) Reflection in teacher education: issues emerging from a review of current literature. *Reflective Practice* 16.1, 123–141.

Bulley, C. et al. (2005) Sports physiotherapy competencies and standards. https://www.physiosinsport.org/media/wysiwyg/SPTCompetencies_Standards.pdf (accessed 17 December 2016).

Cameron, D. et al. (2008) Expressing voice and developing practical wisdom on social justice through art. In C. Delmar and C. Johns (eds.), *The good, the wise, and the right clinical nursing practice*. Aalborg Hospital, Arhus University Hospital, Denmark, pp. 59–72.

Clarke, N. M. (2014) A person-centred enquiry into the teaching and learning experiences of reflection and reflective practice — Part one. *Nurse Education Today* 34, 1219–1224.

Cotton, A. (2001) Private thoughts in public spheres: issues in reflection and reflective practices in nursing. *Journal of Advanced Nursing* 36.4, 512–519.

Fay, B. (1987) *Critical social science*. Polity Press, Cambridge.

Gaydos, H. (2008) Collage: an aesthetic process for creating phronesis in nursing. In C. Delmar and C. Johns (eds.), *The good, the wise, and the right clinical nursing practice*. Aalborg Hospital, Arhus University Hospital, Denmark, pp. 163–178.

hooks, b (1994) *Teaching to transgress: education as the practice of freedom*. Routledge, New York.

Johns, C. (2013) *Becoming a reflective practitioner* (4th ed.), Wiley-Blackwell, Oxford.

Johns, C. (2014) An enquiry into the spiritual. *International Practice Development Journal* 3 (2) [9].

Krishnamurti, J. (1996) *Total Freedom*. Harper, San Francisco.

Lewin, K. (1951) *Field Theory in Social Science*. Harper and Row. New York.

Mann, K., Gordon, J. and Macleod, A. (2009) Reflection and reflective practice in health professions education: a systematic review. *Advances in Health Science Education* 14, 595–621.

Mc Carthy J., Cassidy, I. and Tuohy, D. (2013) Lecturers' experiences of facilitating guided group reflection with pre-registration BSc Nursing students. *Nurse Education Today* 33, 36–40.

McGrath, D. and Higgins, A. (2006) Implementing and evaluating reflective practice group sessions. *Nurse Education in Practice* 6.3, 175–181.

Novelestsky-Rosenthal, H. and Solomon, K. (2001) Reflections on the use of Johns' model of structured reflection in nurse-practitioner education. *International Journal for Human Caring* 5.2, 21–26.

Nowlen, P. (1988) *A new approach to continuing education for business and the professions*. Macmillan, Old Tappen, NJ. O'Connor, A., Hyde, A. and Treacey, M. (2003) Nurse teachers' constructions of reflection and reflective practice. (Qualitative research into tutors' perceptions and experiences of using reflection with diploma nursing students in Ireland.) *Reflective Practice* 4.2, 107–119.

O'Donovan, M., (2007) Implementing reflection: insights from pre-registration mental health students. *Nurse Education Today* 27.6, 515–664.

Paterson, C. and Chapman, J. (2013) Enhancing skills of critical reflection to evidence learning in professional practice. *Physical Therapy in Sport* 14, 133–138.

Pirsig, R. (1974) *Zen and the art of motorcycle maintenance.* Vintage, London.

Platzer, H., Blake, D. and Ashford, D. (2000) Barriers to learning from reflection; a study of the use of groupwork with post-registration nurses. *Journal of Advanced Nursing* 31.5, 1001–1008.

Ramsey, S. (2010) Making thinking public: reflection in elementary teacher education. *Reflective Practice: International and Multidisciplinary perspectives* 11, 205–216.

Rolfe, G. (2014) Rethinking reflective education: what would Dewey have done? *Nurse Education Today* 34, 1179–1183.

Russell, T. (2013) Has reflective practice done more harm than good in teacher education? *Phronesis* 2, 80–88.

Ryan, M. (2013) The pedagogical balancing act: teaching reflection in higher education. *Teaching in Higher Education* 18.2, 144–155.

Schön, D. (1983) *The reflective practitioner.* Avebury, Aldershot.

Smith, A. and Jack, K. (2005) Reflective: a meaningful task for students. *Nursing Standard* 19.26, 33-37.

Toffler, A. (1973) *Future Shock.* Pan Books, London.

Chapter 10

A Teaching Dilemma Journal Entry

Christopher Johns

> At every turn I am faced with a dilemma the mind creates and which
> only intuition can resolve

Teaching is never routine. There is always a choice as to the effective approach. Yet knowing the most effective choice is complex. Every teaching session is different, although it may feel similar to previous teaching experiences. In fact, too similar, as I churn out the same old stuff time after time, irrespective of the actual students present. How easy it is to become complacent and unreflective when teaching becomes merely a task to do, a functional exercise, rather than a deeply interactive encounter.

Today I am faced with the *dilemma* of how to best to deliver a session on reflective practice. The session is part of a university's School of Health Professions lecture series. The invitation is from the Professor of Physiotherapy. The audience will be a mixture of practitioners, teachers and researchers spanning healthcare disciplines, including physiotherapy clinical educators who mentor university students in clinical practice where reflection is part of the curriculum. Possibly 50 people are expected to attend. The venue is a lecture theatre. What are their expectations? The professor is vague – the clinical educators would like something on reflective practice. The time slot is one hour. Time is like a void – how to fill it? As I see it, I have three fundamental approaches:

- Give a theory lecture and answer questions
- Give a narrative exemplar that encapsulates reflective practice to open a dialogue
- A mixture of the above – narrative as an exemplar (lecture first or story first?)

Turning over the options, I wonder what approach would work best? I naturally lean towards a narrative approach rather than theory. Narrative is applied theory. It paints a whole picture, enabling the audience to engage with the experience and its insights. However, I am uncertain. I know that the audience often do not respond well to a narrative approach, especially if the audience is large, unknown, has a technical rational background, with vague expectations, and are gathered in a lecture theatre. The limitation

Becoming a Reflective Practitioner, Fifth Edition. Edited by Christopher Johns.
© 2017 John Wiley & Sons Ltd. Published 2017 by John Wiley & Sons Ltd.
Companion Website: www.wiley.com/go/johns/reflectivepractitioner

of time is also problematic. Sometimes a dilemma is so great that the practitioner simply does not know what approach to take. Dilemmas create anxiety, as I have now. Yet I have experience of all three approaches, so why am I having difficulty?

I walk with Jerry, my Labrador retriever, along the flat lode path that twists around Carn Brea. We walk this path most mornings. Walking with Jerry helps me *bring the mind home* to focus on this dilemma. I do not want to grasp the dilemma tightly. If I do, thinking suffocates ideas. Dilemmas need to breathe. It hits me. Perhaps I can start the session with my dilemma of preparing for the session – to reveal the tension between a technical rational (lecture) and professional artistry (narrative) approaches. It is a tension that reverberates at the core of any professional curriculum that aspires towards reflection. Perhaps I shouldn't worry about my audience's expectations given their expected number and diversity, but simply focus on my own expectations. Focusing on the idea of dilemma, I can draw comparison with the dilemmas that face practitioners in everyday practice, as a form of reflective modelling. In this way I can tune the audience to an aspect of their everyday practice and how reflection may help reframe the situation either as anticipatory (as in my case), within practice, or afterwards through reflection-on-experience.

Back at the cottage Jerry curls up on the sofa. I decide to tell the story about my dilemma of preparing for the session. Then what? What theory would be helpful to include? I need to talk about the value of story at some point within the session and key issues with a reflective curriculum, possibly defining reflection and a model of reflection. Theory pressure building! What theory to bring in and what to leave out – pressure on the time space. I have one hour and would like to dialogue for 30 minutes. But will they be a dialogical audience? I imagine being asked questions rather than dialoguing if time is limited. It is the usual pattern of these events. I doodle a PowerPoint slide on the value of story.[1] I have no standard list for this. I let the list settle. More value of story will surface later as if the mind continues to work below the radar.

I need to give my audience some background of my reflective practice roots; being a lecturer-practitioner at Burford Community Hospital and how I reframed the rehabilitation care modules as part of the BSc degree programme at Oxford Polytechnic – linking this reframing from a reflective perspective to my dilemma in preparing the session today.

Key points:

- The modules had ten two-hour sessions over a ten-week placement. The first time I prepared the module I constructed 'typical' or 'archetypal' stories based on patients I had nursed, representing common conditions clinically experienced at the hospital. This approach is similar to a problem-based learning approach.
- The second time I taught the module I prepared students to write and share their own stories of working with patients at Burford. This realisation was like an awakening.
- I asked myself, 'How will the students react if I teach through story?' I imagined the lament, 'Give us the facts.' Students know the lecture approach, and learning outcomes ('By the end of the session the student is able to …') are the bread and butter of teaching. Writing modules at the university is prescribed in such a way, the logic being the student knows what to expect. Yet the risk is that the teacher becomes chained to organising the teaching to meet these outcomes. However, the students reported that learning had become more responsible, more intense and more enjoyable.
- The significance of contracting this approach with the students: surprisingly I met little resistance. I say surprisingly because, as hooks (1994) writes, 'the urge to experiment

with pedagogical practices may not be welcomed by students who often expect us to teach in the manner they are accustomed to'.

Yet, I didn't consider whether the students would appreciate my storied approach, wrapped up as I was in this new reflective paradigm.

- My thinking about a 'story approach' was inspired by reading reflective theory, notably its potential for bridging the theory-practice gap by 'feeding in' theory as context of experience, so that theory became subjective and contextual rather than abstract – experience being the hook to hang theory on. Students reported that theory became more alive and more meaningful.
- The coherence of a reflective approach to learning and supervising the students' clinical practice.
- The students have their own objectives as set by the university. As a reflective teacher I asserted that meeting their learning objectives is the students' responsibility, not mine, and that my role was to service this need. In other words, they must view me as an expert resource.
- As a consequence, teaching from a reflective perspective radically shifts the power differential within the teacher–student relationship by giving voice to the students' experiences. The student sharing her experience holds centre stage and invites the audience's response. However, my authoritative voice cannot be denied. Its presence is always there and yet I can quieten it to enable other voices to powerfully rise. I become the servant, servicing the dialogue in ways that ensure an effective learning experience.
- Guiding learning is a process of caring to enable the students to grow, based on Mayeroff's (1971) idea that caring is enabling the other person to grow. This mirrors listening to the patient's story and enabling the patient to grow through her own illness narrative: coherence between learning process and outcome.

I bullet-point these issues onto a PowerPoint.

Order of play:

- Ask the group their expectations of today's session
- Dilemma; story of preparing the session
- Link dilemma to teaching at Burford and the significant issues that arose
- Link dilemmas to everyday practice and decision making, using a model for clinical judgment (see Figure 4.2)
- Value of writing story (see Table 2.2)
- Definition of reflective practice and points arising
- Key curriculum issues to consider within a reflective curriculum
- General dialogue

The Actual Session

As it was, in the actual session, I fell between two stools. The audience had not thought of their expectations. I immediately sensed a dilemma of whether to dig these out. But I didn't. I sensed the 'time trap'. I let it pass by and moved on to my 'dilemma story'. This was received without comment. Narratives take time. Talking through theory takes time. Surfacing issues takes time. By the time I worked through the above agenda there were just 10 minutes remaining for dialogue. Ploughing through the set of PowerPoints I failed to open any meaningful dialogical space, despite my invitation to dialogue at any point during my presentation. Perhaps the audience, transfixed by PowerPoint, passively sat back to receive the knowledge. I could not adjust within the actual session, as if my plan had wrapped me up. The audience raised two questions which I tried to answer rather than give back to the questioners, as I would normally do from a reflective perspective: the time trap closing.

Could I have done it better? Perhaps I could have used a *dialogical* approach grounded in the audience's own stories, expectations and issues, simply open a dialogical space and keep my own stories, theory and issues on the back burner just in case they were required. In other words, pursuing their expectations and throwing my teaching plan out of the window. *Teaching plans are a trap*, especially when the plan is as unrealistic as mine with its intended narrative and theory input.

There are no prescriptions but there are many paths. Knowing which path to take is fraught with uncertainty. Yet at the end the audience were appreciative. The organisers said the session had helped them to think about reflection within the curriculum. But I was left dissatisfied that I hadn't found the right balance.

Three Months Later

I give a session on reflective practice at a local hospital. A mixed disciplinary group of 12 healthcare practitioners. A small room. One and a half hours. I approach it from a dialogical approach by raising a number of issues presented on a PowerPoint. The practitioners are reticent. In my anxiety, I begin to answer the issues myself, feeding in theory. An hour passes. I sense we are becoming stuck. Reframing, I decide to share a story but then someone shifts the dialogue to another issue. Plenty of unstructured dialogue, but I felt responsible for ensuring it happened. I should have more faith in dialogue, but with an unknown audience it isn't easy.

As with the Plymouth session, should I have commenced with their expectations rather than my issues? Why didn't I do that and keep my issues on the back burner in case their expectations were not forthcoming? I sense my embodiment, brought up on lectures and control, still struggling to break free even after years of effort. Perhaps reflective practice makes me think too much. I risk, experiment and learn. At least I assume I learn. Risk evokes anxiety of getting it right. But then, what is the right way? Is it an embodied sense of fitting in with curriculum objectives or people's expectations? Perhaps it is both, and there is the rub: reflective practices by their very nature are subversive and perhaps engender audience anxiety in that no one quite knows how to respond, especially if it comes 'out of the blue'.

Summary

You might imagine that an experienced teacher and workshop facilitator would take such teaching sessions in his stride. It is as if reflection has disturbed my normal function of the mind, creating mountains from molehills. The shadow of the dominant technical rational approach is long, simply because I always sense, especially with groups I do not know, that that is what they expect, and I remain anxious about failing them. As such I always at risk of falling between two stools, but then no one said that teaching from a reflective perspective is easy.

In Chapter 11 I offer an exemplar of reflective writing as an assignment at degree level and how such work might be graded.

Endnote

1   See Table 2.2.

References

Hooks, B (1994) *Teaching to transgress: education as the practice of freedom.* Routledge, New York.

Mayeroff, M. (1971) *On caring.* Harper Perennial, New York.

Chapter 11

Life Begins at 40

Christopher Johns

Write from the body without fear of the teacher's rod

Introduction

What should a student's written reflective assignment look like? This is a challenging and perhaps vexing question. Assignments are designed to test the student's achievement of curriculum objectives, whether as an essay, portfolio, case study or suchlike, with a deepening criticality through academic levels. From a reflective perspective, criticality means the ability to critique and juxtapose theory with insights gained through reflection, which are assimilated into personal knowing, as evidenced through subsequent experiences.[1] Much of practice knowing is uncertain, where applying theory becomes the professional artistry of interpretation. From a technical rational perspective, criticality refers to the ability to critique theory in an abstract way, with little if any practice evidence to support its value to inform practice.

However, there is much more to learning than applying theory to practice. This may be hard to see if teachers view learning through a technical rational lens. In contrast, professional artistry covers the whole gamut of practice knowing.

One way to consider writing an assignment is through understanding the marking criteria constructed to judge it, usually across a range of grades. However, this demands that the marking criteria adequately reflect the task. For example, Table 11.1 sets out the grading criteria grid for an *essay with reflection at degree level* applied at the University of Bedfordshire. Examining the grid suggests it has been designed from an essentially technical rational perspective and the reflective element added on, with little emphasis given to insights drawn from reflection. Indeed, the grading categories are vague and not easy to interpret. Such profiles are unsatisfactory. Reflective assignments should always be grounded in the exploration of insights. There can be no other approach. There is no need to test the application of a model of reflection. These are *merely* heuristic devices, a means towards an end, although skill in utilising a reflective model is vital towards realising insight.

A specifically designed reflective marking grid is shown in Table 11.2. This grid utilises a fail/pass grading at master's level. You might argue that the ethical and personal influences

Becoming a Reflective Practitioner, Fifth Edition. Edited by Christopher Johns.
© 2017 John Wiley & Sons Ltd. Published 2017 by John Wiley & Sons Ltd.
Companion Website: www.wiley.com/go/johns/reflectivepractitioner

Table 11.1   Example of an inadequate reflective assignment marking grid

University of Bedfordshire

Faculty of Health and Social Sciences
2010 Grading Profile – Essay with reflection   Insert unit code (   )   Level 3   *V3fm 2010*   Form 1 of 1

Weighting as a %	Criteria	Fail 0,1 F 2,3, E4	D- 5 D 6 D+ 7	C- 8 C 9 C+ 10	B- 11 B 12 B+13	A- 14 A 15 A+16	Self grade	Assessor grade
	Focus on the task set	Has addressed the task set in a superficial manner with some evidence of focus & structure	Has focused on the task set in a descriptive but reasonably structured manner	Has focused on the task set in a logical and reasonably structured manner	Has focused clearly on the task set in a structured manner with some evidence of originality	Has focused clearly on the task in an insightful, original and critical manner		
	Issue Handling	Some relevant issues are described and used in a superficial manner	Some relevant issues are described and some understanding of them is evident	A range of relevant issues are selected and handled with evidence of some analysis	A range of issues are handled competently showing skills of analysis and some synthesis	Issues are analysed in a competent and considered manner demonstrating good skills of synthesis		
	Presentation & written expression	Presentation is acceptable but improvements could be made. Meaning generally clear, but does not always get to the point. Some grammatical and spelling errors	Presentation is acceptable. Gets to the point, although clarity could be improved. A few grammatical and/or spelling errors	Presentation acceptable, generally logical & neat, adding to the value of the work. Meaning clear with good written expression. Few grammatical and/or spelling errors seen	Presentation shows care and is logical adding to the value of the work. Meaning clear with an articulate, fluent written style. Only a few grammatical and/or spelling errors seen	Presentation is excellent with significant care and attention to detail. Written expression is also clear, articulate, accurate and to the point. Very few written expression errors seen		
	Reflection	Some evidence that reflection has been achieved but it lacks structure and insight	Evidence that reflection has taken place with limited structure and insight	The reflection has some structure demonstrating limited but useful insight into the value of experience	The reflection shows structure and analysis demonstrating that significant learning has taken place	The reflection is structured, critical, and insightful demonstrating clear evidence of learning		
	Use of current / specific knowledge and theory	Some evidence of relevant knowledge and theory but limited, at times dated, and very descriptive in nature	The knowledge and theory cited is generally relevant but lacks some understanding. Parts of this may be dated	A reasonable understanding of knowledge and theory is demonstrated with relevant recent material included	Understanding and analysis of the knowledge and theory base is clear including recent relevant material	Shows an in-depth understanding of the knowledge and theory base analysed achieving significant levels of synthesis		
	Use and quality of referencing	A barely adequate or relevant number of references with some referencing errors being seen	An adequate number of references. Generally cited correctly but with some errors. More care was required	An appropriate number of references are used and generally cited correctly and integrated well. Few errors	Referencing is correct, consistently supporting & enhancing the quality of the work. Few errors	Referencing is correct. It follows the guidelines given to the letter and consistently supports and enhances the work.		
Students name		First markers name/Date		First markers signature		Total score →	Self =	Assessor =
Student number		2nd markers name		2nd markers signature		Attempt 1 / 2	Weighted score*	

Table 11.2 PD Osteopathy: Assignment criteria for reflective essays

	Weighting	Fail	Pass
		Increasing criticality and creativity →	
Clear expression of insights evidenced through reflections on specific experiences	30	Understanding and analysis of knowledge base is limited and superficial to support claimed insights	The experiences chosen for inclusion are central to the insights. They are analysed competently and creatively to support the emergence of insights
Consideration of ethical factors around the notion of the right thing to do and congruence with my values	10	Little evidence of an ethical understanding for practice. Inadequate reflection on the impact of one's values and intentions to guide practice	A robust insight into the value of ethics and values to guide practice showing a clear appreciation of the nature of ethical dilemmas
Consideration of personal factors, including past experiences, that were influencing my responses	10	Little evidence of appreciating the impact of personal factors and previous experiences in shaping responses	The significance of personal factors and past experiences in influencing clinical judgement and action is critically analysed, revealing a deep sense of self
Critical juxtaposition between an informing literature and insights	20	Limited range of literature explored with over-reliance on secondary sources. Weak dialogue between the literature and insights resulting in unconvincing juxtaposition	A broad range of primary sources is evident, with good critical analysis and juxtaposition leading to compelling and creative insight development
Consideration of how insights will shift my future practice	10	Unconvincing claims as to how insights might shift practice with insubstantial consideration of the ability of self to act on insights	A clear exposition of the way insights might or have shifted practice alongside an appreciation of those factors that might constrain responding in new ways
The paper is presented in a suitable scholarly/esthetic manner	20	The structure is fragmented. Written expression makes some of the arguments difficult to access. Lack of appropriate signposting and planning. Careless referencing.	Written expression and presentation are clear and concise. Arguments put forward succinctly. Paper is well structured and flows coherently throughout around insights.
	100		

Module: Reflective Practice [Code:]

Name of student

1st marker   2nd marker

might be combined into a new category that states something like, 'What influencing factors constrained realising desirable practice?' However, you might also argue that understanding such influencing factors is itself an insight. If so, why use any grading criteria beyond the identification and exploration of insights? A problem with all criteria is that they encourage conformity to fit in with criteria. Rather like viewing a patient through assessment criteria, it limits the view and stifles the imagination, which, from a reflective perspective, is unhelpful to say the least. Perhaps the aesthetic quality of description should be graded, as reflective writing should engage the reader.[2] Insights should be built into narrative to illuminate their context and show how the practitioner grasped and responded to the particular situation, clearly a vital aspect of professional artistry. Insight without description is sterile. Presumably, insights could simply be listed, but this would take them out of context and the 'whole' picture distorted. The other element that may require grading is reflection on the learning process, given the significance of becoming a reflective practitioner. Reflective criticality would be reflected in the exploration of insights.

As such, a potential grading of a reflective assignment might reasonably be:

20 per cent description/construction of narrative

80 per cent exploration of insights

Of course, this is a moveable feast. Designing congruent ways to grade any assignment is complex, and yet it is vital to get it right. Recently I read, 'Passing people by'[3] to fourth-year nursing students. I asked them to grade the work. I was given A1, the highest grade. I asked the students if they wrote assignments like mine. They unequivocally replied, 'No.' Being caught up in grading criteria and the demand for references stifled the creative process. Within universities, it is normal to view all assignments from a technical rational bias, and consequently heavily weight 'theoretical framing'. However, this is just one side of knowing. Of course, such is the dominance of rational thinking that no professional artistry bias exists. A synthesis between technical rationality and professional artistry is akin to the difference between separate and connected knowing, leading to constructed knowing (Belenky et al. 1986), which provides a potentially useful way to balance the whole brain and, as such, to view learning and grading.

What follows is Clare's final written assignment that required her to 'draw insights from reflection on a number of experiences and the learning process'. The assignment was written as the final assignment of 'Becoming a reflective and effective practitioner'.[4]

Skill Box

- Before reading the 'assignment', familiarise yourself with the assignment grids set out in Tables 11.1 and 11.2. Critique them for their relevance to grade degree-level reflective assignments. Compare these profiles with any grading criteria currently in use within your practice and reflect on the differences.

Clare writes,

It was Pitkin (1932) who coined the phrase life begins at forty, and how right he was. The first day I attended the course[5] also happened to be my 40th birthday and where my life as a reflective practitioner was to begin, although at that point in time, I could not have envisaged the significant impact and influence the course would have on me. What follows is the story of how my practice developed as result and an analysis of factors that constrained my development. This will be illustrated through a series of experiences I wrote in my reflective journal, which, when viewed alone are perhaps not of great significance. However, like a children's dot-to-dot picture, it is only when the dots are joined together that a tangible picture becomes clear.

At the beginning of the course I recorded my feelings and thoughts at the end of the day on a separate piece of paper in my journal. I felt I was reflecting. This made me question why I needed to be on an eight-month course to do this. Initially I was silent within the group rather like a passive resister. It was only when I began to share my experiences within the group did I realise that all I was doing was stating what had happened and how I had felt. It was when I was challenged and *forced* to examine my feelings and view the situation from different perspectives that I started to learn from my experiences. However it still took some weeks and a comment from the group's guide who informed me that, 'an effective practitioner is an informed practitioner', for me to ashamedly acknowledge to myself that knowledge acquisition does not happen magically but does in fact require a degree of effort on my part. It wasn't until the fifth session that I took the risk to seriously participate. Before then my participation had been zilch. I had been a passenger. I said something like 'I have something to share.'

Within my current practice one of my clinical responsibilities is to perform Electrocardiographs (ECG) for all the inpatient units of the hospital. Initially I found this interesting. However, once the novelty had worn off I viewed it as a task that had to be done. My lack of enthusiasm was quite evident in my journal entries until one day following an attempt to perform an ECG my journal entry was very different:

'*When I arrived on the ward I was shown in to the ladies bedroom I introduced my self and started to explain the procedure the nurse interrupted me stating that I was wasting my time, 'she doesn't understand a word you are saying, she has dementia'. My anger levels rose but I carried on trying not to let my feelings show, the lady looked at me with watery pale blue eyes and speaking in a language of her own was trying to tell me something but I was unable to understand her, she kept tugging at my arm getting more frustrated with tears falling down her cheeks. I reassured her that I would not be performing the ECG and left the ward. The image of her eyes stayed with me, had they once been sparkling deep blue, full of life and what had those eyes seen in their 82 years of existence. I felt disgust with the nurse for treating her with disparagement and disrespect but I also had to acknowledge the uncomfortable feelings within myself about my view of performing an ECG as an tedious task and had appreciating the privilege of entering into this intimate relationship ...*'

I would have liked to confront the nurse but I let it go. Swallowed my disgust but it left a nasty taste. I must admit I am a conflict avoider but then I guess most nurses are. The impact this experience had on me was immense; it enforced me to examine my attitudes, beliefs and focus my thoughts upon the nurse-patient relationship, especially the challenges faced when the patients' ability to communicate is compromised.

I asked myself – What sense do I make of this? Morse (1991) states that the nurse-patient relationship is established as 'the result of interplay or covert negotiations until a mutually satisfying relationship is reached'. She discusses the types of relationships that exists and divides them into two categories, mutual or unilateral. The latter she describes as being asynchronous with one person unwilling or unable to develop the relationship to the desired level of the other. Morse (1991) provides an example of why mutual involvement is not possible, that is when a patient is unconscious or in a psychotic state. Due to the fact that the lady with blue eyes was suffering from dementia automatically forced her into a unilateral relationship.

Rao (1993) believes the act of communication comprises all the ways that people send and receive messages. However Miller (2002) draws to our attention that most people do not think about the way they communicate on a day-to-day basis and are often unaware of how they relate to others yet communication is essential to our development as social beings and it is the ability to communicate that enables the development of short and long-term relationships. What happens then if the ability to communicate becomes impaired? Bush (2003) suggests that people who cannot communicate, or who communicate inappropriately are often marginalized by society and run the risk of social alienation and diminished function and that as a result of the frustration of being unable to make needs and feelings understood by others challenging behaviour and behavioural disturbances can occur. It has been proposed by Lliffe and Drennan (2001) that communication with the patient suffering from dementia may be the key to understanding and resolving behaviour disturbances. One method of communicating with people with dementia is validation therapy, this was developed by Feil (1993) and attempts to help the person deal with their feelings by validating them, subsequently helping them to move from their inner world to the shared reality of the present. It is claimed that validation therapy promotes communication with the severely confused older person on their own terms, on subjects and issues that are chosen and are important to them, assuming that all the words and actions of a person with dementia have a real sense of purpose and value.

Picking up the story; as a consequence of confronting and examining my feelings my attitude towards performing ECGs altered. I no longer viewed it just a task that had to be done as quickly as possible but recognised that although only brief I was engaging in a relationship with another person which should be given time and respect. Having shifted my viewpoint I found that I once again I found performing ECGs a positive experience. I was mindful of this when I received an ECG request from one of the wards that specialises in treating elderly people who are more severely confused suffering from dementia or other organic brain disorders. The name on the ECG request seemed vaguely familiar however I was not prepared for the shock when I was introduced to the lady. Sitting slumped to one side with saliva dribbling out of the corner of her mouth was a lady with whom I had contact with about a year ago when she received a course of ECT to which she responded well. My last memory of her was of a bright smiling physically fit lady in her 50s who was able to return back to her work, which incidentally was as a health care assistant on one of the other elderly wards. This is an extract from my journal entry for that day.

> '*When I first saw her the shock was immense like a jolt of electricity had surged through my body causing my skin to prickle and take a sharp intake of breath, it took me a moment to recover. What message had my face portrayed and had she seen it? How lonely must it be to be trapped inside a body unable to communicate verbally and how must it feel to be reliant upon nurses, with whom you had once worked along side with, to feed, wash and dress you … what is it about this situation that I find so uncomfortable I perform ECGs on other patients who are unable to communicate verbally and do not feel the same. Perhaps the sadness I feel is that she is too young to be treated on an elderly mental health ward and that her own profession has in some way let her down …*'

I remembered the group's guide had recommended an article about silent advocacy (Gadow 1980) and I set about finding it. However, it was then that I started to question my motives for doing this. Was it, that if by being more informed about a situation helps me to become a more effective practitioner or was it to help me resolve my uncomfortable feelings and feel better in myself?

It was this conflict that I shared with the group at the next session. I began by sharing the experience and discussing the conflicts I faced which was helpful, the focus of the discussion wandered slightly with issues around communicating with patients with communication difficulties examined. One of the group members made a comment about how some nurses without realising it treated people as an object and lost sight of the person.

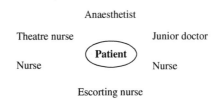

Figure 11.1   People in the treatment room.

That resonated within me. In response I was defensive and categorically stated that within the ECT department people were treated with respect, dignity and as individuals.

But this comment niggled away at me. During the next two ECT sessions I metaphorically took a step back and observed with more critical eyes how we regarded and treated the patients receiving ECT. I was reassured that the mental health nursing team did show respect for the patient, taking time to explain procedures and provide reassurance, although once the patient was asleep the focus of them as a person was lost. One thing that struck me was the amount of people that are present during treatment; on that day seven people, including the patient were in the present in the treatment room [Figure 11.1]. Conversations took place that excluded the patient.

At the next clinical team meeting I shared this experience and my observations, in order to generate discussion I posed some questions. How would you like to be treated if you were to receive ECT, what aspects of our practice are positive and what areas could we improve upon?

In order to gain a better understanding I suggested we recreated the scenario as fully as possible to experience first hand of being on the trolley with people attaching various monitoring equipment to you. Benner (2003) highlights that good nursing practice requires ongoing clinical knowledge development through experiential learning. However, it is not automatic and requires openness, attentiveness and responsible engaged learning on the part of the practitioner. One of the team members was not a willing participant at first but did join in and at the end of the session commented that she had never thought about it from the patient's point of view.

We discussed this exercise within the next team meeting, we all felt it was worthwhile, and that it gave us a better understanding of how the patient feels before they are anaesthetised. What struck us all was how vulnerable and intimidating it felt lying on the trolley with so many people surrounding you. From this we considered ways we could improve our practice, limiting the amount of people surrounding the patient until they are asleep, encouraging the doctors to have discussions about treatment regimes out of earshot of the patients and instead of having the radio on play more soothing and relating music. This exercise was only carried out with the mental health nursing staff who felt it would be beneficial for the whole treatment team to undergo this, particularly with the theatre nurse and the anaesthetist who by the nature of their work spend the majority of the time with unconscious patients.

Morse (1991) highlights, nurses working in operating rooms use a strategy of depersonalisation which includes transforming not only the person into a patient, but of the patient into a case. According to Sisson (1990) hearing is the last sense to go when a person becomes unconscious. Studies of patients' memories of their unconscious state indicate that they heard and understood various conversations that took place while they were unconscious (Tosch, 1998; Podurgiel, 1990; Lawrence, 1995). It is imperative as Leigh (2001) points out that health professionals evaluate the way in which they communicate with unconscious patients. Russell (1999) study concludes that hospitals are often noisy which can make the patient anxious whereas reassurance and explanations by nurses help them to feel safe, secure and feel less vulnerable. This study also found that where nurses became over involved with technical equipment and the physical aspects of care reduced the level of communication with the patient. While Podurgiel (1990), and Green (1996) both recommend that personalised care should be given through the use of effective communication strategies such as speaking directly to the patient and using touch to enhance communication and express emotional support. Dyer (1995) cautions that touch is a two way process and permission should be sought before a nurse invades a patients personal space.

At the end of an ECT session I shared our experiential experience with the theatre nurse, hoping that she would be receptive to the idea of participating in a similar exercise with the anaesthetist. 'Whatever did you want to do a thing like that for?' was her cynical reply. I attempted to explain that I felt it was important to view the care we gave from the patients' perspective. She ridiculed such an idea – 'What a load of poppycock, how do they know what they need, we are the anaesthesiology specialists not them, so how can they possibly know what they need and I certainly do not need to lay on a theatre trolley to know how to do my job.'

She left the department with very ruffled feathers and I felt irritated and disappointed as this extract from my journal entry shows.

'My emotions are all in a muddle like a big ball of spaghetti lying heavy and uncomfortably in the pit of my stomach. I have experienced these feelings before, when I was a child in primary school there was one particular teacher who no matter how hard I tried to please and gain her approval she all ways knocked me back leaving me feeling angry and frustrated and confused. Only now I am not a schoolgirl I am a professional practitioner and believe in what I am trying to achieve. Why do I always let her get to me? Why do I feel intimidated by her and unable to assert myself with her when I can with other people? ...'

When I read this extract in the guided reflection group, Colin [the guide] in his ubiquitous coaxing manner simply asked, 'so why do I let her get to me?' A silence descended over the group as I contemplated this question. Was it a simple identification with a teacher from primary school? How could I know that? I connected this experience to another experience that concerned a junior doctor who was constantly late and on one occasion did not show up at all. I had no hesitation in letting the doctor know my feelings. Colin asked, 'How can you change things?'

I replied, 'I can't imagine how I can.'

He suggested the other group members put themselves in my shoes to imagine how they would like to respond and what might stop them. Like me the group were uncertain. They could feel the conflict.

Colin suggested I use Transactional Analysis [TA] (Berne 1961) to examine the pattern of communication between myself and the theatre nurse. The gist of this theory is that people communicate from learnt ego states – either parent, adult or child. Ideally we should use adult–adult interaction as befits collaborative and responsible professionals. Effective communication is when lines of communication are not crossed – for example adult–adult or parent–child. However, when someone gets anxious they often revert to 'type' and move into either parent or child ego states.

Understanding this theory I discovered the root of the breakdown. The theatre nurse's response was not the adult response I had invited. Instead, it was a cynical dismissive response I linked with the primary school teacher [critical parent]. It conjured up similar feelings that left me seething. I became the 'hurt child'. I had spoken to her as an adult, she responded as a critical parent. Stewart and Joines (1987) describe this as a 'crossed transaction'. *Cross* is an apt description of how I felt! Looking again at how I communicate with the theatre nurse it became evident that I often revert into 'child mode' in response to her 'critical parent mode'.

Colin then talked through TA theory based on parent– adult–child interactions.

'So how can you stop reverting to a hurt child mode?'

I confessed, 'I don't know.'

Colin asked, 'Imagine the situation again – how might you respond differently?'

I mused, 'He's using the MSR cues.' It reminded me of Star Wars and using the force. Uncanny. I smiled, 'Smack her in the teeth!' The group laughed. The spell was broken.

One of the group suggested I might have said, 'You sound just like my primary school teacher' and walk away. A subtle confrontation that keeps my integrity.

Applying the transactional analysis framework was most helpful using the labels of critical parent and hurt child- it enabled me to visualise the relationship between myself and the theatre nurse, and, perhaps most significantly engendered the feelings associated with those labels. It was illuminating and challenging, and prompted me to examine my patterns of communication with other members of the team towards promoting more effective collaborative working.

Deepening Insight

The point of reflection is gaining insight. Whilst these are laced within the above description, I have been starkly reminded of my vision to realise person-centred nursing. I had become complacent! Practice had become routinised as if I was on auto-pilot most of the time. What a wake-up call! My concern for patients was relit. I learnt something about myself and my communication skills improved. Perhaps, most significantly, I acted to create a more therapeutic environment. Checking out insights is significant, because it helps to solidify learning.

One of the biggest factors that hindered my development was myself. At the beginning my attitude was arrogant and the reasons for attending the course were influenced by the educational credits that could be obtained. Although I consistently kept a reflective journal my entries were descriptive, inexpressive and, once written, were not returned to. I am not sure when exactly my transformation happened as it was a gradual process. However I remember feeling uncomfortable when other members of the group shared their journal entries. The words of a teacher who taught spelling came back to me, he said, 'If you cheat you are only deceiving yourself and it will be you who has to face the consequences.' I felt like an impostor, and my atheism would be exposed at any minute. Writing my journal was finding my voice. The emphasis on rich description focused me to pay attention, notably those things I had taken for granted, that had become part of the wallpaper. Perhaps that was why I had initially nothing to say. My lack of voice rendered me silent. Finding voice gave vent to thoughts and feelings, opening my mind to ideas, what Belenky et al. (1986) describe as the subjective voice – 'the quest for self'. Then I could explore, critique and juxtapose a literature to inform my emerging insights – the synthesis of what Belenky et al. term the separate and connected procedural voices [see Table 5.1]. This synthesis moulds the connected voice. It was empowering and led to action. The world became a better place for myself and for patients.

Finding my voiced in my journal empowered me to find my voice in practice to question and challenge. I felt I had shed some dark fear lurking in me, implanted aeons ago during my childhood, schooling and nurse training –'be a good girl- good girls are seen but not heard'. No longer will I be silent or silenced. It is an insult to my integrity to act for the good.

This journey has been lonely at times, but having undergone a complete transformation of my attitude and realised the power that reflection has to change and improve practice, I wanted to share this enlightenment and sought after converting my colleagues to my newfound faith. However in my passionate and over-zealous approach, what I in fact achieved was to alienate my colleagues, not bring them on board. I realised that in order for me to have any influence, a drastic modification of my approach was needed. Put another way, it's no good having a voice if it isn't heard!

There were times on this journey that I became exhausted and on occasions I wished I could remove my reflective lenses and view things through my old eyes. Reflecting daily on my practice constantly highlighted areas that need modification or change. Like a rolling stone gathering moss.

For me one of the immense values of this course was that the process of reflection was guided. Being in the reflective group helped me to remain focused and motivated me to continue on my journey. If my reflective journey had not have been guided, then I feel it may well have been more of a magical mystery tour.

Has attending this course helped me to become an effective practitioner? The answer is unequivocally yes. Although I am a novice in the world of reflection, I realise the potential reflective practice has on shaping the future of our profession whereby we can begin to value our practical expertise as a profession (Bulman 2004).

Grading

Clare's descriptions from her reflective journal gives her narrative richness and authenticity as does the evocative richness of her language, '*the lady looked at me with watery pale blue eyes and speaking in a language of her own, was trying to tell me something ...*'. And later in the same passage, '*the image of those eyes stayed with me: had they once been sparkling and deep blue, full of life, and what had those eyes seen in their 82 years of existence?*' Again in the same passage , '*I felt disgust with the nurse for treating her with disparagement and disrespect but I had to acknowledge the uncomfortable feelings within myself ...*'. In this passage I sense the cathartic and creative impact of writing. It engages the reader. The use of reflective questions is also useful, as they immediately engage the reader put herself in Clare's shoes: '*Why do I always let her get at me?*' I am sure many readers will identify with this sentiment leading to the reader's own reflection.

Skill Box

> Grade Clare's work at degree level
>
> - *What feedback would you give Clare to justify the grade and your own ideas about how her insights could have been developed?*
> - *Consider what insights you gain from engaging with Clare's work.*
> - *Construct a grading criteria you feel would be most appropriate for grading reflective assignments.*
> - *Reflect again on the dichotomy between a technical rational and professional artistry approach and how each perspective might frame reflective grading differently.*
> - *And ask yourself and your colleagues, do we in fact need grading criteria?*
> - *What would be the academic fallout of scrapping them?*

Summary

Clare's narrative is a good example of reflective writing to meet academic requirement. Constructing narrative (as the fifth dialogical movement) is a significant aspect of reflective practice, whether for self-interest or performance, professional portfolio or reflective essays. Yet grading reflective assignments is problematic when the assessment is viewed differently from technical rational or professional artistry perspectives. Indeed the whole issue of grading becomes problematic with an emphasis on meeting specific criteria.

In Chapter 12, I offer Jill's reflective writing as a further exemplar of reflective writing written as an academic requirement.

Endnotes

1 See Chapter 5.
2 See Chapter 6.
3 As set out in Chapter 6.
4 Becoming a reflective and effective practitioner (see Appendix 3 for details).
5 Becoming a reflective and effective practitioner (see Appendix 3 for details).

References

Basford, L. and Slevin, O. (eds.) *Theory and practice of nursing: an integrated approach to caring practice*. Nelson Thornes, Cheltenham.

Belenky, M. F., Clinchy, B. M., Goldberger, N. R. and Tarule, J. M. (1986) *Women's ways of knowing: the development of self, voice, and mind*. Basic Books, New York.

Benner, P. (2003) [1961] Clinical reasoning: articulating experiential learning in nursing practice. In E. Berne, *Transactional analysis in psychotherapy: the classic guide to its principles*. Grove Press, New York.

Berne, E. (2003) [1961] *Transactional analysis in psychotherapy: the classic guide to its principles*. Grove Press, New York.

Bulman, C. (2004) An introduction to reflection. In C. Bulman and S. Schultz (eds.), *Reflective practice in nursing* (3rd ed.). Blackwell, Oxford.

Bush, T. (2003) Communicating with patients who have dementia. *Nursing Times* 99.48, 42–45.

Dyer, I. (1995) Preventing the ITU syndrome or how not to torture an ITU patient (part 2). *Intensive and Critical Care Nursing* 11.4, 223–232.

Feil, N. (1993) *The validation breakthrough: simple techniques for communicating with people with Alzheimer's-type dementia*. Health Profession's Press, Baltimore, MD.

Gadow, S. (1980) Existential advocacy. In S. Spickler and S. Gadow (eds.), *Nursing: image and ideals*. Springer, New York, pp. 79–101.

Green, A. (1996) An explorative study of patients' memory of their stay in an acute intensive therapy unit. *Intensive and Critical Care Nursing* 12.3, 131–137.

Lawrence, M. (1995) The unconscious experience. *American Journal of Critical Care* 4.3, 227–232.

Leigh, K. (2001) Communicating with unconscious patients. *Nursing Times* 97.48, 35–36.

Lliffe, S. and Drennan, V. (2001) *Primary care and dementia*. Jessica Kingsley, London.

Miller, L. (2002) Effective communication with older people. *Nursing Standard* 17.9, 45–50, 53, 55.

Morse, J. (1991) Negotiating commitment and involvement in the nurse–patient relationship. *Journal of Advanced Nursing* 16, 552–558.

Pitkin, W. B. (1932) *Life begins at forty*. McGraw-Hill, New York.

Podurgiel, M. (1990) The unconscious experience: a pilot study. *Journal of Neuroscience Nursing* 22.1, 52–53.

Rao, M. T. (1993) *Coping with communication challenges in Alzheimer's disease.* Singular Publishing, San Diego, CA.

Russell, F. (1999) An exploratory study of patient perception, memories and experiences of an intensive care unit. *Journal of Advanced Nursing* 29.4, 783–791.

Stewart, I. and Joines, V. (1987) *TA today: a new introduction to Transactional Analysis.* Russell Press, Nottingham.

Tosch, P. (1988) Patients' recollections of their post-traumatic coma. *Journal of Neuroscience Nursing* 20.4, 223–228.

Chapter 12

Reflection on Touch and the Environment

Christopher Johns and Jill Jarvis

Effective narrative is aesthetically and emotionally engaging

Introduction

Jill Jarvis undertook the BSc Palliative Care programme at the University of Bedfordshire.[1] The assignment for the holistic practice module asked her *to reflect on and draw insight around three aspects of her practice*. She works as a night staff nurse in a hospice and chose to write three exemplars around one patient, Sally, concerning touch, the environment and spirituality – all concerned with a broader plot – 'How can we create places of healing?' Touch and environment are the focus of these two brief narratives. I include this narrative to illuminate the aesthetic quality of Jill's writing and her juxtaposition with a relevant theory.

As with all reflective texts, Jill invites you to engage with her insights in context of reflecting on your own clinical and educational experiences.

Touch

Jill writes:

This narrative concerns my experience with Sally who struggled to accept her horrific circumstances as life slipped away. Sally was diagnosed with acute lymphoblastic leukaemia two years ago. She underwent a bone marrow transplant, which completely cured her illness. Eighteen months later she developed cutaneous T-cell lymphoma caused by graft versus host disease. There has only been one other case like this reported in the world! Filled with astounded disbelief, Sally was left to suffer the consequences of this devastating condition with the knowledge that no curative treatment is available.

Becoming a Reflective Practitioner, Fifth Edition. Edited by Christopher Johns.
© 2017 John Wiley & Sons Ltd. Published 2017 by John Wiley & Sons Ltd.
Companion Website: www.wiley.com/go/johns/reflectivepractitioner

On admission to the hospice Sally is in the terminal phase of her illness. Using selective literature, I enhance and substantiate my intuitive awareness that many skills used in palliative care are not formally taught in nursing school but acquired during life experience and personal study. I aim to explore the depths and meaning of touch to gain insight into its therapeutic value. By reflecting on my thoughts, feelings, and reactions of the care I administer, I aim to gain insight to improve my nursing.

The evening reports continues, 'Her skin is burnt all over; each movement causes pain creating many difficulties with her care. She is having trouble coming to terms with her condition.'

The words reverberate – perhaps it is us who is having the difficulty. But I say nothing.

My mind troubled, I leave the office and wander along the corridor greeting patients and informing them that I am here tonight. A penetrating, nauseous vapour fills the air leading towards an open door. Standing at the doorway my eyes are transfixed by the small wispy figure covered only by a thin linen sheet. Her face is peaceful in sleep, disfigured by ferocious, sore red patches which connect and weave their way into every crease and feature of beauty. The main attack centres on her eyes, producing a monstrous appearance of two cracked, shivering starfish oozing from tentacles. Small mounds of decaying skin cling desperately all around her head, reluctant to completely give up and let go. Goosepimples emerge on my arms; my body shudders coldly, ending the momentary glance.

On auto-pilot, I continue to the next room. Disgust and horror overwhelm my mind as I smile at the clean-shaven, unblemished tanned face of the gentleman sitting comfortably reading. Conversation readily flows, we discuss the beautiful view from the window, but my brain struggles to dismiss the suffering in the previous room.

Sally calls for assistance. She requests I cream a very sensitive sore area on her back. As my hand approaches, an invisible layer of heat three inches from her body penetrates my skin. Like entering a hot oven I carefully make contact with her slippery flesh. The cream dissolves into oil and trickles onto the sheets. With gentle circular movements my fingers attempt to coat the raw burning tissues of Sally's back, lubricating the rippled surfaces. Feelings of sadness and hesitance are replaced by pleasurable sensations. The moist warmth infuses through the dryness of my hands, creating suppleness and ease. In silence, I continue covering any area of need, enjoying the experience of Sally's relaxation radiating through my fingertips.

'That's wonderful,'she whispers, 'You're not wearing gloves.'

Startled, I question, 'Should I be?'

'Well, I'm not contagious, but everyone wears them because it's so revolting.'

Sally's reply is nonchalant.

Checking for approval, I ask, 'Would you prefer that I wear gloves?'

With eyes closed Sally relaxes, smiles and mouths, 'No, no it's lovely.'

Continuing our intimate interaction until the peacefulness of sleep encompasses Sally, I leave feeling enriched by this encounter.

Returning to the office, thoughts of gratitude swell my mind. How privileged I am to work in an environment that values and prioritises time with patients. Gone are the days when I was considered a time-waster! De Hennezel (1998: 61) speaks to me, 'how often are nurses rebuked for wasting time when they follow their heart's natural instinct and give a little of their simply presence to the sick'. Even in a hospice I sense the underlying culture that we do things to people rather than essentially be with people.

As morning slowly emerges, I draw back the curtains, enabling Sally to witness the beauty of the sunrise over the lake. She smiles whilst beckoning me to her, and taking my arm, she thanks me for last night. Our eyes meet as I reassure her that I also benefited by creaming my neglected hands.

Sally rushes into conversation about her history and prognosis. As if frightened that I might leave her, she holds my hand tight. With resentfulness she recounts her story, bewildered how or why she has to suffer such torment. Restrained by her grasp I can only listen; no words are available to explain or bring comfort. Normal responses of hair-stroking or hugging are inappropriate due to the excruciating pain they cause. Motionless, I stand as the painful darts of information enter my heart and compassion is portrayed through facial expression and contact. Consumed into the depths of reality and truth, I feel Sally's pain opening, disturbing craters in my soul. My mind wanders to things I should put right and others that I want to do before I die (Autton 1996). Slowly an awareness of death is expressed, as De Hennezel (1998) observed many times. Like panning for gold, I sieve through each word. Trickling down the mountains of despair is a tiny but clear meandering stream of hope and desire. The simplicity of Sally's needs bring tears to my eyes. Lowering my head, a spontaneous kiss reaches her erupting cheek; fragments of her scabby skin cohere to my lips but I only feel love. Sally mouths a return gesture, and smiling, we squeeze hands and disengage. 'See you later,' I whisper, leaving her space. Sally nods, closing her eyes.

Sally's history in report left me dumbstruck. What could I say to her that would make a difference, alleviate anguish and help her find peace? As Autton (1996: 121) agrees, 'In some circumstances words can be more of a hindrance than a help.' By using touch, I relayed my feelings to Sally (Talton 1995). I had the intention of achieving connection with Sally through physical contact. Sympathy and empathy can be exchanged by touch, as Edwards (1998) explains, citing Wyschogrod [p. 801], 'fellow feelings that you and I are one'. I wanted Sally to know I cared, to break down the barriers of being strangers and facilitate her journey of acceptance. Estabrooks and Morse (1992) use the beautiful phrase 'bumping souls', which sums up what I wanted to achieve. Sally and I 'tuned in' to each other through the caring touch (Fredriksson 1999). I find amazing peace inside me that so much can be gained without the use of words!

Touch has been categorised as task-oriented, caring and protective (Fredriksson 1999, Talton 1995). Task touch is the most commonly used by nurses and does not always have the intent to communicate in a positive manner. It can be defined by 'hurried, rough, jarred movements' relaying 'frustration, anger, or impatience' (Fredriksson 1999: 2). I find this comment disturbing and not true in the hospice. Because of the horrific condition of Sally's skin I was very wary of how I apply the cream. Taking time to register Sally's reaction to my contact and constantly reassessing our intention, I was able to ensure that we understood each other. To make the mistake of hurting Sally would create fear of me administering treatment and in turn cause anxiety instead of ease (Davidhizar and Giger, 1997).

The disgust I felt on first seeing Sally produced intense guilt. The T-cell lymphoma had totally consumed her skin into a revolting, stinking mess. I suppose it would have been normal to reach for gloves. However, I felt they would create a barrier within the touching process, preventing skin-to-skin contact. I wanted to communicate my acceptance of Sally despite her disfigured body. Autton (1996) describes how reassuring physical contact can be transferred by healing massage. Transmissions of pain and touch have joint nerve pathways (Talton 1995). The gentle movements of my fingers on Sally's back initiated relaxation and eventually sleep. What better way, during the night, can there be of dealing with personal mental trauma? So often, as hospice nurses, we turn to sedatives to induce sleep, but I am learning that giving time to patients is more effective and rewarding. This can be demonstrated clearly in the way that Sally acted in the morning.

If I had created a barrier by wearing gloves, would Sally have received my message? No, I think it would have intensified her feelings of self-repulsion and ugliness. I didn't even consider using gloves. Sadly, when I tried to discuss this with my colleagues, they dismissed the idea and requested that we should all wear aprons as well to protect our clothes! My words fell on stony ground, as if I had touched something deeply threatening they inherently recoiled from. When they look at Sally do they only see disgust rather than this suffering woman? The disgust expressed by my colleagues disturbs me. It resonates with the idea of body work as dirty – the body work behind the screens (Lawler 1991), with the need to protect self from both its physical and emotional impact. The apron protects not just the body but forms an emotional barrier, as if it is death itself touching them. If we choose to work in a hospice then such attitude must be confronted, yet with compassion and understanding that this is not easy work. De Hennezel (1998 61) writes,

> Many of the people I've met at the bedside of the dying feel themselves to be useless and ill at ease in this situation of just being there and not doing anything. You might wonder where such attitudes stem from. We need to reorient our values to being with rather than doing to.

Writing this reflective narrative has heightened my awareness of the physical and therapeutic areas of touch. Chang (2001: 2) observes, 'touching is an integral part of human life'. Within the nursing environment using touch is a normal, frequent method of administering care both physically and psychologically. Nurses are also allowed to enter the private zones of the individual through intimate touch due to societal agreement (Hickman and Holmes 1994). However, consideration must always be given to ethnic background, personal history and social connotations to ensure that touch is appropriate and authentic (Talton 1995). Turton (1989) reminds practitioners to be mindful of their use of touch and its therapeutic impact. Ochs (2001) suggests that we should always ask permission before touching patients or family. I find it more agreeable to continually assess the person's reactions (Talton 1995). The meaning of touch is personal and can only be translated by the recipient (Chang 2001).

Surprisingly, Estabrooks and Morse (1991) note, 'One of the most neglected areas of touch in nursing research is the investigation of the touching behaviours of nurses.' These authors suggest that nurses develop their own touching style through individual life experience and training. It is a comfort to know that touching can be a learned behaviour, especially when observing those who appear to have a comfortable natural ability of its proper use (Estabrooks and Morse 1991).

Environment

Slowly washing my hands in the cream enamel basin, my eyes wander around Sally's room through the mirror above the sink. Wilting, shrivelled stems interspersed by youthful blooms hang from vases. Stagnating in discoloured water, they silently scream for attention. Twisted chocolate wrappers hide between magazines haphazardly balanced on the bedside table. Walkman cables, compact discs and tubes of cream create a 'modern' work of art. 'Get well' cards lie abandoned, children's drawings huddle in a corner and photos of loved ones faces face the window.

An unintentional arena of chaos faces me as I turn around, feelings of claustrophobia creep inside my body. I need some space. Each item of furniture is overburdened with unnecessary clutter. The floor extends storage pads and dressings, red 'infected' linen bags openly display their contents.

Reaching for a paper towel, I dry my hands carefully, ensuring that nothing is knocked from the nearby shelf. Gadgets of hygiene engulf the small washing area whilst the sad magnolia walls absorb the atmosphere of dull isolation and neglect. Sally is asleep, so I tiptoe away.

Standing outside the hospice, a refreshing night breeze hits my skin. A stabbing tightness restricts my chest, Sally finds even ripples of air painful on her burning flesh. She is cocooned in the moist, foul-smelling warmth of her room. Aromas of freshly mown grass fill my nostrils but Sally's sense of smell has become numbed by a continuous stench. Confined to her bed through weakness but craving independence, she is rendered helpless in personally changing her surroundings. I wonder how she would arrange things if she were able?

At the main entrance a beautiful arrangement of fresh flowers adorns the foyer. 'Welcome' signs invite my arrival and homely décor instils comfort. Windows proudly display wonderful views of nature, a lake, gardens, wildlife and an abundance of glorious, towering, protective trees. The corridor turns, revealing a quiet area of cosiness to relax, chat with family or befriend other patients. Visually nothing to fear is apparent except the word 'hospice' all around the building!

An intoxicating, foetid odour invisibly digests the air, as I get closer to Sally's room. 'Can't sleep,' she whispers, as I move blankets and clothes by her bedside. 'Can I tidy your room?' slips from my mouth. Sally giggles, 'Where will you start?'

Mesmerised by activity, Sally remains quiet. Within half an hour her environment evokes order, cleanliness and thoughtful comfort. Nursing supplies are secretly hidden in cupboards. Smeared surfaces now shine with approval. Photos smile at Sally from wardrobe doors and cards hang appreciably overhead, displaying their messages of comfort. Wiping tears of joy from Sally's eyes, I ask if the room is to her liking. Nodding contentedly, Sally pours herself into conversation centred on memorabilia. Time rushes by, twilight creeps across the sky bringing a new day. Exhausted, Sally drifts leisurely into the land of dreams.

How many times do I ignore the irritating untidiness of patient's rooms? Actually the answer is never. Mess constantly annoys me but I don't always clean it up! Neither do I consistently take time to consider how a patient feels about their surroundings.

Sally craved her independence but it had been snatched from her. She would have loved to keep her room tidy, bright and cheerful. Her pleasure when seeing her room tidy and family photos smiling at her confirmed it. Yet why had we allowed her room to get in such a mess? It suggests we do not pay much attention to the impact of the environment on her wellbeing. Florence Nightingale turns in her grave.

Sally is vulnerable and silent. The intra-subjective world of the patient is discussed by Summer, who claims the patient becomes vulnerable, in need of help due to illness. Summer states (2001: 4), 'the patient comes to the illness-induced interaction hopeful that this exquisite vulnerability will be acknowledged'. Hope that this will happen comes from 'a yearning for a recognition or consideration by others of unmet needs' (4). Morse and Dobernect (1995) mention the determination of the patient to endure the unpleasant 'side effects' of illness (cited by Summer 2001: 4), in this case the mess in her room. I felt she had lost something of her identity in the mess and that she had become part of the mess.

Loss is described by Robinson and McKenna (1998: 7) as having three attributes:

- Loss signifies that someone or something one has had or ought to have had in the future, has been taken away;

- that which is taken away must have been valued by the person experiencing the loss;
- the meaning of loss is determined individually, subjectively and contextually by the person experiencing it.

Each point is salient as regards Sally. A sense of guilt burdens me that we had let her room get into such a mess. Chris challenges me in the group, 'How do I ensure that all staff respect the patient's environment?' 'Can I be influential in changing attitudes?' I like to think so, but I already have a reputation for complaining about care issues. People tend to agree with me but nothing gets changed, as if the place is infected with inertia. A focus for future experiences, that is, if I persist with reflection after the course is completed. The value of reflection is to lift these things into consciousness, things we take for granted or get complacent about, but then we also get complacent about reflection. We need to establish a regular reflection group at the hospice where such issues can be aired openly and acted upon.

The daily nursing rituals of ward rounds, checking that everything is 'shipshape' has long gone (Biley and Wright 1997). In an investigation by Rogers et al. (2000) on the sources of dissatisfaction with hospital care, the environment comes right at the bottom of the list! This research included 229 people but only 6 complained about untidiness, or dirty bathrooms. Am I to believe that hospitals and hospices are very tidy, clean places? Unfortunately we nearly all have personal stories to tell, or have heard disturbing reports to the contrary. Is it good that people are so grateful of our care that they feel unable to express their concerns? Sometimes I feel that in nursing we have gone from one extreme to another. For example, identifying the task of cleaning to a particular person usually, in my opinion, gets the job done, whereas relying on individual commitment unfortunately often doesn't! This is a good example of why the stench from Sally's room had not been dealt with. Everyone had to be aware of its existence, with the exception of Sally, but nobody took responsibility to act.

The sense of smell is the most immediate of our senses due to the olfactory nerve being directly connected to the brain (Davis 2000). Smell is also the most fleeting of the senses; fading occurs when one is exposed to a smell for a long time (Davis 2000: 279). Sally sadly had become a victim of this. I know that bergamot is one of the most effective deodorising oils (Davis 2000), so why didn't I take the time to discover this oil and use it? Davis also informs that bergamot is an 'uplifting' oil producing a relaxing atmosphere for the anxious, depressed person (2000: 57). Although Sally had lost her sense of smell she still could have absorbed the oil into her bloodstream through inhalation (Davis 2000: 281). Music can be used to improve the nursing environment and has been demonstrated to decrease pain, reduce anxiety and promote relaxation (McCaffrey 2002). Sally obviously appreciated music, as a Walkman and compact discs were in her room. Given the potential effectiveness of this non-invasive pleasure, 'it should be offered to all hospital patients in all situations that are known to be stressful' (Evans 2002: 9). Music improves the mood of patients and may reduce the need for sedatives (Evans 2002: 9).

My mind fills with a picture of Sally's room. The light is dimmed, bergamot penetrates the air and soft sounds ripple in the background. Serenity. How easy it is to produce a peaceful haven. So why didn't I achieve this for Sally?

The environment has an enormous impact on both patients and their families. Wuest (1997) argues that a broader conceptualisation of environment needs to become a focus for nursing action. I second that!

Commentary

Does the text inspire your own practice and writing? Jill, no doubt prompted by a technical rational background, dialogues with a considerable literature to make sense of touch. I sense that Jill's practice with Sally is an act of remoralisation (Frank 2002). Frank, who was being treated for cancer, describes his experience with a blood technician (Frank 2002: 18),

> As this technician went about her work I remarked how skilful she was compared to some other technicians. She then said something to me that had a direct reference to my complaint but also elevated the occasion to a wholly different plane – 'Remember,' she said slowly, 'everyone who touches you affects your healing'. That technician [amongst many] is the one who drew me into a relation of care, in the full sense of *remoralisation*. She recognised, and she found a way to express that recognition, that she was not just extracting blood as a part of a diagnostic procedure, but was also affecting a change in who I was as a result of touching me.

Frank makes the point that caring 'is not a substance or thing ... not merely the taking of blood but is possible only within "relations of caring" ... not as a puzzle to be solved but as a mystery' (2002: 13). Frank asks what the technician meant by using the words 'touch' and 'healing'. The words capture the sense of caring: the mutual exchange as something in Frank touched the technician, that she was open to and could listen to his suffering. From this perspective, touch to be recognised as caring, is more than a technical thing. Indeed, being touched without a sense of being cared for, without a sense of intimacy, is demoralising, the sense of being treated as an object. It is the antithesis of caring. For Frank, this experience was remoralising – that the technician placed him firmly on his healing journey. In other words, the role of any caregiver is to remoralise the patient, to help him or her grow through the illness experience, to emerge as more whole having been cut to pieces by the cancer experience, even for patients who are dying, who feel torn apart. Touch is then healing.

I also sense that Jill's writing is her own act of remoralisation, a way of honouring her work with Sally and dispersing both an individual and collective sense of guilt, that somehow the hospice had failed Sally.

Skill Box

- *Reflect on an experience where you use touch in a deliberate way with therapeutic intent. How does Jill's text impact on your own experience?*
- *Do you resist touching people? Why is that? Does it impede your caring practice?*
- *Next time you are at work look about you. Is the patients' environment tidy? Does it matter?*
- *Would you describe your practice as an environment of healing? How could it become more so?*

Summary

Reflective writing enables you to express yourself in meaningful ways. It is a way of finding yourself, of bringing the threads of reflection together to draw insight. It is easy to see that such writing will have a significant impact on readers and prompts reflection on the readers' own practice, especially concerning controversial issues such as wearing gloves and intimacy.

In Chapter 13 Margaret Graham picks up the theme of sharing stories within an educational setting.

Endnote

1   The BSc palliative care programme (latterly the BSc End of Life Care programme) is a 60-credit (or two double modules) at level 3 consisting of one 'holistic ' module that was very reflective and one more theory-driven module dealing with symptom management. Assignments for both modules were case studies, reflecting on patient care that illuminated the critical application of ideas to patient care.

References

Autton, N. (1996) The use of touch in palliative care. *European Journal of Palliative Care* 3.3, 121–124.

Biley, F. and Wright, S. (1997) Towards a defence of nursing routine and ritual. *Journal of Clinical Nursing* 6.2, 115–119.

Chang Ok Sung (2001) The conceptual structure of physical touch in caring. *Journal of Advanced Nursing* 33.6, 820–827.

Davidhizar, R. and Giger, J. (1997) When touch is not the best approach. *Journal of Clinical Nursing* 6.3, 203–206.

Davis, P. (2000) *Aromatherapy A–Z.* C.W. Daniel & Co, Saffron Walden.

De Hennezel, M. (1998) *Intimate death* (trans C. Janeway). Warner Books, London.

Edwards, S. (1998) An anthropological interpretation of nurses' and patients' perceptions of the use of space and touch. *Journal of Advanced Nursing* 28, 809–817.

Estabrooks, C. and Morse, J. (1992) Toward a theory of touch: the touching process and acquiring a touching style. *Journal of Advanced Nursing* 17, 448–456.

Evans, D. (2002) The effectiveness of music as an intervention for hospital patients: a systematic review. *Journal of Advanced Nursing* 37.1, 8–18.

Frank, A. (2002) Relations of caring: demoralization and remoralization in the clinic. *International Journal of Human Caring* 6.2, 13–19.

Fredriksson, L. (1999) Modes of relating in a caring conversation: a research synthesis on presence, touch and listening. *Journal of Advanced Nursing* 30.5, 1167–1176.

Hickman, P. and Holmes, C. (1994) Nursing the post-modern body: a touching case. *Nursing Inquiry* 1, 3–14.

Lawler, J. (1991) *Behind the scenes: nursing, somology and the problems of the body.* Churchill Livingstone, Melbourne.

McCaffrey, R. (2002) Music listening as a nursing intervention A symphony of practice. *Holistic Nursing Practice* 16.3, 70–77.

Morse, J. and Doberneck, B. (1995) Delineating the concept of hope. *Image: Journal of Nursing Scholarship* 27, 277–285.

   Ochs 2001

Robinson, D. & Mckenna, H. (1998) Loss: an analysis of a concept of particular interest to nursing. *Journal of Advanced Nursing* 27.4, 779–74.

Rogers, A. et al. (2000) All the services were excellent. It is when the human element comes in that things go wrong': dissatisfaction with hospital care in the last year of life. *Journal of Advanced Nursing* 31.40, 768–774.

Sumner, J. (2001) Caring in nursing: a different interpretation. *Journal of Advanced Nursing* 35.60, 926–932.

Talton, C. (1995) Complementary therapies: touch-of-all-kinds is therapeutic. *Registered Nurse* 58.2, 61-4.

Turton, P. (1989) Touch me, feel me, heal me. *Nursing Times*, 85.19, 42–44.

Wuest, J. (1997) Illuminating environmental influences on women's caring. *Journal of Advanced Nursing* 26.1, 49–58.

Chapter 13

'Opening My Mind': The Ripples of Story

Margaret Graham

Introduction

I am a reflective nurse educator working in Ireland at the University of Limerick. Being a reflective practitioner, I am committed to continuously developing myself and my teaching practice. I aim to create learning spaces that foster the potential for students to make connections between life experience and practice. For me, narrative and experience go hand in hand – telling, listening to and reading stories stimulate our senses and imagination, encouraging us to see our reality more clearly.

Storytelling and narrative are core to reflection, and some authors use these terms interchangeably (Freshwater 2011). However, storytelling is a spontaneous expression of experience, either in oral or written form, whereas narrative is reflexively constructed to communicate insights (Johns 2010). Narrative contributes to unfolding meaning and significance of reflections, through cognitive, symbolic and affective means (Charon 2006). Such knowledge contributes to expressing vision, guiding my practice as narrative mirrors the reality of a 'concrete life space' (Polkinghorne 2010: 296).

In this way narrative helps me seek ways to realise my beliefs about reflection as a foundation for nurse education (Graham 2015). I strive to embed reflective spaces in my work rather than making them an addendum or afterthought. I move from a traditional teaching style to exploring more creative pedagogies. I share stories and reflection in the classroom, using narratives like *Reflection on my mother dying: a story of crying shame* (Johns 2009), *Honour thy mother* (Graham 2013) and presentations based on my reflection, *Holding a hand: an expression of intent* (Graham 2013).

Illustration of Learning

I illustrate how my work evolves, sharing a learning experience with third-year undergraduate nursing students with their feedback that they engage and learn through this process. These students are studying an introductory module on maternity and child nursing. I have

Becoming a Reflective Practitioner, Fifth Edition. Edited by Christopher Johns.
© 2017 John Wiley & Sons Ltd. Published 2017 by John Wiley & Sons Ltd.
Companion Website: www.wiley.com/go/johns/reflectivepractitioner

mulled over how best to facilitate the achievement of a learning outcome requiring students to 'demonstrate an appreciation of the role of the nurse in protecting women'. The World Health Organization (WHO; 2013) identifies the importance of domestic abuse (also referred to as domestic violence or intimate partner violence) as a universal phenomenon that crosses demographic boundaries. In an Irish context, Watson and Parsons (2005), in a nationwide study, report that 15 per cent of women have experienced severely abusive behaviour of a physical, sexual or emotional nature from a partner at some time in their lives.

My intention is to facilitate learning about this sensitive topic through sharing a story from a published text to open a dialogical space. I happen across a short story, *A colourful marriage*, by Catherine Barry (2005) that illustrates the sombre and complex nature of domestic violence. It gives us glimpses of the challenges and difficulties for women coming forward to report abuse and the effects on family. First I share small snippets to give an inkling of the writing style.

A colourful marriage tells of Heather, an 8-year-old girl, experiencing difficulties in school, who has stopped speaking, is not engaging with peers and has been bed-wetting. Heather and her mother Clare are on their fourth visit to a child guidance clinic.

Clare begins, 'Heather won't speak to me; I am resigned to the fact that she may never speak to me again.' And again: 'I need valium to think straight. I can talk without feeling the pain in my cheek where last night Miles [her husband] repeatedly beat me … I can pretend he didn't say, "The only thing that you are good for is sex."'

Clare picks up Heather's stress, noting, 'I feel the tiny hand grip mine … I feel her anxiety.'

Later Clare wonders, 'Can the psychologist see the yellow and purple bruise under my right eye that I have so meticulously covered up with concealer and make-up?'

As the story unfolds we see glimpses of how the psychologist probes, using therapeutic skills of space and silence, in developing rapport with Clare and then ultimately asking, 'Has Miles ever assaulted you?'

The story continues, 'We [psychology team] know, Clare, what is going on … Heather told us.'

Mention is made of a poster on the clinic wall proclaiming, 'When home is where the hurt is', with contact details for supports and legal aid.

Sharing the Story

Within the module I facilitate several small-group sessions comprising 15 students per group. At each session we read the story and then gather in the spirit of a community of inquiry (Johns 2013). We begin a conversation that ebbs and flows, giving everyone an opportunity to contribute. Towards the end of the session we spend a few minutes looking at the website of *Adapt*,[1] an Irish group that supports women experiencing abuse. This site offers guidance and contact details for women about domestic violence. Prevalence, symptoms, protection and reporting are detailed. I circulate a summary of the resources.

Nevertheless it is critical that I turn to consider students' thoughts about the experience. I ask:

- What did you learn today?
- What struck you about the story?

Students' written feedback follows:

- Today we covered domestic abuse and the support available for women; we read a story which really pulled me into the scene.
- I have learned about domestic abuse and the effect on children, although parents believe children are unaware of the effect it has on children in everyday life – such as withdrawal from school and participation in activities.
- From reading the short story I learned what it must be like to be in an awful situation like that.
- I learnt about how a women experiencing domestic violence thinks and feels about the situation. She pretended that everything was OK, blaming herself. I was concerned for her psychological health and wellbeing.
- The anxiety caused by the self-doubt made it very hard for Clare to build up enough confidence to take a stand for herself and her daughter.
- I think that it is a good way for learning because everyone takes something different from the story and it makes the experiences more rounded, allowing you to view it from different angles.
- It struck me how prevalent abuse is in Ireland, how it is not restricted to lower social-class families.
- I found the story beneficial because it covered the main points and picked up on abuse in a way that involved us, and everyone interacted in the class.
- Very thought-provoking, easy to relate to. Keeping me focused, I learned a lot.
- Reading stories can help me as a student nurse to see the patient as a person, not just another statistic.
- I found narrative to be a good perspective to look from the character; it seems to depict life through their experience; it feels real and relevant.
- It was sad to read about how worthless this woman felt. How she tried to hide it from her daughter. The daughter was the strong one in the story, speaking up to protect both of them. As a learning strategy this was an excellent way to learn about how women will react in this situation, the signs to look for. It was interesting how the counsellor teased it out of her gently.
- I learned about how you can never judge a book by its cover, that when caring for patients we should always remember we don't know what happens behind closed doors.
- The story form was very beneficial as it really struck home the severity of domestic abuse.
- Reading the short story was ideal instead of someone reeling off facts and giving lots of information that you don't understand and can't relate to, so this story sticks in your mind. The short story put it all into perspective, as one girl said how much goes on behind closed doors and no one has any idea of how someone is living at home. The atmosphere created in the lab showed the interest and benefit of short story.
- The short story helped 'open my mind'. I became more focused on the situation being portrayed in the story, I felt the language in the story was quite good and made the situation real, which made me more focused on all characters. It's strange – we feel the daughter needs protection, but she is the protector.
- I found the short story a good way of learning about the topic as it expressed both the mother and the child's views and feelings and had all the symptoms of abuse.
- Learning about signs and symptoms and learning about communicating with these women, I saw how she praised her abuser [her husband was member of the golf club] It was eye-opening.

- I now see nursing assessment as much more than getting facts; there are so many layers to be aware of. It's crazy busy [placement], we just want to get the jobs done. I need to appreciate that there is a vulnerable person who is a victim.
- What scares me is that women who are abused don't simply walk out. There are many factors influencing them; fear, loss of confidence – I can't begin to imagine how bad it must be.
- During this session I found the story a much easier way and interesting way of learning. The thing that I enjoyed most was how the author shows the chaos of Clare's life. The way of writing, along with the language she chose, drew me in in as a reader. It showed me first-hand how domestic violence can occur rather than just learning about the signs and symptoms and ways to prevent it. As for my own knowledge and understanding I will be more aware to think about these situations when I am on practice. I thoroughly enjoyed the learning method though it was awful situation.
- I thought that the language in the story was so descriptive I could sense the fear and anxiety. What really struck me was how Clare was in denial trying to cover up the abuse, yet she is also aware of the effects of the abuse on herself. The line where she says, 'I am used to living life out of the corner of my eye', really sticks with me.
- I learned about the facts of domestic abuse and the effects on the child.
- As nurses this will help us to look out for the smallest clues of abuse. I learned that support is needed for women and children. I learned that someone needs a lot of support and courage to stand up to abuse.
- I thought that the session was helpful, reading the story and listening to what others learned, also as you pick up and learn things that you may not have thought of yourself. I learned that it requires a lot of steps before women will actually come forward about abusive situations in the home.
- I learned that one woman in 11 has experienced severe physical abuse in a relationship. I learn that it may take up to 35 abusive incidents before a woman comes forward I have learnt that domestic abuse can make a woman very anxious. I learned that a child may know everything, no matter how hard parents try to hide the violence.
- Found the use of the story was very beneficial, it gave me an insight in how women can be emotionally affected by domestic abuse and the way which they try to hide the situation.
- I have learned about the legal aspects and how hard it is to leave someone. It am shocked by the WHO stats [15–71 per cent of women had experienced physical or sexual violence from their husband or partner; WHO 2009)]. Tips to protect a woman in the home when she is under threat were shocking [website information].
- The story was very real, learning about domestic violence put it all into perspective and made it a reality. It is not something abstract any more. I need to be aware of this in practice.
- It has made me realise that there is likely to be a woman that is abused that I know in college or at home. I need to listen for the unsaid.
- It got us thinking and to begin to understand the true nature of violence, be it social, psychological, physical or financial. Barry's story enabled the class to rally think and try to understand all aspects. Providing such a real-life scenario in the story showed that domestic abuse can occur anywhere and could be happening all around us without us even knowing; in the story her husband, the abuser, was a successful businessman.
- It must be hard to put on a face that all is well in a relationship when inside life is terrible.

- Story is a great learning tool as we are learning with each other and from each other and hearing each other's opinions.
- It put into context in a relatable story. The language used was simple and clear with strategies like open questioning and reflection included. It is easily understandable for the public or academic students. It strikes me that in nursing so many patient interactions include partners and family members. There may be problems that are well hidden but responses by an abused person may result in consequences later.
- It was frightening to see how women suffer the panic. The fear, the despair was tangible, how women try to cover up the situation and the impact on the family.
- How difficult it is for women to leave abusive relationships – this is empathy up close.
- I am more aware of the resources for women if I ever do encounter abuse – women's aid Adapt house [Irish websites]. I was shocked to learn about the importance of planning to leave and escape a home that is unsafe.
- I also learned about communication techniques used when speaking with a woman who is suffering from domestic abuse.
- I can now use these communication skills in practice.
- I will attempt to be gentle in my interviewing and be aware of the importance of non-verbal cues in patient and family interactions.
- The story was excellent. It made it really easy to fall into the scene and absorb what was happening and then think and reflect on the events rather than have facts talked at me and then try to remember.
- I found today's session an excellent means of learning and gaining understanding of women child and therapist services. It was perfect but a scary and sad, sad fact.

Now, I share with permission the words of a student who has experienced abuse in her family – 'A perfect way to learn. I have come from a family where abuse prevailed. The story brought it back and now I realise what a wonderful woman my mother was.'

I ask, 'Do you find the story distressing?'

'No not at all … This is what we need to do, this will help other children and mothers.'

Reflection

I am energised by these sessions. They are dynamic for me, and student feedback speaks for the way these sessions create a meaningful learning opportunity. This feedback resonates with Bradbury-Jones and Broadhurst's (2015) findings, for example, 'People just think it's physical don't they? But it's more than that, it's emotional and financial '(5).

This short story illustrates 'we live in the midst of unfolding stories over which we have partial control '(Mattingly, 1994: 813). Reflection reveals the chaos of lives but also the inherent order within chaos around meaning. Reflective learning becomes meaningful for students. They see its value and want more.

Bradbury-Jones and Broadhurst (2015) report that students are not prepared to deal with domestic abuse, therefore in using this short story I question myself,

- Is this useful?
- Am I trying to be novel at worst entertaining or is the learning meaningful?
- Does my session raise awareness of domestic abuse?

But is reflection on such a story enough? Previously, I have facilitated student-led visits to a women's refuge, with positive feedback. This approach is in keeping with recommendations by Bradbury-Jones and Broadhurst (2015) that students would benefit from experiential learning opportunities to interact with women and services dealing with domestic abuse. However, that visit involved a small student group in a programme with a flexible schedule. Unfortunately this is not possible with this student cohort due to numbers (50), structure and timetable constraints. However, I have opened the door for them to explore the resources if they feel compelled to. It becomes their responsibility. For me I sense an increasing tension between maximising learning and limited resources. Rolfe (2013) describes these dilemmas as part of a crisis within university systems increasingly dominated by business models, struggling with increased student numbers, increased class size and less contact with students. It's a world where curriculum is content-packed, where there are competing demands and needs with increased emphasis on technical skills acquisition at the expenses of student development. Such technical rationality differs from Barnett's (2005: 142) belief that learning and change in human beings has a 'time horizon' varying for different students, as they learn 'self-belief' and the ability to 'communicate, think and write'. Barnett challenges the business model in higher education, advocating for a curriculum that engages students with learning spaces, where self can expand and flourish. If Barnett's ideas have value, curriculum structures need to be both creative and flexible in accommodating and engaging student groups throughout education programmes. When considering such abstract ideas on learning, I read a research paper by Pratt- Eriksson, Bergom and Lyckage (2014) highlighting the importance of rising awareness for healthcare professions on the 'hidden' nature of the impact of domestic abuse on women and families.

Brookfield (1995) leads me to explore and develop my work, aiming to provide meaningful learning opportunities away from large lecture theatres to sitting together discussing practice in a circle or community of inquiry (Johns 2013). I seek to engage with students to create and open spaces and conversations. To do this I 'power down' and seek to move into a more collaborative posture as befits the community ideal. Sometimes, I am uncertain where this will lead. This is part of the thrill, the roller-coaster, the privilege of working together. Significantly, supporting students to grow and develop calls for a different kind of relationship in the classroom. My vision is in keeping with a humanistic approach to teaching, informed by educationalist Paulo Freire (1990: 67), 'through dialogue, the teacher-of-the students and the students-of-the-teacher cease to exist and a new term emerges: teacher-student with students-teachers'.

In staying close to these educational approaches I recognise and value self-care. Previously I would not take time to do this, with a negative impact on energy. It is easy to fall back on old ways, when tired, and simply deliver the dreaded PowerPoint presentation. Through reflection paying attention to my feelings, I take time to prepare. I pay attention to any feelings of weariness or busyness caught up in a maelstrom of academia. I aim to be *poised* as a way of both engaging and being in control of its consequences. Johns (2013) identifies poise as vital to being available to patients/students. The *poised teacher* or even better, *the poised guide*, perhaps I should shed the teacher label because it is so power-infused. Poise was not learnt in teacher training or even in teaching with its dominant need to control the classroom. High anxiety and accumulated stress are the antithesis of poise.

Critically, I, too, reflect simply it's my way of being. I constantly ask myself, How do I manage this sense of academic dissonance between my beliefs and values? How do I move from the frustration whereby I am numbed by a system that places more and more demands and pressures and performance outputs? I do not question efficiency, but it is easy to get lost and soulless, desensitised to a core belief of engaging with students in dialogue towards reaching their potential as people as practitioners contributing to the health of communities. So I believe a story about domestic abuse can contribute to student learning. It has its parallel in educational abuse. What stories could I write about that!

I turn to the words of Kearney (2002: 156), which have resonance, 'Every tale has a teller, a tale and a reader of the tale, whereby there is an open-ended invitation and interconnection between all the elements … every story shares a purpose, in this way, stories tell us something about who we are.'

I continue my quest. Johns (2013) advocates a curriculum revolution which embeds reflection as the core learning strategy. I differ from Johns in continuing to believe in a 'velvet glove',[2] taking a more incremental change rather than a curriculum revolution within my sphere of practice. For the moment, my quiet 'evolution' continues. However, I resonate with Johns (2013, who argues that we must start with ourselves and send out ripples to engage the whole community. I endeavour to champion reflection but appreciate that resources, both human and structural, are critical in sustaining change. As such I must become political and chip away at the organisational constraints. I must find my voice and speak out, but be wary of marginalising myself (Brookfield 1995).

But organisational change is always on the horizon. A major curriculum revision is due. A new approach to practice placements offering potential for integration of learning experiences through guided reflection may enhance sense making of such experiences.

I return to Johns's (2013) suggestion that bringing about transformation demands four fundamental elements; intelligence, curiosity, reflectiveness and wilfulness. Wheatley (2006), too, uses the word curiosity and the need to discover 'your own questions' (ix) and see if personal experience confirms or disconfirms new science. I keep dwelling with the questions as little ripples of change extend beyond the moment of co-creation. My vision is an approach; being with students I can be available, self-caring and care for the others as a way of being in a relationship with students as a foundation for learning.

Learning to dialogue through story and reflection is a spiral of becoming student-kind with individual students, in class, across landscapes and horizons of learning, generating conversations and ripples of possibilities in avoiding the 'culpability of producing future generations of graduates who are ill-prepared to deal with such an important area of nursing practice' (Bradbury-Jones and Broadhurst 2015: 2071).

Skills Box

- *If you are a teacher and have not used story as a focus for teaching a topic, then try this. Find a suitable text, as Margaret did with Clare, or reflect on your own experience of that topic, for example your own abuse or the story of someone who has been abused. Perhaps even invite an abused person to tell their story.*
- *Evaluate the students' learning experience of learning through story. How do these measure up against Margaret's students?*
- *As a student, seek out narratives of patients and relatives reflecting on their health–illness experience, and consider their significance in informing your learning journey.*

Ripples Continue

Building on my insights, a moment of serendipity ripples through my work. I take up an invitation to prepare a soliloquy, contributing to a faculty-wide teaching and learning symposium.

In the past, feelings of apprehension would have bubbled forth when sharing my reflective writing with peers. I describe myself as a reluctant 'performer'.

This new invitation demands I refine my text for a two-minute soliloquy. I am on a merry-go-round. Lunging from 'Can do this ...' to an inner voice, whispering, 'my story will become meaningless, devoid of many threads'.

Drawing on previous insights, I take a breath, noticing myself, aware of my growing composure.

I use my new-found *poise* a self-management practice, ensuring that such personal concerns and tensions do not hinder my ability to develop my practice (Johns 2013).

I begin to see the soliloquy as a happenstance for sharing my insights, a chance akin to what Senge (2004: 159) describes as synchronicity 'about being open to what wants to happen'.

I seize the moment. Now the task becomes exhilarating A sense of excitement, a disciplined opportunity, I carve and strip back the text. A soliloquy is created.

A week later I read *'To be or not to be' – a soliloquy on learning* at the symposium. We gather in a round-table discussion.

A scribe records the following feedback,

- Margaret opened with a powerful soliloquy that she wrote based on student reflections of a short story on domestic violence.
- All agreed that there was significant emotional impact of the reading on the group and immediately opened up a space for discussion.
- Margaret outlined how she used Brookfield's reflective lens as a device for students to reflect and describe learning through engaging with the story. This forms part of the module evaluation. This enabled students to connect to the human story as opposed to superficially engaging with material. Noted how important it is in many professions to see the person in front of you rather that the symptom or the disease.
- There was a long conversation on the possibilities that such an approach offered to both student and lecturer.
- Group members noted that often material is 'packaged' for students, but activities such as the one outlined offered students the opportunity to engage at a deeper level.
- Group members saw the method as a very useful way to raise awareness of sensitive topics, e.g. domestic violence and mental health.
- Links were made to the work of Eric Fromm
- psychoanalyst and social philosopher, who viewed love/compassion as skill that can be taught and developed.

A colleague from another department notes,

- I could cry it is so powerful.

Another colleague continues,

- A conversation that was motivating and an inspirational way of teaching.
- Made me [colleague] feel revitalised and how we could use innovative ways to teach.
- It shows a way forward for me so that I can be proactive in developing my teaching strategies.

Rippling Outwards

So far, my reflective dialogue shares feedback from self, from students, and ripples outward to colleagues and peers, in a never-ending quest within reflexive narrative in developing self and practice.

Conversational spaces beyond my familiar classroom landscape gather momentum. Taking such a step, with others across the broader academe, is a further step towards collective social action. Such an approach is inherent in Johns's (2010: 28) sixth dialogical movement of narrative construction and expanding my practice, critical in continuing a journey of transformation. Using dialogue in this way, we aim to move towards a better world for students, women and educators (Bohm 1996).

For now, I pause, returning to Okri (1997: 63), and consider 'without extending some hidden or visible frontier of the possible, without disturbing something of the incomplete order of things, there is no challenge and no pleasure and certainly no joy'.

The journey continues.

Endnotes

1   http://www.adaptservices.ie.
2   A term that I used to explain my approach in an earlier reflection.

References

Barnett, R. and Coate, K. (2005) *Engaging the curriculum in higher education*. SRHE and Open University Press, Maidenhead.

Bohm, D. (1996) *On Dialogue*. Routledge, New York.

Bradbury-Jones, C. and Broadhurst, K. (2015) Are we failing to prepare nursing and midwifery students to deal with domestic abuse? Findings from a qualitative study. *Journal of Advanced Nursing* 71.9, 2062–2072.

Brookfield, S. (1995) *The critically reflective teacher*. Jossey-Bass, San Francisco.

Charon, R. (2006) *Narrative medicine: honoring the stories of illness*. Oxford University Press, Oxford.

Chase, S. (2005) Narrative inquiry: multiple lens, approaches and voices. In N. Denzin and Y. S. Lincoln (eds.), *The Sage handbook of qualitative research* (3rd ed.). Sage, Thousand Oaks, CA.

Freire, P. (1990) *Pedagogy of the oppressed* (trans. M. B. Raos), Continuum, New York.

Freshwater, D. (2011) Clinical supervision and reflective practice. In G. Rolfe and M. Freshwater (eds.), *Critical reflection in practice: generating knowledge for care* (3rd ed.). Palgrave Macmillan, Basingstoke.

Gadamer, H. G. (1989) *Truth and method*. Continuum, New York.

Graham, M. M. (2010) Finding my voice. Presentation at the 16th International Reflective Practice Conference, University of Bedfordshire, June.

Graham, M. M. (2013) Holding a hand: an expression of intent. Presentation at the 17th International Reflective Practice Conference, Swansea University, September.

Graham, M. M. (2015) Becoming available, becoming student kind: a nurse educator's reflexive narrative. PhD Dissertation, University of Bedfordshire.

http://womenshealth.gov/violence-against-women/types-of-violence/domestic-intimate-partner-violence.html

Johns, C. (2009) Reflection on my mother dying: a story of crying shame. *Journal of Holistic Nursing* 27.2, 136–140.

Johns, C. (2010) The basic scheme. In *Guided reflection: a narrative approach to advancing practice* (2nd ed.). Wiley-Blackwell, Oxford, pp. 1–26.

Johns, C. (2013) *Becoming a reflective practitioner* (4th ed.). Wiley-Blackwell, Oxford.

Kearney, R. (2002) *On Stories: Thinking in Action*. Routledge, London.

Mattingly, C. (1994) The concept of therapeutic 'employment'. *Social Sciences and Medicine* 38.6, 811–822.

Mid-West Regional Advisory Committee for the Prevention of Violence Against Women (2013) They should not be allowed to get away with it: voices of women who have experienced domestic abuse.

Okri, B. (1997) *A way of being free*. Phoenix House, London.

Polkinghorne, D. E. (2010) The practice of narrative. *Narrative Inquiry* 20.2, 392–396.

Pratt-Eriksson, D., Bergom, I. and Lyckage, E. D. (2014) Don't ask, don't tell: battered women living in Sweden encounter with healthcare personnel and their experience of the care given. *International Journal of Qualitative Studies in Health and Well-being* 9. 23 (accessed 3 November 2015).

Rolfe, G. (2013) *The University in Dissent: Scholarship in the Corporate University*. Routledge, London.

Senge, P. (2004) *Presence: an exploration of profound change in people, organisation and society*. Doubleday, New York.

Watson, D. and Parsons, S. (2005) Report on the National Study of Domestic Abuse: Domestic Abuse of Women and Men in Ireland. Stationery Office, Dublin.

Wheatley, M. J. (2006) *Leadership and the new science: discovering order in a chaotic world* (3rd ed.). Berett-Koehler, San Francisco, CA.

World Health Organization (2013) Global and Regional Estimates of Violence against Women. World Health Organization, Geneva.

Chapter 14

Guiding First-year Nursing Students in Guided Reflection

Christopher Johns

Guidance is creating a learning community

Introduction

So now we must put on our imagination hats and contemplate how guiding reflection within the professional curriculum might work. Of course, many readers experience guided reflection or clinical supervision either as a guide or as a practitioner/student. So, as you read, reflect on your own experiences. Remember these are first-year student nurses with limited experience of being in guided reflection. Lucy, their guide, is also relatively inexperienced at facilitating learning in this way.

Michelle's Experience

Michelle is a first-year degree student nurse placed on her first surgical ward. Her previous placement had been on a medical ward. She has been in training for eight months. The school of nursing had bought in consultation at the time of a periodic revalidation to see how reflective practice could be more meaningfully utilised as a learning approach (see Chapter 8).[1] One consequence was to implement group guided reflection arranged in groups of ten students who met twice weekly for two-hour sessions throughout the three years of training. These groups were guided by the students' personal mentor. It was a bold move, not without criticism from teachers, who were anxious about the resources required to make it work and, of course, their own involvement. The guides attended an ongoing peer-guided reflection group to reflect on and develop their guidance skills,

Becoming a Reflective Practitioner, Fifth Edition. Edited by Christopher Johns.
© 2017 John Wiley & Sons Ltd. Published 2017 by John Wiley & Sons Ltd.
Companion Website: www.wiley.com/go/johns/reflectivepractitioner

facilitated by Marcia, the director of student placements. This group met for two hours every two months.

The guided reflection group commenced four weeks into the students' training. The group was contracted. The contract set out the expectation that by the end of three years, practitioners would be reflective practitioners adept in professional artistry. The students' rota sharing of experiences. Early work in the group focused on appreciating models of reflection and appreciating dialogue.

Michelle's group is guided by Lucy. It is Michelle's turn to share an experience. However, before Michelle can commence, Lucy reminds the group of their contract,

> OK, some key points about dialogue. First, listen with an open mind and respect to what Michelle shares. As you listen become aware of your reaction to her words. Try and suspend any emotional response. Also become aware of your own opinions. Try to suspend these as well so they don't interfere with listening to what Michelle says. Later we can explore our reactions and opinions constructively to gain insight.

Michelle: 'Mrs Morris was admitted for a breast biopsy. She had been a nurse, which made me feel slightly on edge wondering if she would judge me. But not to worry, she was a pleasant lady. The next morning I was doing the drugs with Katie, a senior staff nurse who is also my practice mentor. Katie can be rather brusque when anxious and that morning we were hectic chasing the clock. It became a task to rush through, which I know is not good practice when it concerns patients' medications.'

Michelle paused as if waiting for comment. She looked at Lucy for permission to continue. Lucy simply smiled and nodded.

'OK, when we got to Mrs Morris I asked her whether she had any pain. She was written up for some paracetamol if required. She was due home later that afternoon after the consultant reviewed her results and explored treatment options. She said, 'No ... oh I feel weepy,' and then she burst into tears. I said, 'What's up, Mrs Morris?' She said, 'My friends were saying how scared they would be if it was them having a breast biopsy. I hadn't appreciated these feelings until now. Oh, my husband and my children!' It made me think – she's a nurse and she's so vulnerable. I just stood there, not knowing what to do. What to say that would help? I looked at Katie, uncertain what to do, but she had moved on with the medicine trolley and I knew she expected me to rejoin her. I said to Katie, 'Hold on a moment.' I pulled up a chair and sat with her. I said, 'I'm sorry you feel so weepy. I passed her a tissue. I know that sounds clichéd. I said, "I'll come back later if you like."' Mrs Morris said, 'Yes, I know you're busy.' I expect she'd been watching us.

I told Katie what had happened. She said it must be awful for Mrs Morris and that she would go back later and talk with her. I felt so sad for her. She could have been my mum. We have quite a few women undergoing breast biopsy. I get the impression nurses are not as sensitive to these women as we should be. They look jolly and jovial outside but inside it's like a bombshell!'

Lucy: 'Finding an upset patient whilst doing the medicine round is a common occurrence on hospital wards. It's often one of the few times patients get direct attention, especially for short-stay patients like having a biopsy. Put yourself in her shoes. You spent just a few minutes with her. What were you trying to achieve?'

Michelle: 'To help her. I mean to respond to her distress. I couldn't have walked by. I had to do something. Maybe Katie could have closed the cart for a few minutes and come over. I thought it was insensitive of her. I know she was anxious about time. It's difficult to balance things. Blow the pills, no one will come to any harm. It made me feel so vulnerable – what do you say?'

Lucy: 'Did you have to say anything?'

Michelle: 'Silence is difficult. It's keeping quiet I find the hardest. Did we give her the opportunity to chat? Did we keep away because she was a nurse? Are we frightened of being patronising? Should she be treated any differently?'

Lucy: 'Can you answer your own questions?'

Michelle: 'I don't know. I was afraid of making things worse.'

Lucy: 'I understand that. It's not easy.'

Lucy: 'Evidence suggests that nurses aren't very good at sitting and listening' [Kopp 2000: 47-49].[2]

Anita: 'I can really relate to your story, Michelle. I can see why we need counselling skills. I would also be at a loss to know what to say to her – worrying if I'm helping or hindering.'

Other students then shared brief descriptions of situations where they had felt clumsy talking to patients who were angry or emotional in some way.

Patricia: 'It makes you want to avoid them. The other day in shift report, this staff nurse labelled one patient "a real pain". The charge nurse sympathised with her and said, we know "she can be difficult" but it's not her fault, so let's be positive about helping her. Staff can be so judgemental and lose compassion for patients. It's like turning your head away and pretending not to see them. It's almost you can't afford to care because it takes time!'

Lucy: 'Well spoken, Pat. It is a sobering thought to consider how many women suffer in silence and how nurses are ill equipped to respond to suffering and as a consequence avoid it. Michelle, did you use the cue, "given the situation again how could I respond more effectively?"'

Michelle: 'I did think about this cue but my mind went blank. I think I was too caught up in the emotion of it I couldn't see another way. I think it's more difficult when you do not know the patient. It's not easy when patients have such a quick turnover.'

Connie: 'Maybe we set our relational expectations too high?"

Roy: 'But then how do you help someone like Mrs Morris when caught on the hop?'

Lucy: 'OK. Each of you consider – if you were in Michelle's shoes how you would have liked to respond, and the likely consequences. Make a note of these responses and then we can feed back to Michelle and let her choose what response, if any, would have helped her.'

The group spend about ten minutes writing.
Responses included:

- 'Ask Katie to get someone to take over the medication round with her. That's about making a stand. It becomes an ethical thing – about how to set priorities and use time, although Katie might be put out as a consequence. I mean Katie's priorities were different to Katie's and Katie has the power. She could make it difficult for Michelle if she resisted her.'

- 'Tell Katie you need to spend some time with Mrs Morris. That's what you did anyway, so I'm agreeing with you.'

- 'Have definitely gone back to talk with her no matter what Katie had said. You would have felt better for doing that and Mrs Morris would have more trust in us as a consequence.'

Michelle: 'Thanks, guys. I agree with going back to talk with her later rather than disrupt the medicine round but in the moment it's tough to walk away.'

Lucy: 'Our responses are very much focused on the event itself – finding Mrs Morris tearful. Could staff have done something earlier in the day to support Mrs Morris?'

Michelle: 'We could have been more available to her pre-operatively and more empathic of what the biopsy meant to her. I know I couldn't have made it better for her, change what was wrong. I don't think the pre-operative planning is very good at psychological care. It's all rather processed. Another one on the conveyor belt!'

Lilly: 'As if she is an object. Maybe it's easier for staff not to see the person. That's shocking, saying that!'

Lucy: 'You can't take compassion and empathy for granted, especially if you are busy. You said, Michelle, that it had been a busy morning?'
Lilly jumps in, 'Maybe when you do the same thing day after day you get into a routine and not pay attention to how the person is feeling?'

Michelle: 'Yes, I can see your point, although I wouldn't like to say Katie or other staff are like that. I like to think that if Katie had not put pressure on me to continue the drugs I wouldn't have left her but I wouldn't have been so calm. I'd have been thinking more about other work that needed to be done; pre-meds, eye drops, and things, thinking I wish you'd hurry up. That's really wrong- how do we get over that?'

Lucy: 'I don't really know? Perhaps as practitioners we need to be more prepared to defend our actions.'

Michelle: 'It's true I am worried what others think of me, being relatively new to the ward. I don't like conflict, so conform to expectations on me. But this experience challenges that – I would have felt guilty if I hadn't responded to Mrs Morris in the moment. I felt better having spent just a few minutes with her.'

Lucy: 'I think it is an opportune time to consider communication skills if Michelle was to go back. We have previously mentioned Heron's "Six Category Intervention Analysis" as a reflective communication typology.'
Lucy then talked through the six categories (see Chapter 5). She then asked each group member to apply each of these for use with Mrs Morris – the point being to immediately apply the theory to practice to help the students critique and assimilate it.

Annie: 'I can see that cathartic and catalytic skills were vital – "*How are you feeling now, Mrs Morris?*" "*I'm here if you want to talk about it.*". Lucy, I remember you saying about glib reassurance[3] [Johns 2004: 200] – how it is used to make us feel more comfortable but unhelpful to the patient.'

Lucy: 'Yes, like saying something like, "*Come along, Mrs Morris, it's not so bad.*"'

Roy: 'Also information skills – about who Mrs Morris could talk with from a more authoritative perspective. I don't see any value in giving advice or confrontation – just imagine saying, "*Stop crying. It doesn't help,*" or something like that. How perverse would that have been?'

Martha: 'And supportive skills like eye contact are vital in order to communicate compassion. Perhaps touch might also be helpful?'

Michelle: 'I did put my hand on her arm when she apologised for crying. Not knowing her well enough stopped me from holding her hand. I love the story of touch by Jill Jarvis in "Becoming a reflective practitioner" [Johns 2013],[4] but touch is not yet something I really appreciate or feel comfortable with.'

Mark: 'I haven't read that, but it reminds me of the experience I shared a few sessions back when I touched a distressed young female patient on the shoulder and she recoiled. Ouch! I recoiled back. You must be sensitive about using touch, especially if you are a male nurse. I did read up the research Lucy had listed for us about the use of touch. It is problematic for men[5] (Evans 2002). Evans (pp. 12, 15) concludes,

> The gendered nature of men nurses' caring interactions reveals the ways in which gender stereotypes create contradictory and complex situations of acceptance, rejection and suspicion of men as nurturers and caregivers. Here the stereotype of men as sexual aggressors creates suspicion that men are at the bedside for reasons other than a genuine desire to help others. When this stereotype is compounded by the stereotype of men as gay, the caring practices of men nurses are viewed with suspicion in situations where there is intimate touching, not only of women patients, but of men and children as well. In each of these patient situations, men nurses are caught up in complex and contradictory gender relations that situate them in stigmatizing roles vulnerable to accusations of inappropriate touch.

Ouch!'

Lucy: 'That's helpful, Mark. We've had several experiences concerning touch, so maybe we can explore it more deeply in a later session. OK, where are we with alternative options?'

Clare: 'Did you go back and see Mrs Morris later, as you suggested you would?'

Michelle: 'I said to Katie, "Shall I go and talk with her?" I felt I needed permission after Katie had suggested she would have a word with her. Katie affirmed she would when it was quieter, so I didn't. I did go to say goodbye when she went home. I don't know if Katie had a word with her or not. I feel a bit awkward about that now. Bit guilty that I let her down. If it happened again I would certainly go back and talk with her, irrespective of Katie.'

Lucy: 'Did you find any literature that might have informed you?'

Michelle: 'I did do a literature search around breast biopsy and found an informative paper by Woodward and Webb dated 2001.[6] I wrote this down,

> The quality of life a woman experiences during the process of investigation and treatment for breast disorders is linked with the communication and support provided by others, and includes family members, friends and clinic personnel.

Another paper by Knopf dated 1994[7] recommends that nurses working with breast cancer develop strategies to help patients clarify, interpret and process information. They say that greater attention should be given to the emotional experiences of all women during the diagnostic phase of breast disease, that breast biopsy is not a benign experience – citing Northouse et al. [1995].'[8]

Roy: 'Wow, that's impressive, Michelle – can you give us those references?'

Lucy: 'Let's summarise. Michelle, what's been useful?'

Michelle: 'Without doubt reflecting on using Heron's work, especially the cathartic and catalytic skills. I can really see how I could have used them with Mrs Morris. Reflecting on my own emotional response has also been good. It links with previous shared experiences by people – that it's more difficult to be available to people who are emotional if we are not poised. How do others feel?'
The other members of the group then summarised what insights they had gained.

Lucy: 'The ethical dimension is significant – how we manage time and set priorities. Also autonomy – Michelle feeling able to make her own decisions, even as a student nurse, although I appreciate that can be tricky. But learning to read the politics of ward culture is useful. Seeing things for what they are even if our hands feel tied. Let's consider Katie's position more carefully – her dilemma that if she stopped, then other patients might suffer by having their medication delayed.'

Michelle: 'Gosh, I hadn't seen Katie's perspective clouded by Mrs Morris's upset.'

Lucy: 'Let's apply ethical mapping [see Table 14.1].'

Rona: 'I think it's so easy to glibly reassure people. I hope I don't, but like Michelle has said, what do you say to them? Perhaps letting Katie respond would have been better if we feel we lack skills rather than make a mess of it?'

Michelle: 'Yes, but she said it to me, not to Katie – I felt I had to respond – I would have felt stupid if I just asked Katie to help!'

Lucy: 'How do you feel now, Michelle?'

Michelle: 'So much better. I know I've got to be more confident with my communication skills. I shouldn't be so anxious about messing it up. Maybe I shouldn't have judged Katie so harshly, saying she was insensitive. I hope she did go back and have a word with her. I can ask her tomorrow. We don't find time to talk much.'

Lucy: 'Yes, it's good to follow up events and discuss more with your ward mentors. Does Katie have any supervision?'

Michelle: 'I did ask about clinical supervision but no, there is nothing to support and develop ward staff. I think maybe they did once but it petered out. They need it. You hear so many complaints from patients and relatives about poor care.'

Lucy: 'Mentors are meant to support you although, as you say, they also need support. Perhaps the school could do more? I'll raise that again in my next team meeting. We can pick up your feedback with Katie when we meet next Friday. Mark – I believe it is your turn to share an experience?'

Lucy's Reflection

Lucy shared this session within her own guided reflection group.
She says,

What did I learn about dialogue today?

1 What we do in our groups is to facilitate student growth. I take the idea of growth from Mayeroff [1971 :1], who notes [reading],[9] 'To care for another person, in the most significant sense, is to help him grow and actualise himself.' That growth is a reciprocal thing – I also

Table 14.1 Ethical mapping: Should Michelle stop the drug round or continue it?

Patient's / family's perspective/ other patients	Who had authority to make the decision/ act within the situation?	The doctor's perspective
Mrs Morris was visibly upset and needed care at that moment. Other patients may be watching and expect nurses to be caring yet also know they are busy. They may also expect Katie and Michelle to give them their drugs first and then see Mrs Morris.	Within-the-moment Michelle felt she did not have the authority to respond as she felt best – i.e. spend more than a few moments with Mrs Morris	Most likely to see Michelle's primary role to ensure all patients received medication on time. Perhaps some sympathy for Michelle's plight? We can only speculate.
If there is conflict of perspectives/ values - how might it be resolved?	**The situation/ dilemma**	**What ethical principles inform this situation?**
Michelle experienced intrapersonal conflict, uncertain in her own mind what's best. Michelle's options: 1 just let Katie respond; 2 spend more time with Mrs Morris and delay the medicine round; 3 go back to Mrs Morris after the drug round as she had promised; 4 glibly reassured her; 5 get someone else to speak to Mrs Morris.	Should Michelle delay the drug round by responding to Mrs Morris's outburst?	Michelle had to weigh up the needs of Mrs Morris against the needs of the other patients awaiting their medication. Would other patients have come to harm? Virtue – what should a caring nurse do?
The nurse[s]' perspective	**Consider the power relationships/ factors that determined the way the decision/ action was actually taken.**	**The organisation's perspective**
Michelle was confronted with Mrs Morris's suffering. Her caring instinct ruled that she should stop the drug round and comfort her. However she felt she should also continue the drug round – that her colleagues would criticise her for neglecting her task. Michelle also felt she lacked the skills to comfort Mrs Morris. This made her feel uncomfortable and fearful of not knowing how to respond. She had not experienced similar situations previously.	Michelle felt she should continue the medicine round within the boundaries of normal practice. She did fear sanction from Katie if she hadn't.	Anxious to avoid complaint from patients not receiving their drugs on time or medical angst about 'irresponsible' nurse behaviour not giving out medication at prescribed times. Tasks are appealing because they reinforce the primary value of 'smooth running' of the organisation.

grow through dialogue because it's a development curve for all of us. I don't set myself up as 'expert'.

2 My role as a 'servant-leader' and being of service to the students [Greenleaf 1975].[10] It reflects a shift from 'teaching at them' to 'learning with them'. The students have become more responsible for their learning, even in the short time the group has been together. In fact,

I'm surprised at just how much the group works together. I know some of the students are quiet and others talk a lot. Peter, for example, tends to dominate and be quite opinionated. But he's changing. I don't tend to interfere or censure because I sense the group will find its synergy. Also the structures we use – students taking it in turns and 'being in the other's shoes' facilitates participation from quieter members.

3   This leads on to the idea of 'community' – that what is nurtured in group-guided reflection is community. It develops from moving from an individual consciousness to a group consciousness or coherence where the whole is greater than the sum of the parts. Bohm suggests that coherence has a very high creative energy that we put to work through reflection and dialogue.

4   I used Heron's Six Category Intervention Analysis as a way to help the students see communication skills. It reminded me of the way I try to use facilitative skills in de-emphasising my authority as 'teacher'. Using facilitative skills role-models them for the students – what Johns terms 'parallel process framing' [Stewart and Joines 1987].[11] I thought I would be giving more advice or confronting actions that I felt weren't appropriate, but it hasn't been generally necessary. Again, the technique 'of being in the other's shoes' creates options that are essentially confrontational but in a safe and non-authoritative way.

5   I am convinced that attributes of being available to the patient such as concern for the person and poise can be meaningfully developed through guided reflection. They are relevant within every situation and emerge as a vital aspect of professional artistry.

6   The whole issue of authority is challenging. We, as teachers, are so used to being in authority with students that it's difficult for us to shift, and yet it is vital. As Bohm [1996: 42] states [reading],[12] 'the school is a very authoritative structure. It has its value but it is a structure within which it might be difficult to get dialogue going … there is no place in the dialogue for the principle of authority and hierarchy.' I replaced 'family' in Bohm's text with 'school'. This is the fundamental assumption that has to change – that if we are going to work through dialogue than we must adopt the assumption that our role is to serve students to grow, and that requires a radical shift in the teacher–student relationship, moving into an adult–adult mode using a TA perspective. I know this is contentious because of the resistance some teachers have to such a shift, especially a maternal attitude towards first-years. I've often heard it said that students are irresponsible children, but perhaps that's because we don't let them grow?'

Stella: 'Are you suggesting I'm maternalistic? I'm telling you, girl, that I have been managing first-year student groups for the past 15 years. I do not need telling that my approach to teaching is wrong, especially by the likes of you, still wet behind the ears. I will admit I do not like new-fangled ideas such as reflective practice. There is no proof it works. I teach it in a didactic way, as with any other theory.

Marcia: 'OK, let's look constructively at how we teach reflective practice. Perhaps we do not need any lectures but accommodate such teaching within the guided reflection groups? However, we need to be consistent. Stella, frankly I am anxious – your reaction and attitude are unhelpful. However, I do acknowledge that change is never rational and we need to explore our emotional responses in a respectful way.'

Skills Box

- Review 'Guidance' in Chapter 5. What would you say were Lucy's strengths and weaknesses as a guide? If you are a guide, how does this narrative inform you?
- Reflect on one experience where you struggled to know how best to respond. What insights do you gain in dialogue with Michelle's experience?

- Use ethical mapping in a systematic way to facilitate an appreciation of ethics.
- Google Six Category Intervention Analysis – is this a useful approach to learning about communication skills? Test it in practice and reflect on outcomes.
- To what extent do you think Michelle was 'available' [using the Being Available template – Table 4.3] to Mrs Morris? To what extent do you think you are available to patients and relatives? What is your reflective evidence to support your assertion?

Summary

Perhaps it is only through group -guided reflection that such aspects of professional artistry as concern for patients, poise and communication skills can be understood and developed. These are not cognitive skills. As Michelle's experience illuminates, these attributes are not easy in the face of experiencing another's suffering. They are the essence of personality and, as such, take time to develop through constant attention and care. In Chapter 14 I offer a further illustration of guiding nursing students working with third-year students.

Endnotes

1 See chapter 8.
2 Kopp, P. (2000) Overcoming difficulties in communicating with other professionals. *Nursing Times*. 96 (28) 47–49.
3 Johns, C. (2004) *Being mindful, easing suffering*. Jessica Kingsley, p. 200.
4 Johns, C. (2013) Reflection on touch and the environment. In C. Johns, *Becoming a reflective practitioner* [4th edition] Wiley-Blackwell, Oxford, pp. 117–124.
5 Evans, J. (2002) Cautious caregivers: gender stereotypes and the sexualisation of men nurses' touch. *Journal of Advanced Nursing*, 40.4, 441–448.
6 Woodward, V. and Webb, C. (2001) Women's anxieties surrounding breast disorders: a systematic review of the literature. *Journal of Advanced Nursing* 33.1, 29–41.
7 Knopf, M. (1994) Treatment options for early stage breast cancer. *MEDSURG Nursing* 3, 249–257.
8 Northouse, I., et al. (1995) Emotional distress reported by women and husbands prior to breast biopsy. *Nursing Research* 44, 196–201.
9 Mayeroff, M. (1971) *On caring*. Harper Perennial, New York, p. 1.
10 Greenleaf, R. (1975) *Servant-leadership*. Paulist Press, New York.
11 Stewart, I. and Joines, V. (1987) *TA today: a new introduction to transactional analysis*. Russell Press, Nottingham.
12 Bohm, D. (1996 edited by Lee Nichol) *On dialogue*, Routledge, London, p. 42

References

Bohm, D. (1996) (ed. L. Nichol) *On dialogue*. Routledge, London.
Evans, J. (2002) Cautious caregivers: gender stereotypes and the sexualisation of men nurses' touch. *Journal of Advanced Nursing* 40.4, 441–448.
Greenleaf, R. (1975) *Servant-leadership*. Paulist Press, New York.
Johns, C. (2004) *Being mindful, easing suffering*. Jessica Kingsley, London.

Johns, C. (2013) Reflection on touch and the environment. In C. Johns, *Becoming a reflective practitioner* (4th ed.). Wiley-Blackwell, Oxford, pp. 117–124.

Knopf, M. (1994) Treatment options for early stage breast cancer. *MEDSURG Nursing* 3, 249–257.

Kopp, P. (2000) Overcoming difficulties in communicating with other professionals. *Nursing Times* 96.28, 47–49.

Mayeroff, M. (1971) *On caring*. Harper Perennial, New York.

Northouse, I. et al. (1995) Emotional distress reported by women and husbands prior to breast biopsy. *Nursing Research* 44, 196–201.

Stewart, I. and Joines, V. (1987), *TA today: a new introduction to Transactional Analysis*. Russell Press, Nottingham.

Woodward, V. and Webb, C. (2001) Women's anxieties surrounding breast disorders: a systematic review of the literature. *Journal of Advanced Nursing* 33.1, 29–41.

Chapter 15

Guiding Third-Year Nursing Students in Guided Reflection

Christopher Johns

Guidance is service to enable others to succeed

Introduction

In chapter 14 I explored guiding first-year nursing students. In this chapter I explore guiding third-year students. As you might expect, the tone of the session is different working with students who have been in guided reflection for over two years.

Karen

Karen is a third-year student nurse on her professional practice placement. She has chosen an elderly care unit where she has been provisionally accepted for a staff nurse position. The ward has an established clinical supervision project whereby Karen receives individual supervision from Toni, the ward sister.

Karen studies with her guided reflection group that meets twice weekly at the university for two hours. This forms the basis for the professional practice module. There are eight students in her group, supervised by Gary.

Today, Karen shares: 'One night last week Hank, one of the patients, complained to me about the actions of one of the night care assistants. Evidently she was very rude when he asked for help. She told him he would have to wait, that he wasn't the only patient on the ward. He was very angry and distressed about it. I felt awful for him. Somewhat impetuously I wrote about his complaint in the notes. I did this because I felt angry on his behalf and also to cover my own back in case something happened because of that, if he had got worked up and had a heart attack or he made a formal complaint. I didn't state who was involved or the nature of the incident. Christine, the staff nurse on duty that

Becoming a Reflective Practitioner, Fifth Edition. Edited by Christopher Johns.
© 2017 John Wiley & Sons Ltd. Published 2017 by John Wiley & Sons Ltd.
Companion Website: www.wiley.com/go/johns/reflectivepractitioner

night, picked up what I had written in the notes and said that she felt "very sad that I had to write that, that some things were better said, not written". She didn't deny the incident happened but criticised my documenting it.'

Karen paused, clearly upset recounting the situation.

Gary responded:	'I can see you are upset by the event. Is that because of the way you handled it or because you still feel angry on Hank's behalf or both?'
Tom interjected:	'I'd feel angry if I had been in your shoes.'
Pauline:	'Me too! Some of these care assistants shouldn't be allowed loose!'
Karen:	'Thanks guys. I was anxious about Christine's remarks as if it was me who was the villain. I re-read my notes of the incident because I had written them in a hurry. You know, in the heat of the moment. I realised I had used a word that could have been replaced by a better one.'
Gary:	'An antagonistic word?'
Karen:	'Yes. I made a further comment and replaced my initial note to make it clearer to people reading it. What got me was Christine criticising me about my way of documenting it when *Nursing Times* and the government bang on about "whistle blowing" and how complaints should be documented. I felt she was trying to cover for the person involved, though she did acknowledge the event had happened.'
Gary:	'And now?'
Karen:	'I pointed it out to Leslie as he was the charge nurse on duty that morning. He was working a long day and said he would have a word with the person involved when she came on for the night shift. I went home and worried about it all night, worried how she would take it, what she would say.'
Gary:	'You were worried about comeback – that somehow you had broken some unwritten rule about being loyal to colleagues rather than acting in the patient's best interests? I sense your anxiety about this incident. What would you do differently if you found yourself in the same situation again? It might be helpful if the whole group considered what they would do if in your shoes. I'm certain we all experience such events to some degree.'

After a few minutes pause Karen said: 'This is a hard one. The only thing I could have done differently would have been to ring the care assistant and ask her to explain from her point of view.'

Louise:	'What response might you have got?'
Karen:	'From my perspective, if it was me I would have appreciated it.'
Gary:	'And knowing the person involved?'
Karen:	'I can't say. She could nearly be my grandmother.'
Tom:	'How do you normally get on with her?'
Karen:	'I see her in the evenings and nights when she works but I don't have much to do with her. I suppose my relationship with her is superficial.'
Gary:	'Do you think this action against Hank was out of character for her?'
Karen:	'I think it was an exaggeration of her normal character.'
Gary:	'You think?'

Karen:	'I don't work with her. It's difficult to know how she is with other patients. The event itself was quite trivial, it's Hank's anger that got to me.'
Lil:	'Do you think Hank's anger was reasonable? I mean is he always giving staff grief?'
Karen:	'If it had been me on the receiving end then I would have been upset and angry. She was inflicting her values on him, not respecting him.'
Gary:	'I sense you feel you didn't handle Hank's complaint in the best way. Have you shared this in your practice supervision?'
Karen:	'No, not yet. It's helpful to work it through here first.'
Gary:	'Do you think writing a complaint in the notes is the best way of reporting patient distress?'
Karen:	'I'm not sure. Do you think it was the wrong approach?'
Gary:	'Let's open that up.'
Pauline:	'I guess that altering the notes might be construed as unprofessional. Perhaps other staff should have picked that up. I know you were trying to dampen down the conflict.'
Karen:	'Yes I was. What would you have done?'
Pauline:	'Umm, tricky. I know you were emotional because of Hank and the hostile feedback. Maybe discussing the situation at shift report would have been better? Reporting the incident to the charge nurse sounds good. It's not unreasonable to expect him to deal with it.'
Karen:	'He's a conflict avoider! He would have conveniently forgotten about it and brushed it under the carpet. That would have made it worse. I can imagine them saying I went running to mother and got them into trouble.'
Gary:	'Reporting it to the charge nurse was an option. What other options do you have? Think about what would have been the "right" response – use ethical mapping.'
Karen:	'Clearly Mandy, that's the care assistant, was in the wrong – she abused a patient and that cannot be tolerated. She has no defence for this except to play down the incident or accuse Hank of lying. I know I should have been more mindful of the consequences of writing as I did in the notes. It wasn't the best way of reporting this. Altering the notes was not a good response as it looked as if I was trying to cover up my mistake. Everyone is so fearful of conflict. I do need to talk this through with Mandy. If it isn't possible face to face then I could ring her at home. I could have asked Hank if he wanted me to report the situation – I rather took that for granted. I have a moral duty to care and expose situations of abuse.'
Ann:	'Yeah, so many experiences we reflect on involves conflict and yet it seems we are not good at dealing with it. It would it be useful to frame Karen's situation in the Thomas–Kilmann conflict mode instrument.[1]'
Peter:	'Yes that would be cool.'
Gary:	'OK Peter – talk us through it.'
Peter:	'I can draw it on the screen. Basically it posits five styles of conflict management along the two axes of assertiveness and cooperation. The five styles are avoidance, accommodation, compromise, competition and collaboration. So avoidance is non-assertive/non-cooperation. Accommodation is non-assertive/ cooperation – where you give way to the other's demand. Compromise is partly assertive/cooperative – finding a way to move through the conflict. Competition is assertive but non-cooperative – the struggle to see

who wins and loses! Collaboration is both assertive and cooperative – the ideal professional mode although rarely realised as personal agendas always interfere. Cavanagh's research indicated that nurses and nurse managers most used avoidance, then accommodation, then compromise, then collaboration and then competition.[2] The research is quite old so maybe it's changed now.'

Gary: 'Thanks Peter, succinctly put. Can we understand why nurses are most likely to avoid conflict? As Karen said – the charge nurse tends to brush conflict under the carpet.'

Pauline: 'Does it relate to the harmonious team in which staff are more loyal to their colleagues than to their patients and as such sacrifice the patient's best interests in favour of avoiding conflict with their colleagues to maintain a harmonious façade?[3] From this perspective Karen, not the care assistant, becomes the problem because she broke this "rule".'

Karen: 'That's really uncomfortable. How do we overcome this and achieve collaboration? We have to shed fear of consequences and that's exactly what I fear to the extent I wouldn't report the complaint again, especially as I'm going to work on the ward as a staff nurse.'

Gary: 'But then you do not act for the best and sacrifice your integrity.'

Lil: 'Ouch. That's tough but true.'

Karen: 'Any tips for speaking with the care assistant?'

Gary: 'OK. Remind yourself what style of managing conflict you want to be.'

Karen: 'Collaborative. There is no other desirable mode when you examine each of them.'

Gary: ' I agree. Now, imagine I am the care assistant. The key factor is to keep the situation grounded in the situation rather than it becoming a secondary situation of interpersonal conflict, as indeed it has already become. Remember the maxim "tough on the issues, soft on the person". See taking action as an act of personal integrity as fearful as you are of its potential consequences of ostracism.'

[After rehearsal] *Karen:* 'OK I can try that.'

Next Session

Karen reported: 'I went home and phoned her!'

Lil: 'Good for you. How did you feel when you picked up the receiver?'

Karen: 'Terrified! She was angry but she didn't get as angry as she possibly could have done. I think she was also feeling guilty.'

Gary: 'Have you learnt that it pays to belong to the harmonious team? If so, if a similar situation occurs, you will think twice before confronting it?'

Karen: 'I don't know. I'm really dejected and yet I can sense it's vital that I am not intimidated. If we can't raise issues because of fear of conflict then we all go about as if wearing masks. I can't simply sweep this under the carpet.'

Peter: 'You haven't – you did phone her and refused to play the harmonious team game. When is your practice supervision?'

Karen: 'Tomorrow! I feel like a chicken at the prospect of talking about this situation but I must. I must be assertive and not a coward. Why did

	Hank wait to see me!? He was probably just thinking about it when he saw me.'
Lil:	'Perhaps he trusted you?'
Karen:	'I like to think so. It's important patients can trust nurses to act for them as necessary.'
Lil:	'How do you think the care assistant might be feeling now?'
Karen:	'I hope she appreciates that I had the courage to ring her.'
Gary:	'So be positive about this – your phone call to Mandy was an act of integrity. Her anger was her guilt. You enabled her to release that energy, yet she was also confronted with the fact that she did not act appropriately towards Hank. You can rationalise her anger in this way. It's imperative that you do not see yourself in the wrong. It's easier with the charge nurse because that's what supervision is about – a non-judgmental space to reflect on and learn through experience.'
Karen:	'I hear what you say but it's not easy. I'm not assertive.'
Gary:	'Let's talk about assertiveness. It links well with conflict management. What do we know about it?'
Peter:	'Johns sets out the assertiveness action ladder, which offers a practical approach to reflecting on self being assertive and where we might get stuck.'
Gary:	'Thanks again Peter. You are good at pulling out these reflective frameworks. Let's look at it [turning to page 247 of the fourth edition of *Becoming a reflective practitioner*] [see Figure 15.1].'[4]
Karen:	'I can see myself getting stuck at rung 3 – "Authority to assert self". Being a student and not wanting to upset the apple cart. I've got a good argument and supervision is the optimum space. JDI!'

10	Treading the fine line between pushing and yielding	
9	Playing the power game	
8	Staying in adult mode	
7	Being skilful enough to be heard	
6	'Just do it!' [JDI]	
5	Creating the optimum conditions to assert self	
4	Making a good argument	
3	Authority to assert self	
2	Ethically right to assert self	
1	Feeing the need to assert self	

Figure 15.1   The assertive action ladder (Adapted from Johns 2013: 247). The assertive action ladder was designed by analysing the pattern of becoming assertive with practitioners within guided reflection. It was apparent that nurses are not equipped to manage conflict positively, leading to a huge wastage of energy and a low sense of self-esteem. It is true to say that the effective practitioner is an assertive practitioner and yet, in a culture where nurses are not expected to be assertive, this may itself cause conflict. The ladder has been adapted in light of reflection on its use in guided reflection although its basic tenets remains unchanged.

Gary:	'It's worth thinking about levels 7 to 10 on the ladder. The idea of "being heard" or as Johns noted in an earlier edition[5] "being adept at interaction skills". Don't know why he changed it. He was referring in particular to using Heron's Six Category Intervention Analysis.[6] It would also have been good to consider it last session with Karen anticipating phoning the care assistant.'
Ann:	'I like the idea of being forthright – giving the charge nurse information – that Hank complained and how Karen dealt with it. Then, depending on how he responded to be confrontational- "What is he going to do about it?" There seems little room to use the more facilitative skills of catharsis or catalysis although I imagine if he is any good at supervision he would respond with those techniques.'
Peter:	'If I was the charge nurse I would want to intercede and confront the care assistant's and the night staff nurse's behaviour.'
Gary:	'Rung 8 "Staying in adult mode" reflects how the normal pattern of communication between people is adult–adult from a Transactional Analysis perspective. Perhaps I should say "ideal" rather than "normal" as people so often do not communicate from these ego levels. TA theory goes something like this – people communicate from ego levels – parent, adult, child. As I noted, adult–adult is ideal – the position of responsible and collaborative professionals. However, when people get anxious they can flip into either learnt parent or child mode. When the situation is with someone in authority who is anxious – for example, the charge nurse anxious about the complaint or altering the notes, then he is more likely to flip into critical parent mode. That creates anxiety for Karen who is then likely to respond by flipping into child mode. In this way the pattern of communication is reciprocated and doesn't breakdown. The key for Karen is to recognise the pattern of communication and be mindful of staying in adult mode, which means also helping the charge nurse to stay in adult mode. In that way you can have an "adult" conversation, which is the only truly professional model of communication. I suggest we revise Heron and TA theory and link it to any new experiences to explore next time. Have another dekko at Stewart and Joines, "TA Today".[7] Communication is the crux of professional artistry. Time is getting on. Karen, can you summarise what insights you have gained?'
Karen:	'Reflection has reinforced my patient-centred values – the importance of listening to and working with patients like Hank. It involves a moral responsibility. I realise I do care about patients. I'm not good at conflict and felt intimidated, I need to develop a greater sense of poise so I am not so easily rattled by such issues. As a result I feel I have grown through this experience – more grown-up, more adult, less like a frightened panicky child. It has exposed the myth of collaborative relationships. The idea of the harmonious team is compelling – I can see it. My assertive, conflict management and communication skills all need developing, and yet I do feel more assertive. I also need to talk to the charge nurse tomorrow and overcome my hierarchical fear of punishment.'

Practice Supervision

The next afternoon Karen knocks on the charge nurse's door. She sits and tells Ken about Hank's complaint and her response to it. She focuses on giving him information as suggested in her last guided reflection group.

Ken responds: 'What do you want me to do about it?'

Karen is initially flummoxed: 'I want you to deal with it. I'm sorry I changed the notes that was so unprofessional. It won't happen again.'

Ken: 'It wasn't very clever but I understand why you did that. So we can let that go. As for the night staff you have already taken responsibility by confronting Mandy. She isn't easy. She's been on the ward a long time working nights. Taking her on was courageous. I must admit you did me a favour. I have avoided conflict with her. I will have a word with Christine [the night staff nurse] and remind her that any abuse of patients cannot be tolerated. Perhaps then she will be more mindful of her own responsibility and take action with Mandy if she's abusive to patients. How does that sound?'

Karen: 'Good. I was so anxious coming to see you today. Anxious that you would be angry at me and not want me on the ward as a staff nurse. Conflict is so hard and yet it shouldn't be if we were all responsible for our actions and working towards the same values.'

Ken: 'If it's any consolation, you've confronted me to take more role responsibility. So thank you for that. I hope we can be really open with each other in the future. I know it's a cliché to say "my door is always open", but from next month you will no longer be a student but a staff nurse.'

Karen: 'I think we should establish group guided reflection or supervision on the ward. That might help improve dialogue between staff although I expect those you want to attend won't unless it is made compulsory.'

Ken: 'Umm, food for thought.'

Next Session

At their next guided reflection session Gary asked Karen for feedback.

Karen: 'Yes I did talk to him. I was anxious as anticipated. I gave it to him flat as we discussed. He was really receptive. He actually thanked me for helping him deal with his own issue of conflict avoidance. Picking up the assertiveness ladder I can sense the power game.'

Gary: 'Say more?'

Karen: 'How we can easily be intimated by senior staff who have power of sanction over us. I did some homework on French and Raven's sources of social power that we've explored previously.'

Gary: 'Remind us?'

Karen sets out the framework: 'French and Raven set out six sources of social power that are either authoritative or facilitative.[8] Authoritative sources are positional, coercive and reward. Facilitative sources are relational and expert, although reward can also be

Authoritative	Facilitative
Positional power: legitimate power given by the person's position within the organisation.	*Relational power*: power of influence that stems from relationships [for example, charisma]
Coercive power: the power to impose sanction [rife within a blame–shame culture]	*Expert power*: power that stems from knowing and wisdom
Reward power: extrinsic [for example, pay, promotion]	*Reward power*: intrinsic [for example, realising one's values, doing a good job]

Figure 15.2   French and Raven sources of leadership power

facilitative if the reward is intrinsic rather than extrinsic. It's easier if I draw it on the board [see Figure 15.2]. Positioning Ken in this framework I can see how he's been trapped in his own power game. He's been under considerable pressure as a fairly newly promoted charge nurse. It made him anxious and critical of every little thing. He needed to control things to feel safe. For some reason he could let go with me as if he knew he could trust me. I really felt different about him after that – like empathy, knowing how he was feeling and how tough it was for him. He didn't want to appear as if he wasn't coping, hence the tough parental front.'

Peter: 'I've noticed that with charge nurses and sisters I've worked with. They are like critical parents always at you for little things. You're right, it is as if they are anxious and flip into this parental role. It's hard not to respond as a child especially when you rely on them for good reports.'

Gary: 'There is so much pressure on organisations to perform. It is as if the whole organisation is anxious and this gets transmitted down the hierarchy into every member of staff at every level. So no doubt Ken gets treated like a child from his modern matron and all the way to the boardroom. It's like an anxiety infection that is very hard to breakthrough. It requires a transformational leadership throughout the organisation where the blame–shame culture is put to rest. Referring back to French and Raven we can see that most managers are authoritarian, relying on position and sanction power with rewards for good children. We need leaders who are transformational, who emphasise facilitative sources of power notably expert and relational sources of power. However, this demands a shift in the balance of power that must be compensated by responsibility. Yet, how can staff grow into responsibility when they are constantly being treated like children?'

Pauline: 'Wow. I want to be a transformational leader but is it possible within a transactional culture? I sense you would stick out like a sore thumb and be marginalised as being different.'

Gary: 'That's very true. There is great pressure to know your place and conform to social norms. Check out Johns's new book *Mindful leadership*[9] that really addresses the tension of becoming a leader in a transactional culture.'

Lil: 'I have an experience to share that relates to Karen's. It is about me pushing an issue and getting slapped down when I told the senior nurse I couldn't do as she requested as I was talking with a patient. She told me to stop that and do as she requested. I said no. She shouted at me in front of the patient to do as I was told – she had certainly flipped into critical parent. I felt humiliated. I apologised to my patient trying to stay in adult mode and did as she requested. The patient seemed to understand ward politics and gave me a smile so I didn't feel I had failed her.'

Ann: 'Pushing the fine line – rung 10 of the assertiveness ladder. You didn't know when to yield! Ouch.'

Lil: 'Yes it did hurt but I felt outraged. She could see I was with a patient talking about discharge. She said I could do that later as if talking was some low-level task.'

Gary: 'And if it happened again?'

Lil: 'Good question. I know I must keep my cool and not get outraged. Perhaps play the power game knowing she is such a tyrant with student nurses but be mindful I am yielding so that I don't feel such a failure.'

Ann: 'Yielding. Pushing the fine line – treading careful not to overstep the mark and get punished. That's quite some skill, to be that mindful. It's a form of retreat from a situation you can't win to preserve your integrity. Hands up – I yield! '

Peter: 'Surviving to fight another day!'

Gary: 'Thanks Ann. Knowing when to yield is an important professional skill. As Ann says it is about maintaining one's integrity. This sense of outrage, is that healthy or professional?'

Lil: 'No! I can sense stress eating me alive.'

Ann: 'Yeah some days I could do with a suit of armour as protection.'

Gary: 'Managing ourselves within practice is clearly a vital aspect of professional practice. Stress consumes energy and makes us less available to our patients and colleagues. Johns calls this ability to know and manage our emotional selves *poise* as we explored within the "Being Available" template.[10] Goleman and colleagues describe it as emotional intelligence.[11]'

Lil: 'I probably let stress build up in me until it explodes. Obviously I didn't explode with the senior staff nurse. Subdued by her authority over me. Later, Jenny asked me something silly and I exploded at her. I apologised afterwards.'

Peter: 'Is that horizontal violence? Feels like bullying to me.'

Ann: 'Yes, one thing that bothers me about Karen's experience we haven't really touched upon is the notion that she felt bullied by the night staff nurse. Bullying is an insidious and debilitating experience for its victim. It is difficult to resist, possibly the reason why the "bully" has picked on that person. Both bully and victim get caught up in a pattern of behaviour from which neither can easily break free. As I read it, Karen threatens her control and thus becomes a target as if a naughty child being scolded by a critical parent. I wonder – does the staff nurse realise she is a bully?'

Gary: 'This is such an important point. Karen's experience illuminates the aetiology of bullying as systemic NHS managerial behaviour whereby those being bullied stand back too timid to act, as if they too might become victims. It also exposes the somewhat Machiavellian notion that others might benefit from another's bullying. How can we and organisations better resist bullying?'

Peter: 'Well, it shouldn't be tolerated, and yet recognising its endemic nature makes it difficult to tackle. Perhaps organisations turn a blind eye to bullying because they consider nurses like Karen should be docile and accept their subordinate position?'

Ann: ' I googled "bullying" after the last session and got a significant number of hits. One example from NursingTimes.net – "Healthcare commission chair Sir Ian Kennedy has called for renewed focus on nurse leadership and issued a warning about the 'corrosive' nature of bullying in the NHS. Sir Ian said 'bullying was "one of the biggest untalked-about problems in the delivery of good care to patients"'. He felt the problem was caused by the NHS's hierarchical culture and occurred across all staff groups. His comments follow last week's staff survey, in which 8% of respondents said they had experienced bullying, harassment or abuse from a manager or team leader and 12% said they had from colleagues." [3 April 2009]. Turning to scholarly articles we find 16 papers written between 2000 and 2010. One useful example is a paper written by Hutchinson and colleagues[12] – "Workplace bullying in nursing: towards a more organisational perspective". I found links to "whistleblowing", "oppressed group behaviour" and "horizontal violence". Seemingly one thing leads to another into a complex and murky organisational culture. I also found advice on how to stop it but such rational advice falters when placed within a transactional health care organizational culture.'

Gary: 'Good stuff Ann. Horizontal violence is akin to bullying. When we can't focus our outrage at those who are at a higher authority level we find a softer target, people at our own level.'

Lil: 'It would be good to have a session on taking care of ourselves.'

Gary: 'That's a good idea. To help prepare I suggest you each keep a stress diary – using the "Feeling Fluffy, Feeling Drained" scale.[13] The scale consists of a visual analogue scale [VAS] 10 cm long. It asks you to mark along the scale the extent you feel either fluffy or drained at the end of your shift.

The scale then poses three questions:

- What factors contribute to your sense of feeling drained?
- What factors contribute to your sense of feeling light and fluffy?
- What can you do to go home feeling more fluffy and less drained?

We can be stressed for many reasons. The first remedy for dealing with stress is to recognise its aetiology. It leaves us feeling drained. Feeling fluffy is a feeling of lightness at the end of the day where one's energy remains full whereas feeling drained is having no energy at the end of the workday. I am sure you've all experienced such feelings.

At the end of the shift, score the extent you feel either fluffy or drained and explore contributing factors and what you can realistically do to improve your fluffy score by acknowledging enhancing feel-good experiences and working at neutralising energy-draining situations. Johns gives an example of one practitioner's score.'[14]

Lil: 'Looking at the example – it seems a bad day at the office! I can identify with her experience. Dealing with angry relatives scares me, and yet it is such an important part of care. I know we must take responsibility and put our hands up if we are wrong but it's tough when we do our best and still get shit.'

Pauline: 'Yes, I agree. I notice she never scored less than 5. All that stress accumulating. I wonder how she works it off? Perhaps explodes, like you Lil!'

Lil: 'Maybe. But I can see how the scale works, that by becoming more mindful of our stress we can begin to work out ways of dealing with it. For example, next time we are faced with angry relatives we are more likely to handle it better. That in itself is rewarding and stress-breaking. Giving ourselves positive feedback. Sharing here in the group will also be really helpful. Like draining the stress butt before it gets too full and using that energy to stop the butt filling in the first place.'

Peter: 'The water butt theory of stress.[15] I like the way we introduce theory to fit with the experiences we share and then use those theories to develop our reflections as per the cue, "What knowledge did or should have informed our actions?"'

Ann: 'I feel I am just beginning to learn to be a nurse. You can learn all the technical stuff easy, but these professional issues are really tough. The ward is certainly a political and social cauldron.'

And so it went on, the group exploring aspects of professional practice that were all inherently problematic and relevant to each group member.

Skill Box

> - *What would you say are the strengths and weaknesses of Gary's guidance?*
> - *What insights can you draw about your own guidance experience or about guidance in general [revisit Chapter 5]?*
> - *Put yourself in Karen's shoes – how would you have responded? Reflect on an experience of conflict with colleagues using the conflict management mode.*
> - *Apply the reflective frameworks deemed essential to professional artistry: Conflict Management Grid, Assertiveness Action Ladder, Feeling Fluffy-Feeling Drained Scale within your reflections. It is a useful way to position self within theory and learn these aspects of professional artistry that are almost impossible to learn from a theoretical perspective.*

Summary

There is a randomness about the dialogue as it follows its own chaotic path around Karen's reflection of her experience with Hank. And yet, within the apparent chaos order emerges because Gary enables dialogue to flow. Theory is fed in. Insights tumble out. A wealth of professional practice issues are covered, threads picked up from previous sessions, seeds laid for future sessions. It is dynamic, fecund.

It suggests that aspects of professional artistry are not possible to teach from a technical rational approach [for example theory-driven lectures]. They can only be appreciated in practice and developed through reflection.

Endnotes

1   Endnotes Thomas, K. and Kilmann, R. (1974) *Thomas–Kilmann conflict mode instrument.* Xicom, Toledo, OH.

2   Cavanagh, S. (1991) The conflict management style of staff nurses and nurse managers. *Journal of Advanced Nursing* 16, 1254–1260.

3   Horizontal violence: Karen's experience reveals the phenomena of horizontal violence (Duffy 1995; Johns 1992; McKenna, Smith, Poole and Coverdale 2003) – a toxic form of dealing with stress. The idea of 'horizontal' stems from bureaucratic- hierarchical systems, whereby the subordinate person [the nurse] is unable to project her anger or frustration at her more

powerful oppressors. She can only fire at her those on her own level or below her. Yet, even on her own level, this violence is muted within the harmonious team, perhaps because people are motivated to be partially invisible, to keep their heads down to avoid criticism (Street 1992). Hence harmonious is a collusive strategy to contain the team's unresolved angst. See Duffy, E. (1995, April), Horizontal violence: a conundrum for nursing. Collegian. *Journal of the Royal College of Nursing Australia.* 2.2, 5–17; Johns, C (1992) Ownership and the harmonious team: barriers to developing the therapeutic nursing team in primary nursing. *Journal of Clinical Nursing* 1, 89–94; McKenna, B., Smith, N., Poole, S. and Coverdale, J. (2003) Horizontal violence: experiences of Registered Nurses in their first year of practice. *Journal of Advanced Nursing*, 42.1, 90–96, at 91; Street, A. (1992) *Inside nursing: a critical ethnography of clinical nursing*. State University of New York Press, Albany.

4   Johns, C. (2013) *Becoming a reflective practitioner* [4th edition]. Wiley-Blackwell, Oxford.
5   Johns, C. (2009) *Becoming a reflective practitioner* [3rd edition]. Blackwell Scientific Publications, Oxford.
6   Six Category Intervention Analysis is explored in Chapter 5 as an approach to guiding reflection.
7   Stewart, I. and Joines, V. (1987) *TA today: a new introduction to transactional analysis*. Russell Press, Nottingham.
8   French, J. and Raven, B. (1968) The bases of social power. In D. Cartwright and A. Zander [eds.] *Group Dynamics*. Row Peterson, Evanston, IL, pp. 150–167.
9   Johns, C. (2015) *Mindful leadership*. Palgrave Macmillan, London.
10   See Table 4.3.
11   Goleman, D., Boyatzis, R. and Mckee, A. (2008) *The new leaders, transforming the art of leadership into the science of results*. Sphere, London.
12   Hutchinson, M., Vickers, M., Jackson, D., and Wilkes, L. (2006) Workplace bullying in nursing: towards a more critical organisational perspective. *Nursing Inquiry* 13.2, 118–126.
13   See Chapter 3.
14   Table 3.5.
15   See Chapter 3. pp. 50–51.

Chapter 16

A Tale of Two Teachers

Christopher Johns

Performance tones professional artistry

Introduction

Janet and John are two nurse teachers who work in different universities. They both have a remit to teach the management of stroke patients to first-year degree students. The students will be on medical ward placements where care of stroke patients is anticipated.

Janet believes strongly in a reflective practice approach to teaching, whereas John is oriented towards a conventional technical rational approach. The students in both institutions have been introduced to reflective practice earlier in their training. This introduction was rudimentary through offering Gibbs reflective cycle[1] and the Model for Structured Reflection [MSR].[2]

John sets out his teaching plan with aims and measurable objectives.

At the end of this session the students will:

1 Understand the aetiology of cerebral vascular accident [CVA];
2 Recognise its common symptoms;
3 Know the range of investigations to establish diagnosis;
4 Have gained a critical understanding of nursing care alongside other professionals;
5 Appreciate the social and psychological impact on the family.

He reviews this set of objectives. The taunt of reflective practice bothers him so he adds:

6 Be able to frame their learning of CVA within Gibbs learning cycle.

He prepares a PowerPoint presentation to enable him to move smoothly between the objectives supported by references. He has two hours to deliver. All in all a solid lecture with some discussion time built in for students to express any thoughts they might have, recognising that some students may have previous experience of caring for stroke patients.

For the assignment John writes 'A case study reflecting the essential aspects of the nursing care of a stroke patient. It is expected the assignment will show evidence of knowledge

Becoming a Reflective Practitioner, Fifth Edition. Edited by Christopher Johns.
© 2017 John Wiley & Sons Ltd. Published 2017 by John Wiley & Sons Ltd.
Companion Website: www.wiley.com/go/johns/reflectivepractitioner

of stroke aetiology and symptoms, investigations, and nursing care utilising Gibbs's reflective cycle.'

When challenged about his use of Gibbs reflective model he replies 'I prefer Gibbs model as it is easier for students to use than the MSR and it's certainly easier for me to teach and mark.'

When challenged about his rationale he says 'The students find reflection daunting so why make it more complicated than it need be?'

'Perhaps they find it daunting because you and others don't give it due attention?'

'That would take too much time. The curriculum is full as it is.'

Janet sits at her computer wondering how best to deliver this session. She considers her range of options. First, a solid lecture based around a series of objectives. She senses many students would like this approach as it fits with their normal approach to teaching. She imagines their demand - 'give us the facts ' [so that we can reproduce them as necessary]. She also knows that she is 'out on a limb' regards teaching from a reflective paradigm. Of course, there is a curriculum expectation to teach reflective practice. She knows that many of her peers teach reflective practice purely from a technical rational perspective that only gives lip service to its learning potential. There is real confusion over whether reflective practice is a learning strategy or a learning outcome.

She thinks back to curriculum planning sessions where her ideas for a more radical approach to teaching through reflective practice were lampooned. She wants to be innovative but feels the pressure to conform from both her peers and students. How easy to become marginalised when you don't play the dominant game. But she is the module leader and she can claim some authority to interpret the curriculum from a reflective paradigm. Her second option to deliver the session from a reflective perspective through performance.

She drafts her lesson plan. The objective is to understand the needs of the stroke patient and the family and the response of the health care team to meeting these needs. That sounds OK. How best to deliver this session? She poses the paradigmatic tension between a lecture and performance approach. It isn't simply a question of applying learning technologies-lecture, discussion, reflective practice and so on. It is much deeper. It is a fundamental value that governs the whole learning approach to teaching nursing as a practice discipline.

She decides she will share a narrative of caring for a stroke patient and relatives to develop the idea of how to construct a narrative. In doing so she will make herself vulnerable by sharing. Taking a risk. She knows that students will appreciate this. It brings her closer to the students, more *working with them* rather than *talking at them*. Diminish the power differential between them.

Collecting the story should be relatively easy as she works one day a week on a number of medical wards supporting students in practice and staff who mentor them. She can arrange to meet stroke patients and their families and the health professionals involved in their care. She can even arrange to give care herself spanning over several days if necessary. Creating space in her busy workload.

For the assignment she writes 'To explore key insights in dialogue with an informing literature through reflection on nursing a stroke patient'.

She thinks 'Umm, does that work? Should I be more explicit about the insights?

For example: 'three insights about the nurses' impact within the inter-disciplinary team towards easing the stroke patient's and family's experience of suffering.'

Janet says to herself – 'I feel I've covered the scope of the inquiry. The assignment is concerned with patients' and relatives' experiences of suffering stroke and the nurses' and other health professionals' response. This skews the inquiry into the human domain away from the usual predominant biomedical focus. The focus on insights is important as the focus for any reflective assignment rather than a test of the students' ability to apply a reflective model. Perhaps an emphasis on an instrumental approach is appropriate at the beginning of training with the explicit intention of enabling students to assimilate reflective cues into a natural way of thinking about practice. By explicit I mean that students are informed that reflective practice is a developmental process unfolding over the three years of training.'

She phones Peter, one of the few teachers she feels a philosophical rapport with. He can see the bigger picture and the competing assumptions that govern it. She talks through her session idea with him.

'Basically, do you have the balls to stick to your guns?'

'It's not a question of balls Peter otherwise I would be castrated.'

Peter laughs, appreciation the pun. 'Go for it then Janet. I support you. Create some ripples and stir up the pond.'

'Thank you. I need that. Just knowing that at least one other person can see the bigger picture and the options is helpful. In a practice discipline such as nursing, we must focus on practice rather than theory as the primary source of learning. I know it goes against the grain, and that most of my colleagues will reject this claim, but I think their resistance comes from an ignorance – they are not reflective about their own work, so how can they teach reflective practice, except from a technical perspective?'

'That's very true Janet! You inspire me to consider reflective practice beyond the technical rational.'

Janet puts down the phone. More resolute in her intention.

Next morning, she puts on her clinical dress and goes in search.

She arranges to meet April, a teacher from performing arts who has expressed an interest in reflective practice, over lunch to explore how performance might work.

Basically, April will introduce some movement exercises to counter inhibition and some breath and voice-projection exercises. She will then take a couple of scenarios from Janet's narrative to involve the group.

Two weeks later Janet and April enter the classroom. Janet introduces April as a teacher from school of performing arts is joining our session to help prep performance. She commences by 'bringing the mind home' to help the group focus on the task. This itself is a new experience for students. She had assumed they would have experienced 'bringing the mind home' as part of their exposure to the model of structured reflection. Clearly not! But then such practice might make teachers uncomfortable and therefore avoid it. She thinks – 'I must get involved more with teaching reflective practice within the introductory module.'

Just three minutes and the group are quieter, more present.

Janet outlines her plan:

- first hour – explore her narrative of caring for stroke patients;
- second hour – prepare for the follow-up study day in four weeks' time.

Key components:

- This will be organised in six groups of six.
- Go out onto wards and talk with stroke patients, their relatives and health professionals – what are the significant care factors, what investigations have been carried out, what is the resultant aetiology?
- Use the Model for Structured Reflection[3] as a framework to consider the experiences of different people involved in stroke care [patients, relatives, health professionals].

In particular consider how people felt and the reasons for that. Consider – do the actions of health professionals really meet needs of patients and relatives? Be critical – if needs are not met, then why? How might real needs be known and met?

- Identify and critique a list of key texts to explore these issues from a theoretical perspective and juxtapose with experience [see MSR cue].
- Reflect on your findings and construct a 'performance' of findings to illuminate stroke care, together with written commentary based on three five-minute scenarios around insights gained for when we meet at our study day in four weeks' time. In total each group has 20 minutes. Choose a narrator who can link the experiences with relevant theory and research.
- Janet and April will be available for consultation as necessary.

The group buzz with novel excitement, seemingly not fazed by the task. Indeed they seem to relish the creative responsibility. Janet then shares her narrative. Posing questions to engage the group, drawing on their previous nursing experiences, linking with stroke theory and research. She explicitly uses cues from the Model of Structured Reflection to illuminate their value in gaining insight. An hour quickly passes. April takes over and the group play with performance ideas using Janet's narrative as an example of how narrative can be acted out.

John reflects on his session.

'It went fine. I was in control and moved through the objectives seamlessly. We had only a brief time for discussion of previous experience. However, that was useful. It added a learning flavour to the session. Maybe more time would help. No time to frame within Gibbs – but then the students know this model having used it previously. I have not evaluated the session. The students are expected to frame the case study using Gibbs' model showing the reflective ability to apply such a model and show insights gained from using it. However, as first-year students with limited experience of using reflection, I have no great expectation of reflective ability much beyond description. Generally the assignments were descriptive Not very reflective but then that's to be expected from first year students. However the students showed a reasonable understanding of stroke and its nursing care.'

Janet reflects on her session.

'No time to fit it all in. However we are available for ongoing support. Performance is complex and may need more prep time. However they got the gist of it and will learn through the experience of doing it. I checked which wards had stroke patients and were willing to talk with the students. Cleared the ground so to speak. I asked the students to evaluate the session – what would they do differently given the experience again? Is there anything more I [as teacher] could have done to support them? All reflective teaching by its very nature needs a critical evaluation rather than take it for granted.[4] I suggested the students also give me anonymous written feedback for me to consider and discuss with them before we do further performance learning. It's quite emotional – I feel closer to the students as if we have bridged a gap between us. I no longer teach at them but teach with them. Rather like the way we value working with patients rather than nursing at them.'

'The performances were brilliant. I never expected them to rise to the challenge so well. The theatre students would like to be involved next time we do something similar. The assignments were so reflective – really highlighted the core issues especially around emotional and psychological issues, challenging whether stroke care was empathic enough. Will definitely approach other "conditions" in this way. It goes to prove that if you give students responsibility they rise to the challenge. Mind you it is not without some trepidation. I felt very anxious about the "performance" part, knowing little about performance as learning. Without expert help I do not think I would have contemplated it. I would have been exposed as an imposter and looked foolish in front of the students. But I did say – "this is learning for me as well" dropping any pretence of knowing. Risky stuff– does such confession undermine students' confidence especially with something that goes against the grain taking us all out of our comfort zones? I had to trust the students and my own instinct that this approach made good pedagogical sense.'

Feedback from Alan – 'I asked the group about the session. The feedback was positive despite one or two dissenting students who felt "lost" in the task. I said to him "Fancy teaching with me next time? I think it will work better with more than one teacher." He responded – "Perhaps we can set up a 'performance workshop' to explore the milieu more deeply with our performance colleagues?" I know he was hedging his bets, wanting to be open to the idea but cautious. Always this fear of incompetence or peer criticism holding us back, making us fall back on known approaches within our collective comfort zone. I sense a pressure on me to conform as if using a performance approach threatens the status quo. An older colleague who always seems to put others down sarcastically remarked at a team meeting if I was hoping for an Oscar? It caught me off-guard. I tried to explain I was experimenting. With withering scorn she suggested I focus on my real role as a teacher and stop using the school as a playground. Teaching is serious stuff and teachers must control the classroom or anarchy would ensue. I must admit it knocked my confidence being slated in public like that.'

Nursing is a practice discipline. As such, practice must be at the core of any curriculum. Theory and research exist to inform practice. It cannot predict practice because nursing is essentially unpredictable and complex – a consequence of its human nature. Therefore, nursing is always interpreted at the point of contact. Hence, practitioners require professional artistry to navigate the seemingly indeterminate nature of practice. This ability is developed through experience and reflection on experience alongside the ability to dialogue with and critique knowledge for its relevance and value to inform. Because of the partiality of individual reflection, learning through reflection requires peer exposure and skilled guidance. Pedantically reflecting on this teaching experience using the MSR gives me understanding and strengthens my moral conviction and commitment to a reflective curriculum.

What issues seem most important to pay attention to?

The tension between a critical pedagogy approach to teaching nursing practice and the existing dominant biomedical focus in ways that can be justified with a peer group that is wary of innovation yet obliged to adopt reflective teaching

What was I trying to achieve & did I respond effectively?

- enable nurses to learn about stroke care;
- enable students to take an increased responsibility for their own learning;
- make learning dynamic and creative in the belief that this will aid learning [is there research to support this??];
- show possibilities of a more creative approach to reflection beyond its normal instrumental application;
- extend the focus of reflection into narrative and performance.

I believe I responded effectively within the limits of my ability. However, narrative/performance is a steep learning curve for me.

What were the consequences of my actions on the patient, others and myself?

- the experience has reinforced my believe in a critical pedagogy approach;
- a new way of working WITH students, opening new curriculum possibilities [the risk was worth it even had it not gone so well].

What factors influence the way I was/ am feeling, thinking and responding to this situation? Resisting forces:

- anxiety about teaching through narrative performance – do I have the skills?
- dominant expectations from others – that I fit in with deeply ingrained social norms about the way nursing is taught and relationships between teachers and students;
- anxiety about 'going against the dominant pedagogical ideology of technical rationality-potential sanction? [what if it goes wrong / students complain?] Can I take the risk?
- use of time- session needs follow-up day for performance.

Driving forces:

- disturbing normal order of things;
- setting a precedent for this type of work;
- believe that learning will be more effective through performance;
- opportunity for cross disciplinary teaching;
- my expectations- it is what I want to do! Commitment to a more critical and reflective pedagogy.

Assumptions shift:

- most significantly the tension between what I was trying to achieve and normal [biomedical] way of teaching this topic;
- given the complex and indeterminate nature of practice (Schon 1987) practitioners need to develop professional artistry – in contrast with technical rationality that (erroneously) assumes order can be imposed through application of knowledge. How can an obsolete ideology retain such dominance?
- Will open a new pedagogical vista within the school (ripple effect).

How was I feeling and what made me feel that way?

- A cocktail of emotions. Anxious about it going well. (Ego!!) Excited to be doing it and living my values. I think it is imperative that teaching is value-driven which makes it hard within nursing schools dominated by a traditional and uncritical biomedical approach.
- Lucky to get the chance.
- Fortunate Alan picked up the positive vibe.

How were others feeling and why did they feel that way?

- From session feedback I know some students felt uncomfortable with this approach although working in small groups enabled them to participate at a more comfortable level.

- One or two felt like guinea pigs to an experiment and anxious about learning the facts.
- However, the majority went along with the idea and threw themselves into the task – it shows that if you give people space to explore something new they revel in the opportunity. Feedback comment – it was most meaningful and enjoyable despite its uncertainty.

How does this situation connect with previous experiences?

- It doesn't really. It was an intuitive response to do something different, to break the mold. I had attended a whole day narrative performance workshop at a recent conference that inspired me and opened up the possibility to teach in this way.

To what extent did I act for the best and in tune with my values?

- From a moral perspective it encourages students to take more responsibility for their learning. However, I did not negotiate this approach simply because this approach was new – so acted in their best interests.
- The evaluative process will offer feedback and open a dialogical space between myself and students for future work.
- Certainly in tune with my critical pedagogy values.

What knowledge informed, or might have informed, me?

- Inviting a performance teacher into the session was vital. She introduced us to some theatre theory [Boal??[5]] that gave the idea of performance greater credibility.
- Reading about the possibility of the performance turn as reflective and nursing practice (Johns 2013) opened my mind to its possibility.

How might I reframe the situation and respond more effectively given this situation again? [How do my assumptions need to change?]

- I assumed the students' would appreciate this creative approach and rise to the challenge despite the risks involved with performance.
- Not offer the performance task but instead simply ask them to bring in their own stories for the follow-up day. Would that have been:
  - more effective learning? I had role-modelled constructing and sharing a story but then this had helped them prepare their own stories requisite to construct a meta-narrative of their own experiences. There is known value in role-modelling (Brookfield 1996).
- I could have mixed and matched story with theory – a compromise that would have watered down my initial idea. I do not think compromises are a good teaching strategy.

What would be the consequences of alternative actions for the students and myself?

- Developing reflective abilities and confidence – nursing is itself a performance. Students become more self-aware and self-knowing, and more aware of the bigger picture against which stroke care takes place – roles and attitudes of other professionals.
- Compromise would have been covering the angles so to speak, to cater for those who wanted facts or didn't want to participate in performance.

What factors might constrain me responding in new ways?

- Authority to influence the curriculum more radically against curriculum resistance and backlash, although I feel I do have some support.

Am I more able to support myself and others better as a consequence?

- I want to establish a narrative performance group within the school of nursing and invite other health professionals. [I suddenly see the scope of this being joint teaching with other health professionals involved in stroke care!]
- I feel stronger to resist any backlash and make a rationale and informed case for enhancing reflective teaching in the curriculum.

What insights do I draw from this experience?

- It is a tip of the iceberg phenomenon – the possibilities for transforming curriculum emerge. It requires a movement from little me [small picture] to a collective enterprise within the school [bigger picture] and indeed a radical curriculum shift. Whew! I can do my little thing and make a local difference but then its impact would be minimal – this needs to be sustained through the whole student learning experience.

Endnotes

1   Gibbs, G (1988) *Learning by doing: a guide to teaching and learning methods.* Further Education Unit, Oxford Polytechnic, now Oxford Brookes University. See also Chapter 1.
2   See Table 3.2
3   See Table 3.2
4   Brookfield S (1996) *Becoming a critically reflective teacher.* Josey-Bass, San Francisco.
5   Boal A (1985) *Theatre of the oppressed.* Theatre Communications Group, New York.

Chapter 17

Teaching Teachers about Teaching

Adenike Akinbode

This chapter concerns self-being and becoming a reflective practitioner within the context of teacher education. As a reflective teacher I have always been aware of the dynamic nature of my practice. I have always sought to continuously deepen my understanding of how my learners learn, and to develop and improve my practice in order to better support learning. The experience of deepening my reflective practice through systematic self-inquiry has resulted in gaining insights into some of the cultural and political issues which impact on teaching in general. Through these insights I began to question my established approach to teaching.

I seek to demonstrate my development over time through the narratives of the experiences.[1] The narratives focus on my work in teaching primary PGCE students their first science workshop at the beginning of the academic year. The narratives focus on this event in three consecutive academic years to demonstrate how my insights into teaching and learning deepen and develop over time, as a result of the reflexive nature of my reflective practice.

The first narrative was written around insights that I had gained after one year of in-depth reflection through engagement with Johns' six dialogical movements (Johns 2010). The *Old Story* presents the approach to teaching the introductory primary science workshop. This had been developed within the team and had been successful, and well evaluated by the students. My thinking about teaching successful adult learners, who were also student teachers, had changed as a result of deepening reflection. The *New Story* presents my attempt to address the insights gained.

Narrative: PGCE Science at the Beginning of the Academic Year 1

The Old Story

Once upon a time there lived a Sage. She showed the Novices how to dance by first performing on a stage ...

It is the first science workshop session with the PGCE students. I would like them to begin to understand how children in primary school learn science through practical investigation. Today I will introduce the process skills of scientific enquiry. I model a teacher's approach right from the start. I begin by displaying the learning objectives on the visualiser which the students also have on the handout I have given them:

Students should:

- know the nature of process skills in scientific enquiry;
- begin to understand the importance of process skills in science learning;
- be able to apply process skills in a practical activity.

This models the approach they will be using with children in the classroom. In school it would be:

WALT: *We - are - learning - today*
'Today we are learning how to plan a scientific investigation'.
I display the list of process skills and give a brief overview of each one. I use my set of balls to model the approach.[2]
'What can you tell me about this?' I begin with an open question to get the students observing. I move on to more focused closed questions to get them to use the sense of sight to really look and notice. I go through each process skill in turn, asking focused questions to encourage students to respond.
'Now can you raise questions about the set of balls?'
'Which question can we investigate easily right now?'
'Can you make a prediction about which ball will bounce the highest?'
'What do we need to consider when carrying out the test?'
'Now that we have results, what conclusion can be formed?'
'Can you form a hypothesis, which is a reasonable explanation for the results obtained?'

Now the students can go through the process themselves using the set of materials placed on their tables, and using the structured guidance in the handout. They have a set of five different tea bags which are labelled with a letter. I show them the equipment available to use for the investigation. I let them spend about fifteen minutes working through the process skills in order to plan the investigation. I move among them joining in with their discussions and giving advice when necessary. We come together for feedback on ideas and progress so far. I ask them to negotiate and modify plans so that no two groups are investigating the same question. This will provide a more interesting feedback session later. Before they begin the practical I ask them to check their chosen resources with me. I have to do a lot of direction here to ensure that they make best use of the limited resources, and select those best suited to their purpose. I have had to do so much running around, talking and organising that I am tired now. I engage with each group to ask them to justify what they are doing. I sometimes prompt and lead them in a different direction to improve their scientific method.

It is now time for the plenary session. Groups give a short overview of their investigation and what they have found out. They all agree that they have learned something about tea bags that they did not know before. I explain that I have given them some familiar materials in an unfamiliar context in order to try to get them to consider the child's point of view. As successful adult learners these students have wealth of life experience, and take much for granted in ways that are different to children's points of view. Students say they enjoyed the session. They evaluate the science workshop as one of the most enjoyable during induction week. This has been a successful beginning.

Transforming

I have an idea. I meet with *Y* to consider what we will be doing in science with the PGCE students. We agree that the introductory session works well, but I suggest we do it differently this year. I explain my idea. 'I like it,' he says enthusiastically. 'We are taking a risk though,' he adds. 'I know we are,' I say; 'Let's do it,' we agree.

The New Story

Once upon a time there lived a Meddler. She asked the Novices to begin the dance, and then she joined them in the middle ...[3]

It is the first science workshop session with the PGCE students. I would like them to begin to understand how children in primary school learn science through practical investigation. Today I will introduce the process skills of scientific enquiry. I share the aims with them which are:

- introduction to learning and teaching science in primary school;
- introduction to practical investigation.

These are all successful adult learners who bring a wealth of life experience to this journey of becoming primary school teachers. They all have experience of science from their GCSEs. I tell them that this is my starting point as a teacher; I am beginning by considering what my learners already know and understand. I tell them that the approach I will be using with them is going to be different from that I would use with children in the classroom; I will explain this later. I have decided to give them a handout at the end of the session. I explain that the task is for them to use the set of materials on their tables to plan and carry out a scientific investigation in any way that they choose. The materials are a set of tea bags labelled with letters. I show them the equipment. I put some guidance points on the visualiser, asking them to consider collaboration and negotiation, and to ensure that all group members participate. I give them some brief questions to reflect on when they have finished the investigation. They have an hour to complete the task. I say that there are two aspects of the task that I would like them to consider. One is the actual scientific investigation and what they learn from it; the other is the process and experience of working within a group.

I have arranged the tables so that the students are in groups of four, five or six maximum. I am expecting that they will find collaboration and negotiation quite challenging. I have asked them to decide what assistance they would like from me if any. I intend to observe what happens and only answer direct questions if asked. I go around to the different groups and observe. I resist the urge to intervene and direct the students. Some groups are working easily and smoothly, but others are taking a long time to reach agreement. Sometimes they call me over, but only to ask for another piece of equipment. Sometimes they ask if their approach is correct; I remind them that what they do is entirely their own choice. This feels easy. I am aware that I do not feel tired as I usually do at this stage in the workshop. I have not been running around directing and organising; the students are making their own decisions. I am conscious as I observe that I will be sharing my reflections on the session with students later. I am surprised and pleased that the students have used the resources effectively without any direction or intervention from me.

It is now time for the plenary session. Each group in turn presents what they did and how they experienced the activity. I notice that they have all engaged in systematic scientific investigation. Many identify the challenges of working in a group, and their thoughts on the implications for the teacher when working with a class of children. I share my reflections on the activity, including the reasons for my actions and my observations during the activity. Each group in turn has identified issues related to learning and teaching. Several have realised in this first session the importance of a teacher being well planned, and trying out practical activities before giving them to the children.

I give them the handout during the final ten minutes. They identify the process skills used in the activity. They realise that they have successfully engaged in a systematic scientific investigation using familiar everyday materials. They look pleased. They say that they enjoyed the activity, and feel less anxious about teaching science now. I explain how I used to teach the session, and demonstrate my teacher modelling using the set of balls and the structure from the handout. I feel that the new approach provides them with a much richer experience; they agree with this view, even those who said earlier that they would have liked more direction from me. This first science workshop has been evaluated well again this year. This has been a successful beginning.

Transforming ... To be continued

Teacher Education

Since my current practice is in teacher education and it is valuable to consider what it means to be a teacher of teachers. Korthagen et al. (2005) raise the issue that it is commonly assumed that a good teacher will make a good teacher educator. They discuss studies which suggest that most teacher educators in European countries enter their new profession without formal preparation. These issues relate to my experience of entering teacher education. I had several years of successful school classroom practice to build upon, and I held the view that I had much of value to pass on to the next generation of teachers. Korthagen and colleagues go on to raise the point that there is a difference between teaching adults and teaching children. As a new member of the academic staff I was required to take a course on learning and teaching in higher education; however, I received no specific support and preparation for my role in teaching teachers. I learned to be a teacher educator in the early part of this second career through engaging within a community of more experienced teacher educators. During this time I was beginning to frame and articulate my theories of practice. Schon's (1983) idea of knowing-in-action is a useful way to describe my practice as a teacher when I entered teacher education. When engaging with my students I became aware of the need to question my knowledge about teaching. How did I know what I knew about teaching? In the school classroom I used my tacit knowledge of practice in a skilled way. I could provide evidence of the success of my practice in a number of ways, which included examples of children's work and feedback on observations of my teaching. When I came into teacher education I needed to begin to frame and articulate aspects of my practice in order to be able to support the learning and development of my student teachers.

Although much has been written about the complex nature of learning and teaching, in my experience this is not addressed in any depth, either through discussion in practice, or in initial teacher education programmes. As a result of the in-depth reflection through self-inquiry study, I began to question the practice I had developed during my early years in higher education. I was aware from experience that student teachers often consider the act of teaching as transmission of knowledge. Therefore my expected role as teacher educator was to 'tell them what to tell'. The following from Loughran (2006:15) is important to consider:

> Combined with transmissive view of teaching and learning, it is not difficult to see how some might equate teaching with simply doing rather than seeing teaching as being carefully structured, thoughtfully created and deliberately informed, in order to engage students in learning for understanding; as opposed to learning by rote.

Reflections on the PGCE Sessions in Academic Year 1

I taught the introductory science workshop with three groups of PGCE students during induction week. At first I found not controlling rather challenging; as I went among the small groups, I was aware of wanting to intervene, particularly to encourage students to modify their scientific method. I realised that completely accurate method was less important than what they were learning about teaching and learning. I also discovered that the groups were often able to identify flaws in the method and to change the question in order to address this without intervention from me. I attempted to be more mindful of how I was feeling and responding in an attempt to model differently. Later in the session plenary I shared my reflections with the students about my role as the teacher during the session. This included explaining how I had to stop myself from intervening and directing during the session. Student *A* mentioned that at one point when I came to observe her group she had been concerned that I would interrupt them. She had not wanted this because they were engaged in an interesting discussion. She had been pleased that I had not intervened. She explained that this incident made her realise that she had always felt the need to engage with the learners as much as possible in the classroom, but she now understood the importance of allowing some space and independence in learning. I found this to be an interesting comment, and one to consider and share with colleagues later.

In sharing my reflections I also demonstrated an example of my uncertainty as a teacher. I discovered some minutes into the third session that I had one group of seven students. I had intended that there would be groups of four, five or six. I had missed an extra chair at one of the tables. I asked Student *B* if she wouldn't mind moving to another table to make a group of five. She said the she did not mind, and moved to the other table. After this I worried about whether I had acted correctly. I was controlling again. Did it really matter if there was one group of seven? I knew that the larger groups were likely to be the most challenging, and I had wanted six to be the maximum. I worried that *B* did mind moving, but had decided not to make a fuss. I was concerned that I might have disrupted a group-bonding process. I remained uncertain about this being the correct decision. In deciding to share this uncertainty with the students I was modelling an example of a decision that a teacher needs to make, while being uncertain that it is the most appropriate way to respond to the unexpected unfolding in the classroom.

Before we implemented the new approach to teaching the introductory workshop we felt that we were taking a risk. My colleague and I both agreed that the new approach to teaching the sessions was very successful. The students had gained so much more than knowledge of the process skills for scientific enquiry. They had begun to unpack other issues relating to teaching. During the following academic year my reflections resulted in me considering in more depth the complex nature of classroom practice. The next narrative demonstrates some of the issues that I raised with students generally in all of my teaching sessions.

Narrative: Work with Student Teachers, Beginning of Autumn term

I am aware of my changing approaches to teaching and classroom engagement this term. I find myself speaking more of my truth, which is about what it really means to be a teacher. I ask students to consider us as a learning community right now in this moment. I ask them to consider what it is that we all bring to this common classroom event. We bring who we are, our life experiences and how they have shaped us. We bring the way that we engage with the world. We bring what has happened to us today prior to meeting together in our classroom. I ask students to consciously focus on how they feel right now. Are they excited and eager to experience what will unfold? Are they tired, anxious or feeling uncertain? How do they feel about the peers they are sitting with? How do they feel about me, the teacher? What do they think of the subject we are about to cover? I acknowledge that we are all unique individuals, and we bring this uniqueness to this classroom event. I suggest that each person is likely to experience this event in a different way to everyone else, and this will affect the learning that takes place. I ask students to consider this when faced with the children in their own classrooms.

The above narrative is concerned with how I wished to raise students' awareness of the complexity of classroom practice. This includes a wide range of factors which will impact on what takes place. These insights led me to recognise that despite the dominant discourse, learning outcomes can never be predicted. Classroom outcomes are always uncertain, and dependent on a range of factors. I began to explore ideas about chaos theory, and considered the value of its application to classroom practice and experience. In the next narrative extract I return to the PGCE introductory science workshop at the beginning of the following academic year. We again decided to teach the session using the new approach. In this narrative I demonstrate how my teaching has developed through my insights about the uncertainty of practice.

Narrative: PGCE Science at the Beginning of the Academic Year 2

A year has gone by since I introduced the new approach to this session. What do I think about it now? The majority of students claim to lack confidence in their ability to teach science. I have my learning intentions for this session, and I have put a lot of time and effort into planning and preparing the resources. However, I have decided to let go of the need to control the development and progress of the session. Through addressing my learning intentions I have created a learning environment that I believe will be supportive; however, I acknowledge that the learning outcomes are uncertain; I await the learners' responses.

I observe the students in action, and respond when they ask. This approach allows for chaos to flow. The outcomes are uncertain; however, I know that learning will take place.

An hour passes and we all come together, I ask the students to share experiences in order to 'unpack' what has just happened. Some speak of initial discomfort due to me not giving them specific direction for the investigation. Some speak of feeling surprised at how much science can be gained from such simple everyday materials as teabags; and others speak of how much they have learned about teabags that they had not known before. They speak of what they have learned through making mistakes and having to modify their method. They raise concerns about the appropriateness of using boiling water with children in the primary school classroom. Some speak of the positive collaborative group experience in working together; others speak of tensions in the group with so many different points of view being made. They decide that groups of six or seven are too many for a comfortable learning experience; they will use smaller groups in their own classrooms. A few speak of having got it all wrong; I explain to them why it is that what they did was right. I tell them how pleased I am as a teacher to hear this variety of comments in the feedback. I could have told them all of the points that have been raised. They respond by saying that finding out all of these issues for themselves means that it has greater meaning and will be remembered.

I share my intentions as teacher, by telling them that this is precisely the point I wanted to make. I have observed so much learning taking place. I distribute the handout at this late stage in the workshop session, and ask the students to identify process skills from the list that they used today. Most find that they have used all of them. I tell them that this shows that they have been 'doing science'. This gives reassurance to the majority who claimed to be lacking in knowledge and confidence.

After establishing the learning environment I let go of control. Students learned about the process skills, and much more besides. They learned about science, they learned about learning, and they learned about teaching. Students selected equipment for themselves without my intervention. I allowed for chaos to flow in my classroom. Beauty arose from chaos.

Chaos Theory

Chaos theory arose from the natural sciences but has been used to explain aspects of human behaviour, culture and experience. Wheatley (1999) explains how for three hundred years up until the beginning of the twentieth century, many aspects of Western civilisation were based around ideas from classical Newtonian physics. The predictability and certainty related to cause and effect drove the way societies and organisations were developed and arranged. The certainty and predictability of cause and effect work when dealing with simple linear systems. However, it was discovered that that this principle did not work for complex dynamic systems. Human behaviour and experience are complex and dynamic. Wheatley explained that 'potential' is a valuable alternative to predictability. Classroom experience is complex and dynamic. I consider the idea of each classroom having 'potential' for learning to be more appropriate than having established pre-defined learning outcomes.

Gleick (1998) discusses how chaos theory was developed. Strange attractors in complex non-linear systems seemed to exhibit random and chaotic behaviour; however, if the system was observed as a whole a pattern could be seen. Scientists tried to classify these complex systems and find the constant which connects them all. They found that each system could only be understood individually. I view the idea of teacher as 'strange attractor' as a valuable way to understand what takes place in the classroom. Since no two human beings are the same, no two classes of learners are ever going to be the same. Each classroom episode will be determined by a range of factors including the relationships between learners and teacher, and the learners between each other. Other issues include the subject, the content and the environment. All of these factors will impact on the learning. A classroom episode is deterministic in that changes will take place as a result of the interactions. The teacher's actions in the classroom will result in change. It is possible to have desired learning outcomes and establish the learning environment to try to achieve them. However the teacher needs to be open to observing the pattern of learning that does take place. This differs from the notion that what a teacher does will result in a predictable set of learning outcomes. Teacher as strange attracter allows for the 'potential' of learning in the classroom.

The application of chaos theory to classroom events needs to consider the issue of control. In order for chaos to flow in the classroom the teacher needs to be able to let go of control so that the pattern of learning may unfold. In the next narrative I return to the first PGCE workshop in the third academic year. In this narrative I demonstrate how I have gained insights on who does the learning in any classroom event.

Narrative: PGCE Science at the Beginning of the Academic Year 3

There is an assumption that the good teacher has clearly stated learning intentions matched to clearly established success criteria. Let's suspend that assumption.

It is the beginning of the academic year and my new PGCE students have come to me to teach them how to teach. Some are interested and excited about teaching science; others are anxious and fear that they lack the subject knowledge to teach science. They come to me to 'tell them what to tell'.

I have my learning intentions as a teacher; 'For students to gain knowledge and understanding of the process skills of scientific enquiry, and how these might be applied through practical investigation'. I have planned and set up the learning environment. I have prepared and organised the resources. I give the students an identified starting point, then I let go of control. Yes I do have some desired outcomes, but I know much more will happen.

> sophisticated, skilful teaching practice is often confused with a good performance, a fun activity or an enjoyable experience. (Loughran and Russell 2007: 219).

I do not set out to entertain the students. My intentions are about helping to reframe these beginning teachers' ideas about the nature of teaching. I tell them 'Some of you will be interested and excited about this activity, but others might be anxious or even cross with me for not giving you clear direction. Later we will come back together and "unpack" this experience. Then I will share with you my thinking as a teacher.'

Students use and apply the process skills without me telling them what to do. They also learn so much more. They learn about science, they learn about learning and they learn about teaching.

I ask them, 'Who does the learning in the classroom?'

They reply, 'We all do, teacher and learners.'

I ask a student 'Who does your learning?' He pauses and thinks for a while, a little uncertain if he has understood my meaning. Then he looks at me and replies, 'I do.'

I say, 'Exactly, that is my point. You do your learning and I do my learning. So, the teacher should let the learners do the learning rather than try to control everything that they do.'

The students start writing vigorously, making notes. This suggests that the ideas need to be remembered, maybe to be reflected upon after the session. Loughran (2002: 38) gives more food for thought.

> If the focus is genuinely on the student teacher as learner, then it is their ability to analyse and make meaning from experience that matters most – as opposed to when the teacher educator filters, develops, and shares the knowledge with the student teachers ... The knowledge developed may well be the same, but the process in developing the knowledge is very different. Who is doing the learning really matters.

Shulman (2004:402) seeks to answer the question 'How does somebody who already knows something figure out how to teach it to somebody else?' Through his research he began to notice that what distinguished teaching expertise was having a range of examples to draw upon in practice. Shulman considered that expert teachers had the ability to address an aspect of learning from multiple perspectives. This suggests to me that being open to and able to respond to unexpected outcomes is important in developing expert teaching. As a teacher educator teaching how to teach primary science, I had to be open to a range of factors in my classroom episode. My teaching involved providing a learning environment in which my students could learn about science processes through planning and carrying out a scientific investigation, gaining results and forming a conclusion, and evaluating their method. This was entwined with considering how these actions might be applied to planning science learning in the primary school classroom. Students also had to consider issues relating to planning the learning environment that would be appropriate for the level of the children. As the teacher of teachers in this situation, I had to be open to uncertain and unexpected outcomes which emerged from the session and to respond accordingly.

Through their workshop experience, I wanted to help my students begin to understand that teaching science involves more than simply knowing the subject facts and telling them to children. Through their practical experience in the workshop I wanted the students to be able to put themselves into the children's shoes to consider what they need to plan for, and also to understand that there was more to planning and teaching scientific enquiry than having a set of procedures to deliver in the classroom. Loughran (2006: 30) addresses issues about the nature of teaching that in my view are not often considered by those outside the profession.

> Teaching is problematic. On the surface, teaching can appear to be well-ordered, technically proficient and purposefully directed routine, but, as so much of the growing teacher research literature demonstrates, when teaching is unpacked by teachers, when their voice prevails, then the constant undercurrent of choices, decisions, competing concerns, dilemmas and tensions are made clear for all to see.

A classroom observer does not have access to the teacher's decision-making, and usually considers the act of teaching to be calm and ordered. Through sharing my thinking and decision-making as a teacher I wanted the students to begin to consider some of the many issues that a teacher needs to think about that usually remain hidden. In order to be able to share my thinking with students effectively I had to focus on reflecting on my practice in sufficient depth to be able to become aware of insights into practice and articulate them. In addition to sharing my insights into teaching practice I was also modelling for students my process of reflecting on my teaching. This demonstrated the importance of reflection in developing the practice of teaching.

Skill Box

> - *Reflect on the 'extent of control' in your next teaching experience either as teacher, guide or student.*
> - *If a teacher or guide:*
>   - *Do you try to enable or control?*
>   - *Are you mindful of parallel process between the way you teach and the way you expect students to perform in practice?*
>   - *Do you emphasise outcome or process? [a reflective approach would give emphasis to process]*
>   - *Do you need session objectives? Would session aims be more appropriate for enabling the learners to do their learning?*
> - *If a student:*
>   - *Are you told **what** to learn or are you supported in **how** to learn. What is the place of reflection in learning?*

Endnotes

1   The stories formed part of a larger reflexive narrative constructed over three and half years of doctoral study. Akinbode (2014).

2   I used three different balls to demonstrate how a teacher might use the simple set of objects as a focus for planning a scientific investigation. I would go through all of the process skills of scientific enquiry, such as making observations, raising a question to investigate, predicting, testing and forming conclusions, so that students understood how they can be developed.

3   The idea of the meddler-in-the-middle was devised by McWilliam (2009).

References

Akinbode, A. (2014) Transforming self as reflective teacher: journey of being and becoming a teacher and teacher educator. Unpublished PhD Thesis. University of Bedfordshire.

Brookfield, S. (1995) *Becoming a critically reflective teacher*. Jossey-Bass, San Francisco.

Gleick, J. (1998) *Chaos: the amazing science of the unpredictable*. Vantage, London.

Johns, C. (2010) *Guided reflection: a narrative approach to advancing practice* [2nd edition]. Oxford, Wiley-Blackwell.

Korthagen, F., Loughran, J. and Lunenberg, M. (2005) Teaching teachers – studies into the expertise of teacher educators: an introduction to this theme issue. *Teaching and Teacher Education* 21, 107–115.

Loughran, J. (2002) Effective reflective practice: In search of meaning in learning about teaching. *Journal of Teacher Education* 53, 33–44.

Loughran, J. (2006) *Developing a pedagogy of teacher education: understanding teaching and learning about teaching*. Routledge, London.

Loughran, J. and Russell, T. (2007) Beginning to understand teaching as discipline. *Studying Teacher Education* 3(2), 217–227.

McWilliam, E. (2009) Teaching for creativity: from sage to guide to meddler. *Asia Pacific Journal of Education* 29(3), 281–293

Schön, D. A. (1983) *The reflective practitioner: how professionals think in action*. Ashgate, Aldershot.

Shulman, L. S. (2004) *The wisdom of practice: essays on teaching, learning and learning to teach*. Jossey-Bass, San Francisco.

Wheatley, M. (1999) *Leadership and the new science: discovering order in a chaotic world*. Berrett-Koehler, San Francisco.

Chapter 18

Reflective Teaching as Ethical Practice

Adenike Akinbode

A class of students is composed of a number of individual human beings who each have their own learning styles and needs. As a result of this I need to be concerned with supporting the needs of the individual in the midst of the many. This makes the classroom a very complex environment in which to practice, especially considering that it is usually fast-paced and the teacher often needs to make quick decisions about how to act. Shulman (2004: 266) in his comparison between teaching and medicine suggested the following:

> There is little doubt that, from the perspective of complexity management, teaching is a far more demanding occupation than medicine. Naturally there are many variations in the practice of each. But overall, the diagnosis and treatment of a single patient under circumstances that the physician controls are far easier than the management and teaching of 30 students under constraints of time, materials and multiple sources of unpredictability. If there is a kind of medicine that resembles teaching, it may be emergency medicine on the battlefield.

I am concerned with some of the complex dilemmas that I, as a teacher, might face in the classroom, dilemmas that reflect the artistry of being a teacher using three classroom experiences from my practice. These experiences took place during a time I was engaged in in-depth reflection through systematic self-inquiry.[1]

Linde (1993) argues that narrative is valuable in the social evaluation of people and their actions. She discusses how reflexivity in personal narrative is made possible due to the separation of self as narrator and central character, in order to evaluate self through observation and reflection, resulting in self-correction and development. Self as narrator is always moral even though the central character of action might not be. As a result of this Linde considers reflexivity in personal narratives to be a powerful evaluative process, which needs to be conducted at a distance from the experience being narrated. This idea suggests that reflection through personal narrative is a valuable way for teachers to consider the ethical issues arising from their practice. Through the narration of the practice experience a teacher could recall, review and question actions, considering whether they had been most

Becoming a Reflective Practitioner, Fifth Edition. Edited by Christopher Johns.
© 2017 John Wiley & Sons Ltd. Published 2017 by John Wiley & Sons Ltd.
Companion Website: www.wiley.com/go/johns/reflectivepractitioner

appropriate in the circumstances. As a result of the insights gained through the narrative reflection, a teacher would be able to develop, recreate and transform self in preparation for future classroom actions. Over time this would result in developing a reflexive approach to practice.

Excruciatingly Busy

I have been teaching for seven working days in a row.
Earlier this week:

Monday:	Colleague *A* asked colleague *B* to cover his teaching. Colleague *B* has lots of questions; I have to take time out from my preparations to answer them. Six hours of teaching today.
Tuesday:	Another six hours of teaching today. I must catch up with colleague *C* today about her PowerPoint presentation for Thursday. It is so difficult having to teach another colleague's materials. 4 p.m. and *C* is in a tutorial, I don't know when she will finish. I am so tired I will catch up with her tomorrow.
Wednesday:	*C* is not on campus today, I send her an email requesting a meeting tomorrow morning. At least I know that we both teach the session at 1 p.m. tomorrow. I am teaching this evening until 8 p.m.
Thursday morning:	*C* is teaching *A*'s seminar. I did not know about this. I have to meet with her at 12 noon when she is finished. It is 12.30 before she arrives. I do not understand this session; it is not my area of expertise. I have not seen the materials previously. This is not how I wish to prepare for teaching a session. 12.50 I must now go to my seminar room.
Thursday 1 p.m.:	I start the Professional Studies session. This is my PGCE seminar group; my 'tutor' group. They are a more challenging group than I have had for some years. Half of the students in the group are 'lovely'. I find them interested, motivated and engaged; always willing to make the most of any learning opportunities which they are presented with. However, the other half of the group consists of a number of young women who (in my view) have rather a 'negative attitude'. It seems to me that they feed off each other's negativity. In other words they are not so 'lovely'. Does labelling them in this way reinforce the way I see them?

I am showing the students some examples of English KS2 SATs papers. I give them the spelling task to try. One of the 'girls with attitude' queries what I am asking them to do. I repeat what I said. She tells me it is wrong. Another member of the group agrees with her. A buzz of voices erupts from the others in their group. In this moment I realise that I am unsure. I leave them buzzing and go to see if I can have a word with *C*. I get her attention; she comes to see me. I check the task and realise that I have made a mistake; I have given the wrong instruction to the students. I return to my room wondering how I should deal with this. What should I say? I feel a sick, sinking sensation in my stomach. I go around the room distributing the remaining papers in order to calm myself and take a couple of minutes of thinking time. I notice my positive students getting on with their task, seemingly unconcerned about anything. The 'girls with attitude' continue to buzz and exude negativity. It is time for me to speak. I say 'You are correct about the spelling task; the teacher would read out the missing words'. This acknowledges that what I said before was wrong. The seminar task continues. I am feeling dreadful and long for the session to finish; however, there are two more hours to go.

I made a mistake. This is exactly the reason why I like to prepare well in advance of a session, especially when I have to work with another colleague's materials. I am supposed to be 'modelling' good practice for these students of teaching. They have seen that I am not properly prepared. There were circumstances beyond my control but I cannot explain this to my students. But what is this really all about? I feel that I did not have control of the situation. What happens when a teacher is not in control? Then maybe chaos flows. What then is the result of chaos? Does this mean disaster?

I observe my students now fully engaged with the SATs task. They are writing, discussing, thinking and learning; even the 'girls with attitude'. So where is the disaster? It exists in my head because circumstances resulted in me not having the control that I would wish for, and not living up to my expectations of myself as a teacher.

Berry & Loughran (2004: 17–18) write:

> 'Well what you think you are doing as the teacher is not always what the class think you're doing, and it's good to see that happening with our lecturers because it sure as heck happens to us. I think it's good that we see you struggle in ways just like us. But maybe your experience covers it up so that we just don't see the reality often enough.'

Maybe for some of these PGCE students my mistake demonstrates teacher vulnerability. Maybe this is reassuring since it relates to their own experiences of practice. Previously with this group I have tried to explain more about the complex nature of teaching. I know that some students come looking for certainty. They want to get it right. I tell them that being a teacher is an ongoing process of development. I have admitted that I too am constantly learning and developing. I have told them that I too have sessions that go well and some which seem to be disasters; this is the reality of teaching. Maybe some of the students recall this and it gives them reassurance.

It is time for the break. The 'girls with attitude' choose to sit together outside the seminar room. I sense from their facial expressions and body language that they are having a complaining session; this is what they do. I need a drink (tea) and go upstairs. On my return they stop talking as I walk past them. My positive students continue to smile and chat with me in their usual friendly and enthusiastic way. I feel I am existing between two parallel universes which occupy the same space in time.

In this second part of the seminar the students have been asked to organise themselves into small groups of three or four to discuss their progress with their school-based enquiries. They were asked to come prepared, the intention is to enable sharing and peer support. I facilitate this session by going around the room to listen in and support some discussions. I notice the 'girls with attitude' packing up and looking ready to leave. This should not be happening, there is still 40 minutes remaining in this seminar. I walk over to their table. They say they have nothing to report back on. They argue that they can best use their time in the Learning Resources Centre. In this moment I need to think carefully how to respond to this situation. I WANT TO TELL THEM *NOT* TO LEAVE. I think that they should not leave, but I ask myself why I think this. I know that they are not happy with the seminar; however, this part of the session requires an input from students, which this group have chosen not to come prepared for. I also think that to leave the seminar now would be impolite and inconsiderate of other people in this classroom event;

this means the other students and the tutor. I respond with careful words; still aware of that sinking feeling in my stomach. I remind them that we still have 40 minutes remaining and suggest that they split up and join other groups who seem to be enthusiastically engaged. They might learn something valuable from their peers. I would like them to be able to see the opportunity for learning in this seminar. Two of them argue for going to the LRC. I repeat my request, aware of the tension and how I am feeling, but maintaining my poise. Now they begin to appreciate that my argument is reasonable, and they follow my suggestion. I watch them disperse. Soon I observe them in discussion with other positive members of the seminar group, and it seems to me that the tension dissipates and the atmosphere in the room changes. Now it is 4 p.m. and time to finish. I am relieved.

Reflection

This narrative is written around insights on a range of issues. My emotional condition is foregrounded, my awareness of these feelings and how I sought to work with the tensions. As a result of being unable to live up to my expectations of myself as a teacher I was feeling rather guilty and highly stressed. There was also a sense of injustice and frustration because I had experienced so many challenges during that week which would explain why I was inadequately prepared for the session, but it was not appropriate to discuss this with the students. I had a great concern about how the students might view me as incompetent. In this narrative I also dialogue with the insight that I found a number of the students rather challenging. I label them 'girls with attitude' to signify my perception of their challenging behaviour. A key insight was that of my emotional entanglement involving discomfort about my negative feelings for this group of students, and the stress and guilt about being inadequately prepared. However, in the midst of the emotional turmoil I was aware of the importance of staying calm and maintaining my professional exterior. I also raise the issue that the disaster that I seemed to be living possibly only existed in my mind. The reality was that the seminar proceeded and the students did gain much from it. One of the dilemmas of being a teacher educator is in what I need to demonstrate for my student teachers. On the one hand it would be helpful for them to know about the tensions, challenges and dilemmas that a teacher faces in day-to-day practice, which mostly remain hidden from view. This would be helpful for them to see and begin to understand more about what it means to 'be' a teacher alongside having the knowledge and skills for 'doing' teaching. On the other hand students need to have confidence in their teachers' expertise. Berry (2007) raised this issue and how it is important that teacher educators maintain the right balance when sharing experiences with student teachers. This means making careful decisions about what to 'model' for students. Elbaz-Luwisch (2007) discusses some studies which have focused on being and becoming a teacher. Being a teacher involves more than just the technicalities of planning, teaching and assessing; it is inextricably linked with personal experience, and involves body and emotion. Learning also involves more than assimilating knowledge transmitted by the teacher.

In the next narrative I focus on a different kind of episode from practice concerned with how I went about dealing with a student whose behaviour to me had been inappropriate. This episode generated a range of emotions, and I seek to demonstrate how I raised questions and managed uncertainty as events unfolded. I sought to maintain my professional calm.

The Session on Water

Today I am teaching the session on water. This is a large group of 45 students, and it is a bit of a struggle fitting them all into this room. This is also the most resource-intensive science session that we teach. I ask the students to organise themselves into small groups and then decide which set of resources to focus on for investigation. Most groups do this swiftly and then begin to work on the task. One group is not yet settled. They sit at the table at the end of the room, but they have chosen the Aqua City play equipment that is set up on the side at the other end of the room. I suggest that they move so that they have proper access to their equipment.

'We'll stay here,' says Q

'I think you should move so that you can do the task properly,' I reply.

'We'll stay here, no one in this group wants to move,' says Q rather aggressively and loudly, it seems to me.

I look at the faces of the other five students in this group. I try to concentrate, aware that there are 39 other individuals actively engaged around me. I cannot read what the other students are thinking. I ask them to move again and they comply. I am aware that my heart is thumping and I am feeling cross and hurt by Q's hostility. I think that as the teacher I had made a reasonable request. I calm down and focus on the entire group. I soon begin to enjoy the session, since although it is crowded, hot and noisy, I recognise how enthusiastically most of the students are engaging with the task. Some groups have devised some wonderfully creative approaches to teaching young children science through the theme of Water.

The session ends and I walk up to Q and ask if I could have a word with her. She replies aggressively, 'I want to talk to you too'. We wait until the other students leave, and then I notice that Q has asked Z to stay with her. I want to ask Z to leave, but realise that Q wishes to have her there for support. Q immediately launches into a rather unexpected tirade.

'You shouldn't have asked me to stay behind when everyone could hear. I wanted to apologise because I shouldn't have spoken to you like that earlier, but I got angry.'

Q is standing with her arms by her side and her fists clenched. I find her stance to be aggressive. She keeps talking, repeating the same things again and again. When she pauses for breath I say to her 'Do you really think that you should be speaking to me in that way?'

She says 'I got really angry but I am sorry, and I have trouble with anger management and I am trying to control it'

I am feeling very stressed and uncomfortable. Q's body language to me conveys aggression, not apology. I think that I should end this confrontation. I want to say 'I think we should stop now. I should not have to put up with this kind of behaviour from a student, so I am ending this and walking away.' My heart if thumping and I feel cross and hurt by Q's behaviour. But in the moment I consider what would happen if I did walk away. The situation would not be resolved. In this moment I cannot see how this situation will unfold, but I decide to wait and see. Q is still repeating what she has been saying, then something new comes.

'I am trying to apologise, this is the only way I can do it, but you don't say anything and I don't know what you are thinking,' says Q

'How could I speak when you haven't stopped talking? Also, I have a different way of responding than you, I think things through before I speak,' I reply.

I notice that Q's body seems to relax a bit. It seems that we have reached a level of mutual understanding. In this moment I see Q as a frightened young woman. The aggression was all about fear. She understood that she had behaved inappropriately, and was struggling to contain her anger. She must see me as being in a position of power as her tutor. I hope that what I said helped her to understand my quiet way of being, which is quite different from hers. She starts to talk about her frustrations. She does not like being in such a large group of 45 students. This is how the undergraduates have been organised this year due to the numbers who have chosen the lower primary pathway. A decision was made to have one large group rather than two much smaller groups. Q feels that they are disadvantaged, when the upper primary students are arranged in groups of no more than 30. Z comes to join in the discussion. I ask if they have shared their concerns with their programme leader. They claim that they did but were not heard. Q explains that it was her frustration with the group's situation that resulted in her losing her temper with me. It just seemed another episode of 45 students in a cramped and crowded room.

Z and Q go onto talk about the module, and it becomes clear that they lack an understanding of its nature. I take them for science in a module that includes the other core subjects, English and maths. I think that I must share these views with the other members of the large team of tutors so that we can all address them in our sessions.

Q apologises again and I say that I can now see that she is calm, in a way that she was not to begin with. I tell her that now I can see that she is sincere.

Reflection

A significant insight gained from reflecting within the moment during this teaching episode was that my first feeling when Q was aggressive at the beginning of the workshop was one of fear that I had upset students, and how I might be judged by senior colleagues. I considered whether my request for the group to move was reasonable, and decided that it was. However, I remained uncertain about how the other students felt about it. The following day I happened to meet one of the other four students in the group (other than Q and Z), who stopped me in the corridor to let me know that none of them agreed with Q. She said that they do not usually work with Q and Z, but the two had arrived late and had gone to the table nearest the door.

The significant aspect of my meeting with Q after the session was my decision not to give in to my feelings of outrage to be treated in such an aggressive way by a student, and to put an end to the meeting. It seemed the decision to maintain my calm exterior and stay to see how events would unfold was the wise decision. Eventually the tension dispersed and we were able to have a conversation. We were together for 40 minutes, and by the end Q was calm. Most of the conversation was about general concerns with the progress of their undergraduate programme, and it eventually became clear that Q's original frustration had nothing to do with me or my science session. An interesting outcome from this experience was that in the remaining science workshops for the module, both Q and Z were highly attentive, and engaged. They participated in a way I had not seen before. I did address one of their concerns by explaining more about the nature of the module in my next session. I had the impression that they appreciated the fact that I had listened to their concerns. I wondered whether any other tutor had ever been able to give them the time to listen to their concerns, such is the demanding nature of our roles.

Clegg et al. (2013) discuss the importance of developing practical wisdom in the people professions. They raise the issue that a technical rationalist approach to professional practice is considered of most value in current Western societies. Kinsella and Pitman (2013) discuss how developing practical wisdom is important if professionals are to engage effectively with the uncertainties and complexities of practice experience.

The people professions which deal with human experience and behaviour cannot easily depend on professional knowledge in practice that is predictable, standardised and measurable. This is true of education. The past 25 years have seen much regulation and direction in education policy, with an emphasis on quantified evidence-based practice promoted for classroom and school improvement. This situation demonstrates some of the tensions between notions of technical rationality and the development of professional artistry as suggested by Schon (1983; 1987)

Clegg et al. (2013) suggest that in addition to the technical knowledge of practice, practitioners in the people professions must also be able to develop ethical professional attributes if they are to engage in desirable practice, which demonstrates appropriate concern for human needs and flourishing. Campbell (2013) describes a reflexive approach to teaching as ethical knowledge. This is explained as a teachers' capacity to examine their actions and intentions as they practice. Campbell (2013: 82) writes:

> It requires them to anticipate and understand how moral and ethical values such as justice and fairness, honesty and integrity, kindness and compassion, empathy and respect for others can be either upheld or violated by seemingly routine and normative practices.

Campbell (2013) argues that some specific input in the ethical aspects of practice should be included in initial teacher education programmes. In her study with student teachers, early career teachers and teacher educators she identified that professional ethics is not addressed explicitly and many beginning teachers are unsure about what it is. Beginning teachers tend to focus on rather extreme examples of inappropriate practice they observe in their placement schools, rather than the everyday dilemmas of practice which teachers face. Campbell suggests that it can be difficult for beginning teachers to learn about the ethical until they have experience of practice themselves. Although Campbell considers the need to address professional ethics early, she does not appear to provide an approach to ensuring that this is developed in practice. In my view being a teacher involves an ongoing process of becoming through inquiry into what happens in the classroom. The process of developing reflexivity through the practice of in-depth reflection is a way to develop professional ethical awareness. Beginning teachers first need to develop some of the techniques and skills necessary for 'doing teaching' alongside being supported in reflecting on their actions a teachers. Deepening and developing reflection as a way of practising is the process by which reflexivity can be developed in qualified practice over time.

As teachers we can never know of all of the factors which impact on our students' lives and approaches to learning. It can be challenging to find the time to focus on each individual student in any depth. The above example from my practice demonstrates a positive outcome to some complex issues, and the importance of taking the reflective space to decide how to respond rather than to react.

These two narratives have focused on practice experiences which were complex, and in which I was very aware of the uncertainty of the outcome within the moment. The next narrative focuses on uncertainty, and my concern about responding effectively. I also deal with a dilemma faced regularly by teachers, about concern for being able to meet the needs of all leaners effectively in the classroom.

Managing Behaviour

There is an assumption that a 'good' teacher provides well for all learners effectively in classroom practice. Behaviour management is a focus of much anxiety for student teachers when they begin. This is the focus for our seminar today. We are considering a scenario in which the teacher is in 'full flow' and notices that one child is disengaged. We are discussing approaches which might be taken. Suggestions are being made:

'Ask him/her to come and demonstrate something.'
'Ask her/him to go and help another child who is struggling.'
'Mention that you will be looking for volunteers.'
Then Y mentions a case he witnessed in school; he says 'What if it is a boy who refuses to do dance because he thinks dance is for girls'?

I think that this is a complex example which cannot be addressed easily in the moment. I think to myself, it had to be Y who raises this; I find that he is often rather out of sync with the rest of the group. His example means taking time to 'go off on a different tangent'. I want to say we will move on and focus only on ideas for dealing with disengagement in the moment, even though we have identified that reasons for this type of behaviour might be diverse. I am concerned that this would sound dismissive, and I do not want to do this to Y. At the same time his example raises a number of complex issues, which I feel we do not have time to focus on right now, and this would really be 'going off on a tangent'. Then I think, why should we not do this? My answer is that by spending time responding to this one student's concern I will not be attending to the needs of the other 33 students, who were focusing on the scenario in hand. These are some of the dilemmas of teaching large groups of individuals. In any moment of classroom practice I have to make decisions. I realise that I often do not know if I have acted for the best. What is the best anyway? I cannot meet the needs of all students effectively all of the time. Loughran (2006: 30) writes:

> Teaching is problematic. On the surface, teaching can appear to be well-ordered, technically proficient and purposefully directed routine, but, as so much of the growing teacher research literature demonstrates, when teaching is unpacked by teachers, when their voice prevails, then the constant undercurrent of choices, decisions, competing concerns, dilemmas and tensions are made clear for all to see.

The reality is that a teacher needs to respond as events unfold in the classroom, and this comes with experience. I can discuss some general principles with my student teachers and model for them some aspects of my own thinking as a teacher. However, only they can decide how they will respond in the moment of classroom practice. As Dinkelman et al. (2006: 133–134) write

> The problems beginning teachers face in learning what it means to teach are quite possibly more complex when seen as problems of teacher education, rather than just problems of teaching. In ways that might not happen from the perspective of a classroom teacher, teacher educators ground their decision-making with appreciation for the developmental process of learning to teach, amidst competing advocacy obligations, and foundations of knowledge (derived from both practice and research) germane to the field.

Reflection

Reflection within the moment enabled me to raise questions and consider actions when a fast response was needed. My dilemma became clear although my response less so. The dilemma- whether to 'go off on a tangent' or cover the content of the seminar as I had intended. Previously, I would have been aware of Y but I would not have raised the questions about the different ways in which I could have responded. Reflection within the moment opens a bigger picture, to put competing needs in perspective. It challenges me with my own agendas and listening to and respecting students' individual voices. Of course, the boy who did not want to dance might disengage from the class. Initially I just didn't see the connection. Indeed I labelled Y 'he is often out of sync with the class' as if I can dismiss his voice more easily as a consequence.

Skill Box

- *Reflect on your 'feelings' about individual students in your class*
- *Can you identify and acknowledge students for whom you have positive or negative 'feelings'?*
- *How will this awareness inform your approach to practice?*
- *Reflect on an episode from practice in which events unfolded in unexpected ways*
- *Consider, did you **respond** to the situation or **react**?*
- *How might you aim to respond effectively in future unexpected situations?*

Summary

Being an effective teacher involves developing some of the technicalities of doing teaching, and much more. Being a teacher involves being able to make decisions about how to respond appropriately and effectively within the moment of practice. This means making fast assessments of situations unfolding in the classroom, becoming aware of what one knows and does not know, being aware of one's own emotions, and one's need to control. The ability to achieve this involves being willing and able to find the space to engage in in-depth reflection on classroom action and experience. Over time a teacher ought to develop reflexivity as a way of practising.

Beginning teachers need to gain experience in order to begin to develop reflexive practice. Initial teacher education should support students in developing the ability to reflect on their practice experience effectively. As qualified teachers they should be encouraged to deepen their reflection on practice. In-depth reflection over time would support the development of reflexivity, which is essential in raising awareness of the ethical issues in day to day practice as discussed by Campbell (2013). It is through this process that a teacher might develop the desired practical wisdom.

Endnote

1   Akinbode (2014).

References

Akinbode, A. (2014) Transforming self as reflective teacher: journey of being and becoming a teacher and teacher educator. Unpublished PhD Thesis. University of Bedfordshire.

Berry, A. and Loughran, J. (2004) *Modeling in Teacher Education: Making the Unseen Clear*. Paper presented at the American Educational Research Association, San Diego.

Berry, A. (2007) Reconceptualising teacher educator knowledge as tensions: exploring the tension between valuing and reconstructing experience. *Studying Teacher Education* 3(2), 117–134.

Campbell, E. (2013) Teacher education as a missed opportunity in the professional preparation of ethical practitioners. In Clegg et al. (eds.), *Towards professional wisdom*. (pp 81–93). Ashgate, Farnham.

Clegg, C., Clark, C., Carr, D. and Bondi, L. (2013) *Towards professional wisdom*. Ashgate, Farnham.

Dinkelman, T. Margolis, J. and Sikkenga, K. (2006) From teacher to teacher educator: reframing knowledge in practice. *Studying Teacher Education* 2(2), 119–136.

Elbaz- Luwisch, F. (2007) Studying teachers' lives and experience. In Clandinin, D.J. (ed.), *Handbook of narrative inquiry: mapping a methodology*. (pp. 357–382). Sage, Thousand Oaks, CA.

Linde, C. (1993) *Life stories: the creation of coherence*. New York: Oxford University Press.

Loughran, J. (2006) *Developing a Pedagogy of teacher education: understanding teaching and learning about teaching*. Routledge, London.

Loughran, J. & Russell, T. (2007) Beginning to understand teaching as discipline. *Studying Teacher Education* 3(2), 217–227.

Kinsella, E. A. and Pitman, A. (2012) *Phronesis as professional knowledge: practical wisdom in the professions*. Springer, Dordrecht.

Schön, D. A. (1983) *The reflective practitioner: how professionals think in action*. Ashgate, Aldershot.

Schön, D. A. (1987) *Educating the reflective practitioner*. Jossey-Bass, San Francisco.

Shulman, L. S. (2004) *The wisdom of practice: essays on teaching, learning and learning to teach*. Jossey-Bass, San Francisco.

Chapter 19

A Reflective Framework for Clinical Practice

Christopher Johns

Reflective practitioners need reflective environments in which to flourish

In the preceding chapters I focused on the educational environment. Now I turn to consider the clinical environment. Reflective practitioners require a conducive reflective clinical environment if they are to flourish. It would be a stark contradiction to develop reflective practitioners within the curriculum only for them to experience an unreceptive clinical environment.

Imagine the curriculum development meeting in dialogue with healthcare organisation representatives. Does education impose its perspective on practice or does practice impose its demand on education? Sense the tension being played out. The meeting agrees that reflective practitioners probably enhance practice despite thin evidence. That being agreed, how can practice best accommodate reflective practice? Indeed, what would a reflective clinical environment look like?

The Burford NDU Model: Caring in Practice

Turn the clock back to January 1989. I am appointed general manager of Burford hospital. It is a time when nursing models are fashionable as nursing seeks a professional identity to emerge from the shadows of medical domination. Models are representational of desired practice composed of complex operational assumptions and systems. As such there is little flexibility within them. It is the heyday of theory-driven practice. Such models have since faded away because nursing in the UK has always been primarily perceived in terms of what nurses do rather than in terms of values.

From a reflective perspective I consider that practitioners should construct their own collective vision for practice and a framework to enable them to reflectively live that vision. In response I construct the 'Burford NDU: Caring in practice' model as a reflective and person-centred approach to clinical practice. The overall pattern of the Burford model is illustrated in Figure 19.1. At the core of the model is a valid vision for practice operationalised through four systems set within a supportive organisational culture.

Becoming a Reflective Practitioner, Fifth Edition. Edited by Christopher Johns.
© 2017 John Wiley & Sons Ltd. Published 2017 by John Wiley & Sons Ltd.
Companion Website: www.wiley.com/go/johns/reflectivepractitioner

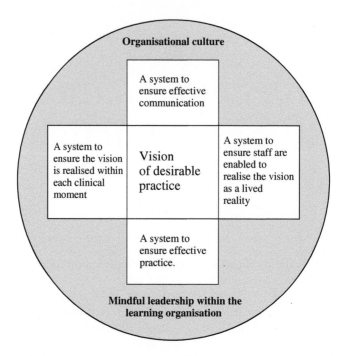

Figure 19.1   The Burford NDU: Caring in practice model

Vision

The Burford model is constructed around a vision of practice that explicitly express its underlying assumptions to govern practice. A vision gives purpose and direction to clinical practice. It is self-evident that practitioners who work together must share practice values to ensure a consistent and coherent approach.

Senge (1990:206/8) writes:

> When people truly share a vision they are connected, bound together by a common aspiration. Visions are exhilarating … they create the 'spark', the excitement that *lifts* an organisation out of the mundane.

In my experience, visions do not profoundly influence practice. They are often written in vague rhetoric, by someone years ago, pinned on office walls covered by layers of organisational memos or buried away in a policy file. The rhetoric is often grounded in caring clichés such as 'we believe in holistic care' that has no meaning for practitioners and is clearly contradicted by even the most casual observation.

Vision, What Vision?

Mandy shared with me what she had written in her journal:

> In one reflective practice workshop Chris has shared his experience of constructing the Burford model vision. This was a sharp wake-up call. I recalled that the department had its own philosophy but if I was challenged as to its contents I would have failed miserably. Once back

in the department, I eventually found the operational policy buried away in a filing cabinet. Included in its contents is the department's philosophy of care; however it did not state who had devised it and when. I asked one of my colleagues who had worked in the department for many years as to the origin and author of the philosophy she looked at me blankly and said 'I am sorry, I did not know we had one duck'.

In my next management supervision I raised this issue with my manager who also was ignorant of these facts but thought it might have been based upon the acute services philosophy. I compared the department's philosophy with one of the acute inpatient wards, only to discover that it was exactly the same. Johns (2013) draws attention to the difficulties caused by having an imported philosophy imposed on a practice: it denies articulation of the practitioner's own beliefs and values and is easily forgotten. What then is the point in having a generic philosophy devised by someone else, locked away in a filing cabinet? None whatsoever. Reflecting upon this, I established that the team believes that we provide a high standard of individualised care for patients within the department. However, we lack evidence to validate this. By not having a philosophy of care constructed on our collective beliefs and objectives of our practice, how do we know where we are going and the rationale for the journey?

I ask the staff to tell me about the hospital's existing philosophy. The philosophy had been 'imported', based on the philosophy of the Loeb Center in New York (Hall 1964, Alfano 1971). Hall's work was a vision of nursing as the primary therapy alongside a complementary role to medicine. In 1982, when Pearson (1983) had introduced this philosophy to Burford, it made sense in terms of his vision to establish nursing beds. However, Pearson had departed three years previous to my appointment. Now, from the nurses' responses, the Loeb vision had faded. It was no longer *alive*. I realise that an imported philosophy imposes a reality on practitioners that denies the expression of their own values or indeed may contradict their own values.

In response, I facilitate the construction a vision to reflect practitioners' values as a statement of collaborative intent to give meaning and direction to our collective practice. I invite all practitioners [not just nurses] to post their values on a public notice board. One month later, I typed the accumulated values and circulated them to each member of staff. I then facilitated a series of community meetings to discuss these value statements, leading to a composite statement that everyone could agree [*The Burford vision for clinical practice*]. I wrote it in a relatively jargon-free language to inform our patients and families.

The Burford vision for clinical practice [4th edition]

We believe that caring is grounded in the core therapeutic of easing suffering and enabling the growth of the other through his/ her health–illness experience whether toward recovery or death. The practitioner is mindful of being available to work with the person and the person's family in relationship, on the basis of empathic connection, compassion and mutual understanding, where the person's life pattern and health needs are appreciated and effectively responded to.

Caring is seamless across health care settings and responds to and promotes both the local community's and society's expectations of effective service. In this respect, we accept a responsibility to develop a culture of reflective leadership and the learning organisation that continually strives to anticipate and develop practice to ensure its efficacy and quality. By appropriate monitoring and sharing, we contribute to the development of the societal value of nursing and health care generally.

Our caring is enhanced when we work in dialogical relationship with our [multi] professional colleagues on the basis of mutual respect and shared values within our respective roles. This means being free to share our feelings openly but appropriately, acknowledging that as persons, we can be stressed and have differences

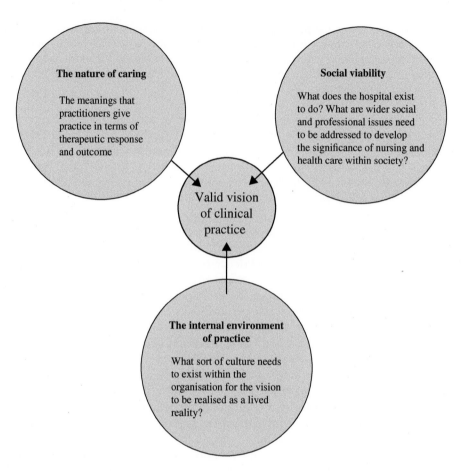

Figure 19.2 The three cornerstones

of opinion at times. This is the basis of the therapeutic team that is essential to reciprocate and support our caring to patients.
[March 2003, amended 2012, 2015]

Valid Vision

To be *valid*, a vision for practice needs to address the three cornerstones [see Figure 19.2]

The Nature of Caring

Illness creates a disruption in the person's normal life patterns, creating anxiety. Person-centred nursing is grounded in the meanings the person gives to their health–illness experience. It respects the person's autonomy and establishes a working-with relationship whereby the nurse is available to enable the person to meet their health needs as much as possible.

The vision acknowledges that people suffer. Suffering can be described as a disruption of the spirit that manifests on the physical, emotional, psychological and spiritual planes.

Working-with the person, the practitioner tunes into their suffering with the intent to help ease it. In doing so, the practitioner is mindful of enabling the person's growth. Mayeroff (1971:1) writes, 'To care for another person, in the most significant sense, is to help him grow and actualise himself.'

To actualise self is to fulfil one's human potential, whatever that might mean for the person (Maslow 1968). Newman (1994) illuminates how suffering creates the opportunity to stand back and take stock of self, especially if suffering is life-threatening. Forced out of our complacency the person may question the very essence of her existence and the things that are really important. Growth is learning new ways of organising self conducive with health. As Remen (1996:156) suggests:

> In the struggle to survive our wounds, we may adapt a strategy for living which gets us through. Life-threatening illness may cause us to re-examine the very premises on which we have based our lives, perhaps freeing ourselves to live more fully for the first time.

This can be difficult for people who are locked into ways of living that are not easily changed.

As suggested above, in writing a vision, practitioners scan a relevant literature to inform and expand their ideas. This adds credibility to the vision by positioning it within the wider professional field. For example, Jean Watson, in her transpersonal model of nursing (1988: 49), states that the goal of nursing

> is to help persons gain a higher degree of harmony within the mind, body, and soul which generates self-knowledge, self-reverence, self-healing, and self-care processes while allowing increasing diversity. This goal is pursued through the human–human encounter caring process and caring transactions that respond to the subjective inner world of the person in such a way that the nurse helps individuals find meaning in their existence, disharmony, suffering, and turmoil, and promote self-control, choice, and self-determination with the health–illness decisions.

These words resonate with the Burford vision but use a very different language. Watson challenges practitioners to think about the role of nursing. It is a far cry from the medical model. Within the medical model, the ill person is reduced to the status of a patient, with a set of symptoms that require investigation, diagnosis and subsequent treatment. Little significance is attributed to emotional, psychological, spiritual and social aspects of being ill or causes of illness. The nursing response is primarily to support the medical task. I am sure many readers will remember being told not to sit on the bed and talk to the patient – there is *work* to be done! The implication being that talking to patients is not work. The rise of technology and squeeze on resources has led to a culture whereby caring has been increasingly subordinated to unqualified staff. When the head is locked into the medical sphere and the medical sphere is most valued within organisations, then practitioners can lose sight of the caring ideal. I know many readers will have experienced this state of affairs when visiting family or friends, or experienced their own heath care.[1] It is important to bring this conflict to the surface because only then can nurses take action to resolve the contradiction to realise caring as a lived reality rather than as an ideal. Yet in a world where the health agenda is dominated by productivity, and a culture of 'more for less', times are hard for caring. Practitioners may switch off their caring self, simply because it is too painful to witness suffering and the failure to ease suffering.

The Internal Environment of Practice

The internal environment of practice concerns the pattern of relationships between healthcare practitioners. The healthcare team develops and sustains collaborative and dialogical ways of working together based on shared purpose, respect and collective responsibility. This may not be easy due to traditional patterns of professional dominance that require surfacing and shifting (Rowe 1996), as indeed was the situation at Burford hospital where some local GPs acted like feudal barons.

Social Utility

Social utility (Johnson 1974) concerns the role of the hospital in responding to and influencing societal expectations, and wider professional issues such as research and teaching. It challenges practitioners to look beyond the immediate context of the practice setting towards the wider social and professional communities. For example, how does the local community view the most appropriate use of beds? Should a quota of beds be set aside for respite care? Should terminally ill patients take priority, considering the nearest hospice is 16 miles away?

The process of writing the vision took four months. It opened a learning space for all practitioners to voice their views and think about their collective practice. It enabled practitioners to become active creators of their own practice and take responsibility for realising their beliefs in practice; to grasp their own destiny rather than have it imposed. It is one thing to hold a vision, it is quite another to realise it as a lived reality. There must be a collective determination to make it happen, otherwise the vision becomes meaningless and deeply frustrating. Old ways are deeply embodied. However the vision opens the contradictory space between vision and practice.

Skill Box

- *Unearth your vision of practice [if indeed you have one]. Who wrote it? Is it valid?*
- *Do all practitioners/ teachers work towards realising it as a lived reality?*
- *Get a group of practitioners together and write a valid vision of practice.*

A System to Ensure the Vision is Realised Within Each Clinical Moment

The hospital had been utilising the Roper, Logan and Tierney activities of living model (1980) that consists of ten activities of living:

- Maintaining a safe environment
- Communication
- Breathing
- Eating and drinking
- Elimination
- Washing and dressing
- Controlling temperature
- Mobilisation

- Working and playing
- Expressing sexuality
- Sleeping
- Death and dying

The 'Activities of Living' model is a reductionist deficit model that reduces a patient to ten activities of living. These activities become the nursing gaze, with the intent of identifying deficit within these activities as the focus of action to return these activities to normal. An audit of its value revealed how practitioners viewed assessment as a task undertaken on the patient's admission with superficial responses to each activity.

For example:

- Eating and drinking – 'likes a cup of tea in the morning';
- Expressing sexuality – ' likes to wear lipstick';
- Death and dying – blank.

One problem with assessment schedules is the demand to fill them in. Hence, if an 'activity of living' box is not completed, it indicates the practitioner has not assessed adequately. The effort becomes to complete the assessment sheet rather than to know the person.[2]

The Roper et al. model is easily understood from a functional perspective because it generally resembles what nurses do. Hence adopting the model requires minimal accommodation. Neither is it written in an obscure intellectual language that characterises many other models of nursing. However, it had no obvious congruence with the Loeb Center philosophy. Pearson (1983:53), in justifying the use of the Roper et al. model at Burford, noted the way the model 'Speaks to nurses in a language which is familiar and related to nursing in this country, and hence its greatest advantage then is its ability to convey meaning to clinical nurses.' Pearson implies that models *should* convey meaning to nurses but this goes against the grain that the nurse must first find meaning for herself and then collectively with her colleagues. Only then are practitioners in a position to consider the value of external prescriptions of nursing to inform their practice. But, if practitioners have developed their own vision for nursing, why would they want to use someone else's?

Hall (1964) challenges the view that nurses can only nurse what the person reveals of himself. As such, the nurse's skill is to create the conditions whereby the person can reveal himself. This may seem obvious in terms of the medical condition, but subtle in terms of being a person and the impact of their medical condition on their life patterns and wellbeing.

I prefer the term *pattern appreciation* (Cowling 2000) to assessment. It better represents the complex interplay of the signs practitioners need to pay attention to in order to know the other person; reading the person's life pattern as a complex whole – a pattern continually shifting moment-to-moment along the person's health–illness journey. This is achieved by reading the signs on the person's surface, for example pain, anxiety, high blood pressure, sadness in the eyes, and pursuing these signs into the deeper self as appropriate. Pattern is always shifting in light of unfolding events. Only when the practitioner is in tune with the person can they appreciate and respond appropriately to the person's unfolding needs. Newman (1994:13) writes:

The new paradigm of health, essential to nursing, embraces a unitary pattern of changing relationships. It is developmental. The task is not to try to change another person's pattern but to recognise it as information that depicts the whole and relate to it as it unfolds.

Clearly 'The Activities of Living' was an inadequate representation of the Buford vision. Hence it was scrapped. The question then – how can practitioners tune into the patient in a manner congruent with the hospital vision? In response I constructed nine *reflective* cues.

The Burford NDU Reflective Cues

Core cue

What information do I need to appreciate the healthcare needs of this person?

The nine reflective cues

- Who is this person?
- What meaning does this health/ illness experience have for the person?
- How is this person feeling?
- How do I feel about this person?
- How has this event affected their usual life pattern and roles?
- How can I help this person?
- What is important for this person to make their stay in the hospice comfortable?
- What support does this person have in life?
- How does this person view the future for themselves and others?

The practitioner internalises these nine cues as a natural reflective lens to appreciate the unfolding clinical situation as a continuous process of assessment, response and evaluation. The cues do not require direct answers. I emphasise this point because the practitioner who has embodied a reductionist systems approach, may miss the reflective point and view the cues as yet another set of boxes to complete. As Sutherland (1994:68) noted:

> Although at first I did find myself going back to Roper et al.'s headings to make sure that I had not missed anything, omitting what was physically important, I did not need to do this for very long.

Sutherland further noted the impact of the reflective cues in changing her mind-set

> Because the emphasis is centred on feelings and the total picture of that person's situation rather than on their ongoing physical needs, it forced me to move away from a need to find things out, fill things in and get things done as soon as possible in an orderly fashion. It forced me to start listening to what patients themselves were saying was important to them and then to plan care with them from this basis. It gradually became a welcome release for me'. [p. 68]

There is something astonishing in Sutherland's words about the way she thought the Burford cues *forced* her to listen to the person, as if she hadn't really listened to the person before. I think it is true, as she suggests, that the 'old model' became the task- hence the effort was to complete it rather than really listen to what the patient or family were saying. As Sutherland suggests, the key is listening and connecting; and then working with the person toward meeting their healthcare needs.

The apparent simplicity of the nine cues disarms people conditioned by complex systems models. Remember that models are merely tools to enable something to be accomplished. As such they must be fit for purpose. Does a carpenter use a spoon to chisel wood? Consider the pattern of the nine cues in my narrative of working with Tony one morning.

Tony

Susan [a staff nurse] asks me to help get Tony up for lunch. I have not met him before. I am informed that he is 53 years old, that he has primary lung cancer with liver metastases. He has been in the hospice for respite care four days.

I ask Susan 'Is there anything in particular I should be mindful of?'

'He's bit moody.'

'Why's that?'

'He's unhappy here and wants to go home. He finds it difficult to co-ordinate himself but doesn't want help.'

I knock on the closed door. No reply. I knock again and enter the room. Hand-drawn cards fixed to the bedroom wall immediately catch my attention.

'Hi Mr Birchall, I'm Chris. How are you this morning?'

He looks at me but doesn't answer. I sense his irritation. Susan's words come to mind. I gaze at the cards pinned to the wall, 'Who made these lovely cards?'

'My grand-daughter.'

'She has talent. Tell me about her?'

'Her name is Michelle. She is four years old.'

He becomes animated talking about her. She is very special to him, adding to his sadness and restlessness. I have opened a door to connect with Tony, talking about the thing that he cares most deeply for and grieves for its forthcoming loss. I reveal I have two young children. We talk about schooling and about his work – he had been a plumber. He knows he is not going to work anymore and accepts this. All the while his anger simmers. Do I let him know I sense this? Such catharsis might prick the tension and yet it might embarrass him. I take the risk 'You seem irritated being here?'

In doing so, I release my own anxiety. As if I have pressed a button, he pointedly says 'I want to be at home. Not that it's unpleasant in here but …'

His words drift off. Patiently I wait.

He adds 'I want to be at home.'

'I sense that … so why are you here?'

'I had no choice because my daughter is away for the week and I need her support.'

He relaxes. He has expressed his irritation - a potent cocktail of anger at the hospice, at me, at himself, at the cancer, at his daughter, that he is dying, grief of anticipatory loss, indeed at the world at large. He moves out of the shadow of his despair more willing to engage with me.

He asks 'Tell me about yourself.'

I sense he needs to know me in order to accept my presence. I explain I work at the hospice to maintain my credibility as a palliative care teacher. He is intrigued. He stands and takes off his pyjamas. His nakedness exposed. I hold him steady as he moves into and out of the shower. Slowly he dresses. I help him with his socks and shoes. I have been with him over an hour.

I ask 'Do you have any pain?'

'No.'

'That's good … I can see you need help with washing and dressing. Do you get this support at home OK?'

'My daughter helps me. We do have a nurse who comes in and monitors me so if things get any worse she's on hand to help.'

We go to lunch in the communal dining room. It is empty. We are late. Everybody else has gone. He invites me to join him for lunch. I stay with him until he has finished. There is something normalising about having a meal with someone. He tells me he was a keen cyclist. I tell him I am a Morris dancer. By the time we finish I am on his wavelength and sense his ease. I too am easier, having worked through my own anxiety of being rejected. I sense the way feelings are reciprocated. It highlights for me the fundamental need to know people in order to respond appropriately to them on a level that is meaningful. We got there but it took an effort.

I imagine it must be difficult for him to deal with yet another nurse. I imagine he would rather have Susan help him, someone he knows. He doesn't say that, at least not in words. Perhaps I could have said to him- 'I'll get Susan to help you,' acknowledging his initial discomfort with me. But then as Susan said he's moody with everyone. Do patients have the right to choose their nurses in hospice? It is a profound question because I cannot impose my idea of relationship on patients. The very nature of suffering and facing dying must always make relationship precarious. In getting to know someone who is suffering I trip along a fine edge of raw emotion.

Perhaps I could have simply connected superficially with him by helping him to wash, dress, escort him to lunch, administer and monitor his pain medication and other symptom relief. But this was not the level of help he really needed. On a deeper level I knew he was in crisis. I could read that, but that was my difficulty. I could not respond easily to the superficial caring issues outside that deeper context. Hence helping him wash and dress became difficult once I had touched his suffering. He also knew that and perhaps resisted me because he needed to protect himself from this intruding stranger. On the other hand he might have preferred my superficial attention. I felt as if I had pushed his limits and challenged his control of the situation.

Later, I share this experience with Susan. She affirms my experience, acknowledging Tony's struggle in facing death. She feels I shouldn't worry unduly as Tony is 'difficult'. In other words my experience is normal. Sensitivity flattened in order to cope with the stress of the day. The patient is the problem not the inadequacy of the nurse.

Before I leave the hospice I go and shake hands with Tony and thank him for accommodating me. He reciprocates my thanks, for having the patience to stay with him. I sense he is lonely here without his daughter and grand-daughter visiting. A week can seem a long time when time is running out and when such relationships are precious.

Who is This Person?

This cue guides me to see Tony as a unique 'whole' person in the context of his world. His family and culture are brought into focus and scope of care. In acknowledging Tony as a person I also acknowledge myself as a person that sets the focus for a patient-centred relationship. It challenges any tendency to reduce Tony to the status of a 'patient' where his humanness may be disregarded.

What Meaning does this Health Event have for the Person?

This cue guides me to listen and be empathic to Tony's experience beneath the surface signs and assumptions that might lead me to assume what it means. My intention is to tune into and flow with Tony's wavelength, opening the door to knowing him and for him to know himself, so he can make sense of his bewildering experience (Figure 19.3). I term this resonance a *synergistic wavelength* – whereby the energy of harmonious wavelengths enhances relational energy. In other words people really feel on each other's wavelength. Newman (1999) describes this as a *rhythm of relating*, acknowledging that the patient's rhythm may be in turmoil due to the illness experience. As Newman notes 'nurses should develop a tolerance for ambiguity and uncertainty and "hang in there" with clients until a new rhythm emerges' [p. 227] more compatible with health.

Flowing with him I am most available to help him sort out his diverse needs and find a healthier wavelength. When people experience crisis in their lives, their wave patterns

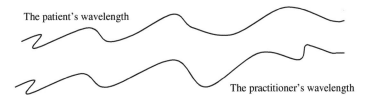

Figure 19.3   Synergy with the patient's wavelength

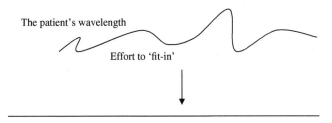

Figure 19.4   Non-synergy with patient's wavelength

become chaotic. Practitioners normally expect the patient to fit into the stereotyped 'good patient' mould- a symbolic straight line that literally flattens humanness (Figure 19.4). In response, the patient tries to 'fit-in' to be accepted and cared for. Failure to 'fit-in' often leads to censure, as characterised by the image of the 'unpopular patient'.[3] Such relationships lack harmony and feel flat.

How is this Person Feeling?

Tony reveals a cocktail of distressing emotions that bubble to the surface. I trip along this cue cautiously, not wanting to intrude inappropriately into his private world but mindful of opening a space whereby these emotions can be safely expressed and discharged as appropriate. Until these emotions are released it is impossible to talk through his experience in any meaningful way.

How do I Feel about this Person?

Initially, I didn't feel comfortable with Tony. His anger lay thick on the surface despite his compliance. My poise was rattled! It is vital I am mindful of my emotional response otherwise I am likely to subconsciously defend myself in order to manage my anxiety. I wanted to convey to Tony my concern and empathy for his predicament; that I wasn't here to oppress him further. To do that he needed to have control of the situation, gained by letting him know me. As his anger eased so did my feeling of discomfort.

How has this Event Affected their Usual Life Pattern and Roles?

Serious illness can prompt a radical reassessment of life-style and what people consider significant within their lives. Disruption of normal patterns can have detrimental consequences if not carefully managed – hence knowing his normal lifestyle is useful so I do not disrupt it unnecessarily or disturb his control over events.

Skill Box

> • *Scan the narrative and identify the extent I explored Tony's lifestyle pattern.*
> • *What other issues might have been beneficial for Tony to explore?*
> • *Do you think a checklist such as the Roper, Logan and Tierney activities would be useful to employ in relation to this cue?*

How can I Help this Person?

My visionary aim is to help Tony ease his suffering. To do this I must understand his suffering as best I can. He did not reveal himself to me easily so to help him I first had to create the conditions where he could reveal himself. Of course, I needed time to do this and fortunately I had it. In the fast pace of clinical practice such time might be at a premium, creating a dilemma for the practitioner in prioritising time for such work.

From a patient-centred perspective creating and sustaining therapeutic relationships is fundamental. It was the background to helping Tony. So I help him by being available to him [see Table 4.3]. To reiterate – the hospital's vision states 'The practitioner is mindful of *being available* to work with the person and the person's family in relationship, on the basis of empathic connection, compassion and mutual understanding, where the person's life pattern and health needs are appreciated and effectively responded to'.

Communication skills such as catharsis, catalysis and confrontation emerge as significant within relationship[4]. Self-disclosure might be seen as controversial- the extent I should disclose myself within relationship. Yet within the human-human relationship he needed to know me as a reciprocal thing.

Skill Box

> • *To what extent was I successful in understanding and easing Tony's suffering?*
> • *Consider suffering from physical, psychological, social, spiritual perspectives.*
> • *Could I have helped him more?*
> • *How available was I to Tony and, as a consequence, identify the strengths and weaknesses of my patient-centred practice.*
> • *Check out the literature on self-disclosure and reflect on your own self-disclosure with patients for its therapeutic impact.[5]*
> • *Reflect on your own availability to a patient or indeed a student if you are a teacher. Do not rush to hasty conclusions.*

What is important for this person to make their stay in the hospice comfortable?

Tony did not want to be at the hospice but felt obliged to because of his social circumstances. The cue raises issues of comfort and control, especially those 'little things' that make a significant difference to the person's comfort and perception of being cared for (Macleod 1994). For Tony I suspect that being understood makes his stay more comfortable, enabling him to flow more easily in this potentially hostile environment. Talking about his granddaughter was clearly significant.

Perhaps I could have challenged Susan's analysis and labelling of Tony as 'difficult'. Labelling is such a perverse act and disrupts any therapeutic potential. It highlights how easily practitioners label people as 'difficult' as a way of dealing with the anxiety these people arouse within them. I recognise my failure to confront Susan reflects a deeper need to avoid conflict, reflecting how practitioners also conform to a social norm of the harmonious team.[6] Knowing what makes people feel comfortable reflects and communicates a deep sensitivity to the person as befits any claim to patient-centred care.

What Support does this Person Have in Life?

I tentatively queried his support at home. I did not meet his daughter so did not gain her perspective. However, the hospice is geared up to social and psychological aspects of care. My role is to collaborate with others if aspects of supporting Tony emerge through our conversation. From a pragmatic perspective, support is vital to mobilise and develop with a view to eventual discharge especially where the person requires support in the community with the risk and associated impact and cost of the person blocking the bed.[7]

How does this Person View the Future?

Tony knew his condition was terminal. His anticipatory loss rippled through our whole encounter. Tony's imminent death is present between us even if we do not mention it. Sometimes I explicitly but sensitively use this cue -- 'Tony- how do you view the future?' as appropriate.

Skill Box

- *Reflect on your usual approach to assessing or appreciating patients. Does it tune you into your vision for practice [if indeed you have one- see previous skill box]*
- *Would the reflective cues enable a different, more effective perspective on the patient? Do the cues facilitate reflective practice?*

A System to Ensure Effective Communication

Communication, whether written or verbal, is necessary to ensure continuity and consistency of negotiated care between practitioners and across different practice settings. Communication is verbal, through language, and non-verbal, through body posture, senses and intonation. Communication is both formal and informal – formal verbal communication takes place through writing notes and reports, through shift reports, ward rounds and various care meetings that may include patients and families. Informal verbal communication takes place in the way practitioners relate to each other and with patients and families throughout the day; corridor conversations, passing remarks, the sluice room conference, coffee chat, etc. I am sure the reader can coin many euphemisms for such informal verbal meetings – all accompanied by a vast range of non-verbal communication that convey positive and negative power messages. Reflective communication on all levels is dialogical[8] alongside the transmission of facts.

Narrative Notes

Since the late 1970s, the nursing process has dominated the approach to thinking and writing about patient care. Essentially, the nursing process is a linear problem-solving approach that structures thinking through four stages:

- Goal setting – an interpretation of assessment in terms of identifying specific actual or potential problems/ patient needs and goals to be achieved in responding to the problem/ need.
- Planning – establishing the response to solve the problem/ need.
- Intervention – carrying out the planned care.

- Evaluation – determining whether the set goal has been met, including re-defining the problem or goal as necessary in light of consequences.

In theory, a practitioner should be able to pick up the care plan and continue the patient's care as a seamless activity. However, most aspects of care cannot be prescribed in advance given the uniqueness of each individual and each caring encounter, at least not without reducing the patient to an object to be manipulated. Some aspects of care may be more amenable to prescription, for example technical solutions to medical problems such as wound dressings, pain management and theatre preparation. These prescriptions can be framed as evidence-based protocols.

The nursing process has attracted much adverse criticism in the 1990s (Howse and Bailey 1992, White 1993, Latimer 1995, McElroy et al. 1995). Although the nursing process was intended to promote a culture of individualised and negotiated care (De la Cuesta 1983), ironically the opposite tended to happen when it was accommodated to fit within the existing dominant medical model culture, resulting in a minimal or lip-service response to the ideology of individualised care (Latimer 1995). The patient became a set of problems or needs diagnosed by the nurse. The nursing diagnosis movement [NANDA] was a natural development from the nursing process in the USA, yet is a process fraught with difficulty because it imposes abstract meanings on 'nursing' concepts in the futile effort to ensure consistency of diagnosis. In this respect this movement mirrors medicine's approach to diagnosis. Practitioners might find come common understanding of what a grade 4 glioma is, but can practitioners find common meaning in using the word suffering, spirituality or agitation?

In an observational study of the impact of primary nursing on the culture of a community hospital (Johns 1989), one practitioner commented- 'much of it is just nursing, you don't have to write that down'. This comment reflects the stereotypical pattern recognition and common sense knowing that this practitioner and her colleagues possessed, and their struggle to write down what was so obvious to them. As another practitioner commented – 'patients we know well don't need care planning'. I asked one staff nurse on her return from holiday if she had read her patients' care plans. She commented, 'I haven't had time because it's so busy', again suggesting that care plans were unnecessary. The human within the machine becomes a contradiction. As Wilber (1998) puts it, systems are the language of 'it' and 'it' is a stark colourless landscape of labels.

From a person-centred perspective, the nursing process is a contradiction, making little allowance for the expert practitioner's intuitive processes in making decisions about complex caring situations (Cioffi 1997). As such, the mechanical linear approach of the nursing process does not fit with expert thinking. Indeed, it is a hindrance, and absurd. Communication systems need to be based on how the expert practitioner thinks. My retrospective audit of nursing notes at Burford revealed the nursing process had no real value either as a comprehensive record of care or enabling the continuity of care. Imagine wasting time doing something that is meaningless!

In response I developed the idea of *narrative notes*. These are descriptive of care given that connects pattern appreciation, clinical judgement, practitioner response and evaluation, highlighting significant moments in the patient's health–illness experience.

Skill Box

- *Consider my narrative of being with Tony. What insightful points would you write in his narrative notes? Remember your intention is to open a dialogical space alongside any transmission of significant facts.*[9]
- *Reflect on your own clinical note writing- is it insightful?*[10]

Talk

To reiterate, verbal communication or *talk* is essentially dialogical, whether with patients, families or colleagues. The manner of practitioner's talk is therapeutic as a caring act in itself.

Reflective Handover

The function of the handover report is to communicate relevant information from one shift to the next to ensure the continuity and effectiveness of planned care. A reflective handover emphasises dialogue between practitioner around key practice issues supplemented by information as appropriate or referral to the notes. With effective facilitation the dialogue takes no longer than the traditional handover of simply imparting information because much of the information can be read in effective narrative notes.

Bedside Handover

However, handovers in closed rooms must be questioned from a patient-centred perspective (Ward 1988). A more reflective approach is to involve patients in dialogue concerning their treatment and care at the bedside. A considerable literature emerged in the 1990s that explored patient participation in decision-making (Ashworth, Longmate and Morrison 1992; Biley 1992; Jewell 1994; Trnobanski 1994; Waterworth and Luker 1990). Working with and negotiating decision-making is congruent with the hospital's vision. Resistance to bedside handover requires appreciation and dialogue:

- fear of breaching patient confidentiality by disclosing information in public areas;
- some patients would not be able to participate;
- some patients would not want to be involved;
- uncomfortable for practitioner used to a more traditional approach of talking about patients behind closed doors.

From a person-centred perspective, the handover is an act of care. Not to involve patients in the handover of their care is an obvious contradiction that reduces them to objects of care rather than active participants in their own healthcare. It may take more time, and may create some risk of public disclosure, but it does lead to greater trust that more than offsets any bureaucratic concern of risk. Unfortunately, organisations, wary of litigation, tend to lean heavily towards risk management even when risk is minimal.[11]

The bedside handover protocol involves the handover staff visiting each patient prior to moving into 'the office' to complete the report. The practitioners greet each patient [and family] inviting them to reflect on their care. It helps practitioners to make better sense of patient information having seen and spoken with the patient beforehand. The protocol emphasises the primacy of narrative notes as the means for continuing care. The notes are stored at the bedside for both patient and practitioner availability. After all, they the patient's notes. The idea of patient-held records is well known in community settings - again reflecting the philosophy of working with the patient in terms of their care. This practice challenges practitioners to be mindful of what they write, knowing that it might be read by the patient or the patient's family.

Tony declines to be involved in his bedside handover. The shift report group enter his room and say hello. We then proceed to the office to dialogue about his care. Susan says Chris has been with Tony this morning. I give a verbal account of what I have written in the notes adding the bit about his 'coktail of emotions' and his granddaughter's cards pinned on the wall. Other staff comment that Tony's irritation has been difficult for them to penetrate but they can understand why he responds like that. I suggest it is us who has the problem not Tony. They agree. I can feel a shift in attitude towards him. As defences drop so compassion rises. One of the group says 'that has been insightful'.

De-briefing

Reflective de-briefing is an opportunity for staff to de-brief as a group at the end of each shift, in recognition of the emotional impact of caring for some patients and issues of misunderstanding. Indeed, it can be part of the reflective handover although at other times it needs more time.

De-briefing has a number of obvious benefits:

- it acknowledges that sometimes, for whatever reasons, practice can be tough;
- it is okay to be distressed, angry – cutting across a culture where practitioners hide their feelings in the [misguided] belief that 'good nurses cope' or not to burden their colleagues;
- where practitioners can be legitimately heard and valued as persons with human needs and human frailties;
- constructing the therapeutic team by bringing staff together to create a new culture of mutual support in their caring quest, bringing vision into clear view;
- confronting inappropriate attitudes, behaviours, assumptions and defence mechanisms that disrupt therapeutic ways of working with patients and colleagues;
- promoting the morale, self-esteem and motivation of colleagues, with organisational consequences of retaining staff, enhancing quality of care and reducing staff sickness;
- defusing toxic stuff and not taking it home with you!
- realising the learning organisation.

Skill Box

- *Rewrite any clinical notes as an unfolding narrative. Commence by telling a story about the patient – 'Tony is a...' Weave your pattern appreciation. Highlight significant issues about the care and treatment he requires [perhaps use the reflective cues as headings until you feel confident to construct more unstructured narrative]. Remember to keep the 'whole person and family' in view rather than reduce them to bits.*

A Reflective System to Live Quality

The reflective practitioner is mindful of *living quality* as part of everyday practice. In doing so, she actively accepts responsibility for the quality of her own performance and for the quality of the whole organisation–'our patients deserve nothing less than the most effective care'. No pressure then!

Quality is lived through individual and collective reflective practices across clinical and organisational practice. Modern day quality is wrapped in the cloak of clinical Governance, defined as

A framework through which Health Service organisations are accountable for continuously improving the *quality* of their services and safeguarding high standards of care by creating an environment in which clinical excellence will flourish.
[DHSS consultation paper- *A first class service*, 1998]

Powerful words, but who takes responsibility for creating this *environment in which clinical excellence can flourish?* Well, any professional practitioner will say – 'it is my responsibility' yet within organisations it requires organisational leadership. Of course, it also requires some grip on what *clinical excellence* means.

Whether or not practitioners take quality seriously, quality systems will be imposed determined by external criteria, most significantly the Care Quality Commission [CQC][12] with draconian powers for failing organisations. The CQC bases its criteria around the patient's experience, patient safety and clinical effectiveness. The CQC emerged on the back of the DH report chaired by Lord Darzi (2008) that set out a vision of the National Health Service that gives patients and the public more information and choices, works in partnership and has quality of care at its heart, quality defined as clinically effective, personal and safe' [DHSS –'High-quality care for all, p. 8]. The Trust is paranoid about negative CQC ratings. It jumps to the CQC tune rather than take a proactive approach in the first place. But then setting standards is time consuming.

The National Centre for Clinical Excellence [NICE] also indicates and dictates the quality agenda. NICE has been integral to clinical governance, setting quality standards for clinical care towards which Trusts work by approving treatments, equipment, interventions and procedures based on current best evidence. It would seem that by adopting such an evidence base, effective and consistent transfer of the lessons of research should be integrated into routine practice, rather than traditional and historical practices that do not improve patient outcome. However, much research and evidence base stems from a technical rational eye whereby the quality of the patient experience is often invisible. This requires a *story* approach. These quality systems impose conformity and compliance and the creative opportunity of lived quality can be lost. The CQC emphasis on improving the patient's experience reflects the central purpose of clinical governance (Halligan and Donaldson 2001). As person-centred clinical practice is developed, so the ensuing dialogues with people and their families will sharpen the care response around meeting peoples' needs and improving quality.

The bureaucratic advantage of external judgement against set criteria measurement is it enables benchmarking- comparing hospitals with other hospitals and the inevitable construction of league tables. But do these tools actually measure quality or simply what it looked for?

Reflective approaches to quality work through triple feedback loops:

Loop 1: Do practitioners' clinical judgement and skilled responses realise desirable practice?
Loop 2: Do the conditions of practice hinder realising desirable practice?
Loop 3: Are the indicators for realising desirable practice adequate?

Three guided reflection approaches to *living quality* implemented at Burford were:

- clinical audit;
- professional supervision;
- standards of care [see chapter 21]

Clinical Audit

Clinical audit is a clinically led initiative which seeks to improve the quality and outcome of patient care through structured peer review whereby clinicians reflect on their practice and results against agreed standards and modify their practice where indicated (*Clinical audit in the NHS* 1996). It offers an opportunity for multi-professional group reflection around specific patients with the primary purpose of answering two fundamental questions:

- Did the patient/ family receive best care?
- Do we know what best care is?

A practitioner prepares and presents an overview of the patient's care using an appropriate reflective framework such as the Model for Reflective Inquiry [Figure 4.2]. The initial focus of inquiry is the practitioners' aesthetic responses, comprising appreciating clinical judgement, clinical action and efficacy. Any personal, ethical, empirical and reflexive factors that influenced the aesthetic response are then considered. The group then re-imagine the situation and explore other, potentially more effective, responses for future action. Insights are summarised and presented to the Clinical Governance Group. At the next Clinical Audit session, the case is reviewed to note its impact on subsequent practice. Of course, each clinical situation is different and learning cannot simply be transferred from one situation to another.

There exists a tension between professional and organisational remit for clinical audit. As *Clinical audit in the NHS* (1996: 4) notes:

> Practitioners are only likely to become involved where they retain a clear sense of ownership of the process of audit and feel it is a safe environment for discussing sensitive details about their professional practice without the fear of provoking management sanction or civil litigation.

Clinical audit is a formal structure that enables practitioners across disciplines to collaborate and demonstrate professional responsibility.

A System to Ensure Staff are Enabled to Realise the Vision as a Lived Reality

In 1990 I established a project at Burford hospital to implement and evaluate what I termed *professional supervision* (Johns 1993) to develop and exercise my leadership role to guide practitioners to develop expert performance in tune with the hospital's vision for practice and take responsibility for their own and collective practice (Johns 1998a.) It is important to note that I viewed my leadership role as one of enabling practitioners, not prescribing or controlling their practice, as befits the philosophy of primary nursing as practised at the hospital whereby a primary nurse takes 24-hour responsibility for the planning and delivery of care to her patients. As such, it is a demanding role that requires particular development and support.

The project involved me guiding primary and associate nurses for one hour approximately every three weeks through sharing their experiences. Sessions were recorded and the data gathered over a four-year period germinated my theories on guided reflection. As explored in Chapter 5, guidance is non-judgemental, the key being that practitioners judge their own performance. However, feedback from these sessions was an understated monitor of quality. I also worked two days a week as an associate nurse following the primary nurses planned care and was able to give more direct feedback from this role.

Clinical Supervision

We were ahead of our time. Guided reflection is often termed clinical supervision when it takes place in clinical practice. In 1993, clinical supervision burst upon the general nursing agenda prompted by the government's concern for greater professional accountability and surveillance to give the public confidence that nurses' and health visitors' practice would be adequately monitored in the aftermath of the Beverly Allitt tragedy. The *Vision for the future* document (National Health Services Management Executive, 1993: 3) defined clinical supervision as:

> a formal process of professional support and learning which enables individual practitioners to develop knowledge and competence, assume responsibility for their own practice and enhance consumer protection and safety of care in complex situations. It is central to the process of learning and to the expansion of the scope of practice and should be seen as a means of encouraging self-assessment and analytical and reflective skills.

This definition was influenced by a psychotherapy and counselling models of supervision, reflecting the backgrounds of the authors of a government-commissioned background paper (Faugier and Butterworth, undated).

It suggests six key aims:

- To develop practitioner competence;
- To safeguard patients;
- Developing or expanding nursing roles [scope of practice];
- To promote practitioner responsibility for ensuring effective performance;
- To promote self- assessment of performance;
- To develop reflective skills.

These aim have a potential tension between, on one hand, the intention to open a learning space for practitioners to develop competence, on the other, a surveillance system to safeguard the public.

If clinical supervision is to be a learning opportunity, then practitioners need to feel safe to reveal their practice. If the clinical supervisor's agenda is to judge performance then practitioners might be cautious of revealing their practice. The contradiction is mediated by the intention of clinical supervision to enable practitioners to develop responsibility to monitor their own performance. The emphasis on developing reflective skills indicates the learning space is structured through reflective practice. This is not straightforward, as many practitioners and supervisors lack reflective and guidance skills, thus limiting the potential of clinical supervision and required an injection of organisational resources to develop effective supervisors. Perhaps this why supervision faded from many organisational agendas, that is until recently when the CQC indicated that they regarded supervision as a measure of organisation quality.

Sustaining Practitioners

The omission of sustaining performance within the clinical supervision definition is problematic given the stressful nature of everyday practice. Low morale, as recent surveys indicate,[13] reflect unsatisfactory working conditions, resulting in high anxiety and stress, with subsequent risk of poor patient care. Such conditions are an abject failure of leadership.

Guided reflection offers the opportunity for practitioners to be heard, to release tension, and take some action although, on an individual basis this is not easy especially if the practitioner is already demoralised.

Skill Box

> - *Google and read 'low morale in NHS' reports.*
> - *How would you rate your own morale [1–10]?*
> - *Do you go home from a shift not satisfied?*
> - *What support systems are in place to develop and sustain individual and collective performance? Are these systems adequate?*
> - *Review the different approaches to guided reflection/ clinical supervision set out in Chapter 5. Be bold and assertive- open a dialogue about supervision in your practice. Is existing supervision adequate? If supervision does not exist- then establish it, preferably from a peer-led group perspective. [This also applies to teachers.]*

Organisational Culture

What sort of organisational culture needs to exist to accommodate a reflective and person-centred approach to clinical practice? I know that existing transactional or bureaucratic cultures cannot accommodate reflective practice simply because they are by their very nature static, reactive and unreflective. Such organisations are overly concerned with risk management at the expense of creativity. What is required is a culture committed to creating and sustaining a *learning organisation* and reflective leadership that serves and invests in people.

Burford was part of a large health authority. However, as its general manager and leader I was able to create a bubble of autonomy aided by its Nursing Development Unit status whilst ever mindful to comply with/ ameliorate the 'bureaucratic demand'. Twenty years later I sense the bureaucratic demand has become ever greater, constricting the autonomy of leaders to create their own learning organisations (Johns 2015).[14]

The Learning Organisation

Creating and sustaining the Learning Organisation is undoubtedly the most significant element of a reflective environment. Senge (1990: 3) describes the Learning Organisation [LO] as

> One where people continually expand their capacities to create the results they truly desire, where new and expansive patterns of thinking are nurtured, where collective aspiration is set free, and where people are continually learning how to learn together.

Organisations learn only through individuals who learn. Individual learning alone does not guarantee organisational learning but without it no organisational learning occurs (Senge 1990).

Senge identified five disciplines that collectively constitute the learning Organisation:

- *Vision* is a collaborative consensual statement of shared beliefs: beliefs that gives meaning and purpose to clinical practice. It sets up creative tension.
- *Personal mastery* is the discipline of holding and resolving creative tension so that one's vision can be realised as a lived reality. It involves clarifying and deepening personal vision and seeing reality objectively. In other words it is reflective practice.
- *Mental models* are the assumptions that govern how the practitioner understands and responds to the world.
- *Systems thinking* is critiquing the pattern of underlying systems that support practice and shifting these systems to enable practitioners to realise desirable practice.

- *Team learning* is collaborating with colleagues to realise a shared vision through dialogue.

In team learning, mental models and systems thinking are aligned to realising this purpose through dialogue and subsequent action and reflection within double feedback loops – do we get the outcomes we desire? Are our vision and our processes adequate?

To these five systems I add *leadership* as the catalyst and driving force to create and sustain the learning organisation. Few healthcare institutions can be described as learning organisations since, in a system largely dominated by highly structured, hierarchical and historically determined professional demarcations, it is an infrequent occurrence that norms or assumptions are challenged or that the required unlearning or relearning take place (Garside 1999). The task of managing these tensions and inspiring and motivating people to learn and contribute to the learning organisation in such a difficult, highly pressurised arena is the primary leadership challenge.

The Chief Executive's Board meeting must itself become a learning organisation, acknowledging its transactional anxiety for what it is and liberating itself from its own tyranny. This requires a decentralising of the organisation and an equalising of power. No easy task for the transactional organisation that seeks to direct and control from the top in order to manage its anxiety and ensure smooth running.

Guided reflection can be aligned with the aims of the learning organisation:

- To clarify and deepen personal and collective visions of best practice.
- To develop personal mastery through holding creative tension between a vision of best practice and an understanding of current practice; it is a commitment to life-long learning to be the best the practitioner can be.
- To scrutinise one's mental models/ assumptions and shift these as necessary towards realising best practice.
- To review and shift organisational systems towards creating the optimum conditions to support best practitioner performance.
- To work collaboratively with colleagues through dialogue to ensure best practice.

Leadership

Leadership is the driving force to create and sustain effective working practices and quality. Yet ideas on leadership vary considerably, depending on your perspective. Healthcare organisations are transactional, where leadership is little more than management to ensure targets are met. The prevailing mantra is 'Command and control'! In this transactional world, people become pawns to be moved around the board. In contrast, the contemporary literature on leadership advocates a transformational style of leadership concerned with creating and sustaining a dynamic and moral learning organisation. (Burns 1978).

In looking at taking the NHS forward to greater quality in a time of limited resources Nicholson (2009) writes:

> Great clinical leadership is fundamental to this. Sustainable health systems are created when clinical leaders are empowered to bring about transformational change supported by managers who back good ideas, remove blockages to progress and provide support.

Nicholson should say 'supported by leaders' simply because managers are focused on tasks not relationships. Wheatley (1999: 164) writes, 'management is getting work done through others. The important thing was the work; the "others" were distractions that needed to be managed into conformity and predictability.'

Leadership spirals all the way down and all the way up the organisation, actively nurtured at every level. My vision of a reflective leadership is inspired by servant leadership (Greenleaf 1978; Johns 2015) with its emphasis on leaders being 'of service' to enable other to accomplish what needs to be done through genuine collaborative relationships that invests in people to enable them to grow and fulfil their potential and 'creating community' to make sure that other people's highest priority needs are being served and grow through community. Servant-leaders are reflective and mindful of self as a leader and the creative tension between leadership vision and the realities of working in a transactional organisation. Leaders are visionary with foresight anticipating what is required based on a firm footing in everyday reality. Leaders are authentic have a strong morality (Bass 1985) acting with integrity towards creating better worlds for others no matter what resistance is encountered, yet yielding graciously as appropriate. Leaders are poised and emotionally intelligent in the face of disturbance and uncertainty, with the ability to sustain self within mutually supportive networks. And without doubt, leaders are inspirational and energetic lifting people to higher levels of motivation and achievement within the learning community. Reviewing these words it is obvious that leadership is complex requiring dedicated development.

Another perspective on leadership is offered by 'front foot thinking' [Table 19.1], that the leader is on the 'front foot'– proactive rather than reactive to situations.

Table 19.1 Front foot–back foot thinking

Front foot thinking							Back foot thinking		
10	9	8	7	6	5	4	3	2	1

Views self as a leader	Views self as follower
Uses initiative/ proactive	Waits for others' command/reactive
Takes responsibility	Shirks responsibility
Assertive/confident	Non-assertive/ hesitant
Mindful of being on 'front foot'	Not aware of being on 'front foot'
Strong sense of purpose/moral/ values	Weak sense of purpose/ moral/ values
Takes initiative	Lets things slide
Alert/is prepared	Not alert/unprepared
Visible to others	Keeps head down
Recognises own value	Need to be valued by others
Focuses on strengths	Focuses on weaknesses
Sees the whole picture	Sees only picture they want to see
Crosses hierarchical lines	Hierarchical bound
Voice is heard	Voice subdued
Expands autonomy	Shrinks autonomy
Foresight	Hindsight
Thinks outside the box/Creative	Thinks inside the box/Conforming
Dynamic sense of relationship	Confined by normal relationships
Poised	Anxious
'In the right place'	'Put in place'
Decisive	Prevaricates
Collaborative style of conflict management	Accommodating/avoiding style of conflict management
Bounces back [resilient]	Falls over [fragile]
Engaged	Detached
Yields	Fails
Takes risks/fearless	Plays safe/defensive

Skill Box

- *Everybody should perceive themselves as a leader through taking responsibility for her own performance and the performance of others. This is the bottom line of professional accountability.*
- *Use Table 19.1 as reflective framework for guiding and reviewing self-becoming either on the front or back foot. Use the table over time to monitor self-becoming increasingly 'front foot'.*
- *Establish an action learning set with leaders from other disciplines and units to develop peer-led leadership.*
- *Lobby management to support genuine leadership development [getting political is a leadership attribute]*

If you are the chief executive then take action NOW!

Summary

The Burford NDU model: caring in practice offers a reflective approach to clinical practice built around four systems set against a conducive organisational background. Systems should be designed to support the clinical approach as stated in a valid vision for practice rather than dictate the approach because they are corporate. The nine reflective cues that pattern *appreciation* are internalised as a natural way of perceiving practice. As such, these cue are always working, breaking down any separation of assessment, planning, intervention and evaluation that has typified the nursing process.

Endnotes

1   See, for example, 'People are not Numbers to Crunch' [Chapter 25]
2   See 'People are not Numbers to Crunch' [Chapter 25].
3   For example, see Johnson and Webb (1995), Kelly and May (1982),
4   Catalysis, catharsis and confrontation are all communication skills within Six Category Intervention Analysis – see Figure 5.1.
5   For example Derlaga and Berg (2014) and Jourard (1971).
6   see also Chapter 15, 'Hank's Conflict'.
7   Delays in discharging patients out of hospital after treatment could be costing the NHS in England £900m a year, an independent review has said. Labour peer Lord Carter's report found nearly one in ten beds was taken by someone medically fit to be released. http://www.bbc.co.uk/news/health-35481849 accessed 16 March 2016.
8   Remind yourself of the significance of dialogue – see Chapter 5
9   I wrote, 'Tony's anger at being in the hospice is difficult to respond to. After helping him wash and dress we lunched together and shared many common interests that helped to lift his despair for the moment. He acknowledges he needs to be here, as difficult as that is for him'.
10 I recently visited a friend in hospital. He complained he couldn't sleep at night. Yet his notes said 'Slept well. No complaints' day after day. Why would the nurses write that?
11 See Chapter 20. pp. 265–266.
12 www.cqc.org.uk
13 For example Google Royal Cornwall Hospitals (Treliske) staff survey: a very low staff morale indicated. 'Cornwall hospitals ranked in worst 20%' (http://www.bbc.co.uk/news/uk-england-cornwall-31621683) 'Staff at RCHT "totally demoralised" but fighting to maintain standards.' Read more: (http://www.westbriton.co.uk/Staff-RCHT-totally-demoralised-fighting-maintain/story-20755542-detail/story.html#ixzz40KutMraK)
14 The development of leadership within the NHS is the focus of my book Mindful leadership (Johns 2015).

References

Alfano, G. (1971) Healing or caretaking – which will it be? *Nursing Clinics of North America* 6.2,273-80.

Ashworth, P., Longmate, M. and Morrison, P. (1992) Patient participation: its meaning and significance in the context of caring. *Journal of Advanced Nursing* 17, 1430–1439.

Bass, B (1990). From transactional to transformational leadership: learning to share the vision. *Organizational Dynamics [winter]*, 19–31.

Biley, F. (1992) Some determinants that affect patient participation in decision-making about nursing care. *Journal of Advanced Nursing* 17, 414–421.

Burns, J. (1978) *Leadership*. Harper & Row, New York.

Cioffi, J. (1997) Heuristics, servants to intuition, in clinical decision making. *Journal of Advanced Nursing* 26, 203–208.

Cowling, W. R. (2000) Healing as appreciating wholeness. *Advances in Nursing Science*, 22.3; 16–32.

De La Cuesta, C. (1983) The nursing process: from development to implementation. *Journal of Advanced Nursing* 8, 365–71.

Department of Health (1996) *Clinical audit in the NHS*. HMSO, London

Department of Health (1998) *A first class service: quality in the new NHS*. HMSO, London.

Department of Health (2008) *High quality care for all*. HMSO, London.

Derlaga, V. J. and Berg, J. H. (2014) *Self-disclosure: theory, research, and therapy*. Springer, New York.

Faugier, J. and Butterworth, T. (undated) *Clinical supervision: a position paper*. School of Nursing Studies, University of Manchester.

Garside, P. (1999) The learning organisation: a necessary setting for improving care? *Quality in Health Care* 8, 211.

Greenleaf, R. (1977/2002) *Servant leadership: a journey into the nature of legitimate power and greatness*. Paulist Press, New Jersey.

Hall, L. (1964) Nursing- what is it? *Canadian Nurse*, 60.2, 150–154.

Halligan, A. and Donaldson, L. J. (2001) Implementing clinical governance: turning vision into reality. *British Medical Journal* 322 (7299), 1413–1417.

Jewell, S. (1994) Patient participation: what does it mean? *Journal of Advanced Nursing* 19, 433–438.

Johns, C. (1989) The impact of introducing primary nursing on the culture of a community hospital. Master of Nursing dissertation, University of Wales College of Medicine, Cardiff.

Johns, C. (1993) Professional supervision. *Journal of Nursing Management* 1.1, 9–18

Johns, C. (2013) *Becoming a reflective practitioner* (4th edition) Wiley-Blackwell, Oxford.

Johns, C. (2015) *Mindful leadership: a guide for health professions*. Palgrave, London.

Johnson, D. (1974) Development of theory: a requisite for nursing as a primary health profession. *Nursing Research* 23.5, 373–357.

Johnson, M. and Webb, C. (1995) Rediscovering unpopular patients: the concept of social judgment. *Journal of Advanced Nursing* 21, 466–475.

Jourard, S. (1971) *The transparent self*. Van Nostrand, Newark, NJ.

Kelly, M. and May, D. (1982) Good and bad patients: a review of the literature and theoretical critique. *Journal of Advanced Nursing* 7, 147–156.

Maslow, A. (1968) *Towards a psychology of being*. Van Nostrand, Princeton, NJ.

Mayeroff, M. (1971) *On caring*. Harper Perennial, New York.

National Health Service Management Executive (NHSME) (1993) *A vision for the future*. HMSO. London.

Newman, M. (1999) The rhythm of relating in a paradigm of wholeness. *Image: Journal of Nursing Scholarship* 31.3, 227–230.

Nicholson, D. (2009) Implementing the next stage review visions: the quality and productivity challenge. Memo to all chief executives of Primary Health Care Trusts in England, all chief executives of NHS Trusts in England, and all chief executives of NHS Foundation Trusts in England [Gateway reference 12396] Department of Health, London.

Pearson, A. (1983) *The clinical nursing unit*. Heinemann Medical Books, London.

Remen, R. (1994) *Kitchen table wisdom*. Riverhead Books, New York.

Roper, N., Logan, W. and Tierney, A. (1980) *The elements of nursing*. Churchill Livingstone, Edinburgh.

Rowe, H. (1996) Multidisciplinary teamwork- myth or reality? *Journal of Nursing Management* 4, 93–101.

Senge, P. M. (1990) *The fifth discipline. the art and practice of the learning organisation*. Doubleday/Currency, New York.

Trnobanski, P. (1994) Nurse–patient dialogue: assumption or reality? *Journal of Advanced Nursing* 19, 733–737.

Ward, K. (1988) Not just the patient in bed three. *Nursing Times* 84.78, 39–50.

Waterworth, S. and Luker, K. (1990) Reluctant collaborators: do patients want to be involved in decisions involving care? *Journal of Advanced Nursing* 15, 971–976.

Watson, J. (1988) *Nursing: human science and human care. a theory of nursing*. National League for Nursing, New York.

Wheatley, M. (1999) *Leadership and the new science: discovering order in a chaotic world*. Berrett-Koehler, San Francisco.

Wilber, K. (1998) *The eye of spirit: an integral vision for a world gone slightly mad*. Shambhala, Boston.

Chapter 20

The Standards Group

Christopher Johns

Reflective practitioners *live* quality

In Chapter 19 I set out the Burford NDU: Caring in Practice model as a reflective approach to structure clinical practice. I noted that standards of care offered a dynamic and creative approach to ensure quality. Standards of care offer a reflective approach to managing quality by focusing on discrete aspects of practice. This approach is based on the Royal College of Nursing Standards of Care project (Kitson 1989). This may seem old hat but, as a reflective approach, it offers a practical and creative approach for practitioners to collaborate to *live quality*. It stands to reason that quality must be monitored against some standard against which 'optimum care' might be known. 'Optimum; reflects the most effective care within available resources, yet always seeking more effective practice whilst staking a claim for more resources.

Consider the midwifery mantra – *be with woman.*[1] How might that be known? Perhaps to simply ask the woman the extent she felt the midwife was with her, what particular factors contributed to her judgement and what might have improved the quality of her experience. From an objective perspective we might construct a series of criteria to make such judgement. Practitioner experience is often discounted as valid 'evidence' even though experience is the most significant determinant for clinical judgment and response (Read 1983).

Standards of Care

A standard of care reflects a local practice situation that is professionally agreed, and both desirable and achievable. *A local practice situation* is a statement of practice sited to the particular practice unit, for example – *patients are cared for in a safe and therapeutic environment.* A midwifery unit may interpret this standard in a very different way to a surgical unit, yet both will pay attention to research and policy that indicate what is therapeutic and what is safe.

Becoming a Reflective Practitioner, Fifth Edition. Edited by Christopher Johns.
© 2017 John Wiley & Sons Ltd. Published 2017 by John Wiley & Sons Ltd.
Companion Website: www.wiley.com/go/johns/reflectivepractitioner

Professionally agreed involves all people involved in meeting the standard of care: nurses, doctors, paramedical staff, cleaners, cooks, pharmacists and so on. The idea of 'professionally agreed' goes against the grain of setting patient-centred standards of care – can professionals and ancillary staff adequately set standards for patients and families? Do patients or patient representative groups need to be involved? At Burford hospital, I invited Age Concern to 'vet' our standards, as most of our patients were elderly. At the hospice, we involve volunteers who have experience of caring for dying relatives as part of the shadow clinical governance committee that oversees the quality initiative.

There is a tension between what is *desirable and what is achievable* that captures the essence of quality. Quality is what is real, what is in front of you. You can feel the fabric of my shirt and sense its quality. However quality is also something relative or comparable with other shirts – i.e., that quality has a desirable element to it. Clearly, standards of care need to be achievable otherwise they are mere pipe dreams and create frustration. Yet, standards also need to reflect desirability, as something to move towards.

A standard of care reduces the practice situation into structure, process and outcome criteria designed to be monitored.

- *Structure* is resources that need to exist to enable the standard to be met.
- *Process* is actions practitioners need to take to meet the standard
- *Outcome* is relevant indictors that inform the standard has been met.

Structural criteria include staffing levels, attitudes and skills of staff; for instance, the complementary therapist undertakes 12 hours professional development yearly, the number of syringe drivers, colours of walls, number of single rooms, maintenance contracts, and the such like. A policy is an example of structure, as is an organisation's mission statement. In contrast, a formulary or protocol is an example of process – actions that practitioners must take usually in a specified order of action; for example, mouth care.

Process criteria might read:

- The practitioner greets each relative on arrival.
- The practitioner gives mouth care as per formulary.

Monitoring tools are designed to be integral with everyday practice – namely observational and interviewing tools. Observational tools are *scanning* and *spotting*. Scanning is a planned monitoring of the standard of care using a designed scan sheet. Spotting is opportunistic observation of criteria during the course of the day, for example- noticing an immobile patient *does not have a drink within easy reach at mealtime*. This example is part of a scanning sheet to monitor a nutrition standard [see Box 20.1]. Student nurses were asked to scan and feedback to staff.

Standards can be built into assessment. The standard on sleep, *Patients are satisfied with their sleep*, used a visual analogue scale [VAS] to both appreciate and monitor the patient's satisfaction with his sleep [Box 20.2]. The VAS can be used over a series of days to monitor satisfaction by identifying and responding to factors that seem to impede sleep – given the therapeutic value of sleep in recovery from illness. Topics such as sleep and nutrition are often taken for granted yet are important determinants of the patient's well-being.

Setting a monitoring schedule is always tentative, especially in the first instance. Perhaps weekly or monthly depending on the particular standard and the extent it is 'spotted' as failing its criteria. Who should monitor? As I suggested with the relatives standard, monitoring techniques that involve asking patients or their families are best slipped into

Box 20.1   Scan sheet 'Patients enjoy a nutritious meal'

	The patient receives a meal ...	Score and comment Yes – 3; so-so – 2; No – 1
1	That he/she has chosen within limits	
2	In an amount he/she can enjoy	
3	That suits their dietary requirements	
4	At the correct temperature	
5	In an environment conducive to eating	
6	On a clean table	
7	With a drink within reach	
8	That they are not rushed to complete	
9	With assistance as required	
10	That isn't unnecessarily interrupted	
11	They were prepared for	
12	Where any underlying symptom that might impair enjoyment has been adequately responded to; constipation, diarrhoea, nausea, fatigue, pain etc.	
13	Other factors - please state	

Box 20.2   Monitoring sleep

The sleep visual analogue scale {VAS} was designed to monitor the Standards of care 'The patient is satisfied with their sleep'. The patient is asked about their usual sleep patterns and mark their normal satisfaction with their sleep. The intention is to improve his satisfaction with sleep. The scale can be used on successive days to see if interventions to improve sleep result in improved satisfaction with sleep.

Sleep VAS	6/11/02
Complete satisfaction with sleep No satisfaction with sleep	
Mark patient's perception on scale. What factors influence this mark? NB: pain, position, hunger, drink, temperature of room, environment, noise, bed, bedclothes, anxiety, emotion, usual sleep pattern, sleeping tablets, full bladder, other?	

Patient:
Date:

normal conversation as part of caring. Obviously questions that suggest judgement on care processes require sensitivity. Visitors may be especially reluctant to give negative feedback when still visiting (Nehring and Geach 1973). As such, questions are better designed as open questions rather than closed questions.

Standards Group

The standards group, as with all guided reflection structures, is a community of inquiry where practitioners come together to collaborate, reflect and dialogue towards improving practice.

The next standards meeting is scheduled for 3 pm – set to overlap the late shift. Potentially it is a quieter time of the day. I say potentially because anything could happen to shatter the quietness. The group meets for two hours every two months to review existing standards and develop new ones chaired by the standards of care facilitator. The off-duty has been planned to accommodate the group, but with staff trimmed to the bone you can feel the pressure.

The group's s eight members are all nursing staff. The meetings are sacrosanct, planned in advance to ensure attendance despite the strain on resources. Some things are too important to neglect, such as clinical practice development and quality of care. Approximately half the group will attend in their own time. Commitment is vital to quality. You must want it! We invite other professionals to join the group as relevant to the topic. For example, a standard of care concerning nutrition will necessarily involve catering staff.

In the spirit of the learning organisation, all practitioners are expected to be a 'standard-keeper'- to manage at least one standard of care around a topic of interest and become resource person for that topic. This includes setting up and maintaining a resource file and ensuring the standard is monitored.

Six staff arrived. As acting coordinator I report a complaint from Mrs James's daughter that she was not informed her mother was being transferred to a community hospital for rehabilitation. Mrs James had suffered a stroke two weeks previously. Her speech had been slightly affected but it seems she told her daughter she was being shoved out and that staff did not care for her. The daughter was angry. Unfortunately one of the staff nurses told her she was lucky her mother was getting this bed otherwise she would have to arrange a nursing home.

Modern matron's remit to the ward manager, 'sort it'. Hence the agenda today to write a standard on relatives.

Jo notes, 'This is not the first time communication has broken down between staff and relatives.'

Exploring the circumstances of this complaint we draft a potential standard statement – '*The family are satisfied with the patient's care.*'

What factors contribute to satisfaction? We brainstorm, using a flipchart and marker pens, ideas based on reflections of both personal and professional experiences. All of us have been 'family' at some time or another.

> Not being involved in decision making
> Being involved in 'hands on' care
> Visiting hours
> information
> Confidentiality

Trust
Not being listened to
Feeling like an outsider
Treated like a nuisance
Knowing who to speak to and who to avoid!
Anger at staff – WHY? All the above!!
Being approached
Sense that staff care about us.
Research?

(Robinson and Thorne's research) (Be proactive!)

We pose the question – 'what research might inform us?'

Rick mentions research by Robinson and Thorne (1986) – 'relatives as interference'.

In this study the researchers posit three positions relatives take with professionals; *Naïve Trusting*, *Disenchantment*, and *Guarded Alliance*. Naive Trusting is an attitude that staff will meet relative's needs. Disenchantment is realising that staff do not meet needs, leading to a breakdown in trust. Guarded Alliance is realising that to get some needs met requires some sort of relationship and tactic. We agree that Naïve Trusting is the ideal, that Disenchantment is unsatisfactory and that Guarded Alliance is probably the most realistic.

I say 'To maintain Naïve Trusting we need to be proactive rather than reactive', and write this on the flipchart.

Rick: 'I'll post this research in a new "Relatives" file within the library and review the literature and put more stuff in the file. In fact, I'll manage this standard if that's OK?'

We explore and connect the ideas strewn across the flip chart and construct a number of process criteria together with matching monitoring questions that can be unobtrusively slipped into dialogue between the practitioner and family member rather than use a formal questionnaire that demands the family's judgement [Box 20.3]. Two spotting [S] events were identified linked to 'concerned interaction' to reflect 'living quality'. The only structural criterion was open visiting times, which already existed. The standard statement is agreed as *'Relatives feel informed and involved in care.'*

When the standard was monitored, it revealed that relatives did generally feel involved prior to the standard being implemented and, although 'results' did not dramatically improve as a consequence, staff were now more proactive and sensitive to relatives, as revealed in handover dialogue.

Skill Box

- *Use the Relatives scan sheet to reflect on your own and collective care of relatives within your practice.*

Triggers for Standards

The standard on 'relatives' was a response to a complaint. Complaints must always be investigated and as such provide a rich learning opportunity. I scan Google for information on complaints. My click on 'patient complaints in NHS' reveals a recent report, *A Review of the NHS Hospitals Complaints System; Putting Patients Back in the Picture* [October 2013].

Box 20.3   Standard statement: 'Relatives feel informed and involved in care'

Relatives standard process scan sheet

The caring team inform the family who they are and how they can be contacted

Q – Do you know the caring team and how to contact them at any time?

The nurse on duty initiates a 'concerned interaction' with the family on each visit

Q - Do the nurses approach you when you visit and ask how things are or do you have to approach them?

S – Does this actually happen?

The nurse responds positively to the family's request for information and nurse informs the relative where she/he, for whatever reason, is unable to disclose information.

Q – Are you adequately informed about the patient's condition and progress?

The nurse is aware of how the family is thinking and feeling about the patient's care.

Q – Do you feel the nurses knew how you think and feel about [the patient's] care?

Q – To what extent are you consulted and listened to in making decisions?

The nurse has explored with the family their desired involvement with the patient's physical care and setting the limits of care-giving.

Q – To what extent do you feel welcomed and involved in caring for [the patient]

The nurse checks out that relatives are satisfied with care

Q – Overall, were your particular needs identified and met?

S – Do the notes reflect the relative's views and needs?

The report states: 'One of the most shocking failures in NHS care was documented on 6th February 2013 when Robert Francis QC published his Public Inquiry into Mid Staffordshire NHS Foundation Trust. He found 'a story of appalling and unnecessary suffering of hundreds of people.' He added:

> They were failed by a system which ignored the warning signs and put corporate self-interest and cost control ahead of patients and their safety. A health service that does not listen to complaints is unlikely to reflect its patients' needs. One that does will be more likely to detect the early warning signs that something requires correction, to address such issues and to protect others from harmful treatment. A complaints system that does not respond flexibly, promptly and effectively to the justifiable concerns of complainants not only allows unacceptable practice to persist, it aggravates the grievance and suffering of the patient and those associated with the complaint, and undermines the public's trust in the service.

This review was co-chaired by the Rt. Hon Ann Clwyd MP for the Cynon Valley and Professor Tricia Hart, Chief Executive, South Tees Hospitals NHS Foundation Trust. In a radio interview on BBC Radio 4's World at One in December 2012, Ann Clwyd described the way in which her husband, Owen Roberts, had died in the University Hospital of Wales. Ann Clwyd spoke of the 'coldness, resentment, indifference and contempt' of some of the nurses who were supposed to be caring for him. She broke down in tears as she recalled his last hours, shivering under flimsy sheets, with an ill-fitting oxygen mask cutting into his face, wedged up against the bars of the hospital bed. She said her husband, a former head of News and Current Affairs for BBC Wales, died *'like a battery hen.'*

Following this programme and others she received letters and emails from hundreds of people who were appalled at such a lapse in standards of basic decency and compassion. Many included accounts of other shocking examples of poor care and of the difficulty people encountered when trying to complain. The report noted that more than 2,500 testimonials were received from patients, their relatives, friends or carers. The majority describe problems with the quality of treatment or care in NHS hospitals.

Key points raised:

- Lack of information – patients said they felt uninformed about their care and treatment.
- Compassion – patients said they felt they had not been treated with the compassion they deserve.
- Dignity and care – patients said they felt neglected and not listened to.
- Staff attitudes – patients said they felt no one was in charge on the ward and the staff were too busy to care for them.
- Resources – patients said there was a lack of basic supplies like extra blankets and pillows.

It seems our complaint fits in with an acknowledged endemic problem within the NHS. It is certainly a salutary moment to read this report, reinforcing in my mind what I know already but had not really assimilated into my practice. It is so easy to blame relatives for being a nuisance or interference (Robinson and Thorne 1986). The above points offer a reflective framework for anyone writing a standard of care. The demanding patient can test the patience of a saint. But then, do we become sinners for being human?

Not all standards of care emanate from complaints, although clearly that is a powerful driving force to take action. A sleep standard emerged from a realisation that a patient preferred to sleep in an armchair than in bed but had not informed us. But then we hadn't asked how he slept at home. He hadn't wanted to be a nuisance [that word again] so hadn't told us. A nutrition standard emanated from observing a patient did not have a glass of water at hand at lunchtime.

Standards can be triggered by an article in a professional journal. For example, a standard on caring might be stimulated by a series of recent papers lamenting the loss of caring in nursing. In one paper Darbyshire and McKenna (2013) write:

> Unless the 'Crisis, what crisis?' dictum guides you, you cannot be oblivious to the seemingly endemic erosion of caring and compassion in nursing. This crisis has been long fermenting but came to a head with the UK revelations in the initial 2010 Francis Report and in the Patients' Association landmark report of 2009.

- All practitioners would purport to care and be compassionate. But are they? How would you make that judgement?

Confidentiality

One morning during bedside handover, I observed the night associate nurse and primary nurse communicate at the bedside of a lady in a three-bed ward. They stood at the foot of the bed as the night nurse informed the primary nurse. The primary nurse was a little deaf, and so the night associate nurse spoke loudly – loud enough for me to hear at the end of the ward and loud enough for the other two patients to hear what was being said. The woman in the bed was also deaf. She was sitting up trying to listen to what was being said. However, she was not involved in the discussion. Clearly the bedside protocol had failed [see Chapter 19] and confidentiality had been broken.

In response, I arranged a teaching session whereby each nurse was talked about in public as per the observed incident. The staff 's reaction was a revelation – they felt very uncomfortable. The standards group took this on board and constructed a standard of care – '*Patients do not have confidential information disclosed about them accidentally.*'

The crux of appreciating confidentiality is to determine the meaning of 'public space' as set out in the UKCC code of professional conduct on confidentiality (1987). Shared ward areas are public spaces, hence the nurse should not reveal things about the patient or family without the patient's permission if others might overhear. As such, any patients unwilling or unable to engage in the report, were not talked about at the bedside. The nurse would cue the patient to self-disclose, for example, 'How are things this morning?' encouraging participation. In this way it was the patient who would disclose information.

To monitor this standard, student nurses were asked to shadow the walk-round handover and feedback their observation using the scan sheet [Box 20.4]. As you might expect, such scrutiny of practice helped staff to become more mindful of patient involvement and confidentiality. It was also an excellent learning experience for students.

Box 20.4   Confidentiality scan sheet

Standard statement: '*Patients do not have confidential information disclosed accidentally*'
Date............................ Handover observed by...

		Score and comment Yes – 3; so-so – 2; No – 1
1	Patients are involved in the handover of their care	
2	Patients control the disclosure of information concerning themselves	
3	The nurses do not talk about the patient outside the patient's hearing	
4	No accidental breach of confidentiality takes place	
5	Patient's notes are not left open in a public space	
6	Ask each patient 'Do you think your nurses have always treated what they know about your health/illness in a confidential manner?' (Sinha and Scherera 1987)	

The Value of Standards of Care

Standards of care are a true quality assurance tool because they do not just monitor quality but seek to develop quality. In summary, standards of care offer practitioners/the organisation:

- A reflective and collaborative approach for developing specific aspects of clinical practice;
- A problem-solving and change-management model;
- A way of realising vision within practice;
- A resource management model – the focus on structure creates the opportunity to reflect on resources available and the way resources are utilised;
- A means for practitioners to demonstrate professional accountability;
- A proactive response to the quality agenda;
- A reflective way to live quality as part of everyday practice.

In Box 20.5 I set out a checklist for writing a standard of care. The last point is rather hopeful because although practitioners are positive about quality as an ideal, in practice they struggle to accommodate this approach with issues of owning quality, time and technique. It sounds easy, but in practice standards are a difficult concept to implement because they may be difficult to write and monitor because of resources.

In Box 20.6 I set out key points in writing a standard of care.

Box 20.5   Checklist for writing standards

- Reflects agreement by all practitioners/ workers involved in meeting the standard statement.
- Reflects patient/ client's rights and needs.
- Reflects optimum quality – i.e., the tension between what is desirable and what is achievable [within resources] [but always have a creative edge].
- Reflects organisational outcomes.
- Reflects professional values and ethics.
- Reflects relevant theory and research.
- Establish a resource file and standard's manager.
- Monitoring strategy designed and review date set [agenda for standards group].
- Avoidance of ambiguous statements or unnecessary jargon.
- Has identified pragmatic monitoring tools [usually observation or questions to ask] and set monitoring schedule and review dates [this will be tentative in the first instance].
- Subsumes relevant policies.
- Has converted process criteria into protocols or care pathways for 'best practice'.

Box 20.6   Key points in developing a standard of care

1 Identify an appropriate topic for writing a standard of care; for example 'patients are comfortable with their pain' – this topic may be a reflection of a current issue or part of a comprehensive list of standards that need to be developed, for example to respond to the National Care Standards Commission's core and specialist standards of care.
2 Write the topic in the centre of a flipchart.
3 Engage the group to brainstorm ideas that relate to this aspect of practice and cluster on the flipchart.
4 Accept all contributions non-judgementally.

5 After approximately ten minutes discuss each brainstormed ideas, led by initiator.
6 Reflect on the experiences of patients around the brainstormed ideas – grounding the activity in actual practice rather than as an abstract idea.
7 Consider all relevant sources of knowledge that might inform the standard [theory, research, policy, etc.] – this will almost certainly require a literature search and review at a later date.
8 Draw relationships between the brainstormed ideas.
9 Reformulate ideas as structure/ process and outcome criteria.
10 Write the definitive standard statement.
11 Design monitoring plan.

Endnote

1   See Department of Health (2007).

References

Darbyshire, P. and McKenna, L. (2013) Nursing's crisis of care: what part does nursing education own? *Nurse Education Today* 33.4, 305–307.

Department of Health (2007) *Maternity matters: choice, access and continuity of care in a safe service*. HMSO, London.

Kitson, A. (1989) *A framework for quality: a patient-centred approach to quality assurance in health care*. Scutari Press, Middlesex.

Nehring, V. and Geach, B. (1973) Why they don't complain: patient's evaluation of their care. *Nursing Outlook* 21.5, 317–321.

Read, S. (1983) Once is enough: causal reasoning from a single instance. *Journal of Personality and Social Psychology* 45.2, 323–334.

Robinson, S. and Thorne, S. (1986) Relatives as interference. *Journal of Advanced Nursing* 9, 597–602.

Chapter 21

Trudy

Christopher Johns

Insights shift the way we perceive and respond to practice

Trudy Smith is a district nurse. She shared her experience of working with Catherine and Gary in guided reflection with me over six consecutive clinical supervision sessions.[1] The narrative illustrates the idea of reflexivity- how insights from one session feed the next session, and how insights create dilemmas as how best to act. The text also illuminates Trudy's growth as a reflective practitioner and how she becomes more aware and sensitive to her practice.

Session 1

Trudy read from her reflective diary:

Catherine is a 47-year-old woman with cancer in her bowel and peritoneal secondaries. She has a colostomy. Her husband called the clinic at 17.45 requesting me to visit. The message was 'wife unwell/ colostomy blocked?' It was taken by another nurse. My dilemma was – do I visit now or do I refer to the evening nurse? I left it to the evening nurse. I rationalised this by thinking that it would be good for her to make Catherine's acquaintance. On my way home I pass nearby this family's house. I was feeling guilty that I had not responded personally, so I popped in. The curtains were drawn upstairs. Catherine was blind, confused, she had 'gone off her legs'. She was lying in the bathroom. I helped to move her onto the bed and she then commenced fitting. Her two sons who were present could not cope with this. They fled. Her husband was shocked. She was fitting for about 15–20 minutes. I called the General practitioner [GP], who suggested I made a 999 emergency call. I resisted this; I was asking myself – 'Do I want her to go to hospital?' I didn't know the preference of the family about managing Catherine's deterioration and eventual death. This had not become a topic of conversation. The GP arrived and gave Catherine some IV valium which worked, although she continued to fit intermittently. Her husband decided on private hospital admission – we had to wait two hours for an ambulance to arrive. I stayed with her during this time. Catherine fitted again on the stretcher going into the ambulance. I felt bad because I hadn't spoken to the boys – was my decision to refer to the night nurse the best decision? I felt I didn't have the full facts of the situation and didn't know the situation well enough to make a good judgement.

Becoming a Reflective Practitioner, Fifth Edition. Edited by Christopher Johns.
© 2017 John Wiley & Sons Ltd. Published 2017 by John Wiley & Sons Ltd.
Companion Website: www.wiley.com/go/johns/reflectivepractitioner

CJ: 'Could you have rung the husband back to explore what was meant by "unwell"?'
TS: '*Yes, I should have done that as Catherine usually managed her colostomy well.*'
I pick up on Trudy's comment about eventual death and asked about her relationship with the family and talking about Catherine's impending death.
TS: '*I have known Catherine for seven months, she knows her condition is terminal.*'
CJ: 'Are you avoiding talking about this situation with the family?'
TS: '*That may be partly true … I need to manage hope and doubt whether I should confront Gary's denial at this time. He is uncomfortable talking about these issues and for these reasons I haven't pushed it. I'm sensitive about a right time to discuss Catherine's death and that right time hasn't presented itself yet … however I do feel this event marks a crisis within Catherine's illness trajectory … I will explore the meaning of this with Gary and discuss the different options for managing the situation when I visit him on Friday.*'
CJ: 'Trudy, do you avoid discussion with Gary and Catherine because it makes you feel uncomfortable?'
TS squirms slightly: '*My relationship is largely with Catherine. Gary has always seemed on the margins, seemingly uncomfortable with the emotional issues and focusing more on managing the physical. As a result I don't know him very well. I blame myself for referring to the evening nurse when I know I should have made the decision to visit myself.*'
CJ: 'Maybe with hindsight we punish ourselves yet maybe at the time that was a reasonable decision. You couldn't have envisaged the way the situation unfolded.'
TS: '*Yes but did I want her at home for my own needs because I would prefer that?*'
CJ: 'If that was true, what would it say? …
       TS is silent.
CJ: 'I sense that Gary and Catherine had different and potentially conflicting needs?'
TS: '*Catherine's needs good symptomatic control right now but in a private hospital? I'm left with a sense that Gary just wants her out of the way.*'
CJ: 'Taking Gary's perspective, perhaps he can't cope with what's happening with Catherine right now?'
TS: 'Yes that's likely …'
As it was nearing the end of our session I asked Trudy 'What has been significant about sharing this experience?'
TS: '*Recognising that my guilt is a reflection of the caring trap[2] … thinking I should be there for my patients at all times. I seem to get entangled in these types of relationships. And secondly, my sense of unease with Gary that goes against my belief of responding to the whole family.*'

Session 2

Twenty days later Trudy and I meet again. She shares her experience of visiting Gary.

He said Catherine couldn't possibly come home as she had a catheter, a syringe driver … a stream of problems. I struggled to respond positively to him. I needed to assess Catherine for myself so I phoned the hospital. They were reluctant to give me any information but they said it was okay to visit. Catherine looked really well. If she had been at a NHS hospital they would have discharged her days ago. She had no memory of fitting. She was no longer fitting but had massive oedema of her abdomen and legs. I was questioning her treatment with the staff. She was not on any steroids. I thought the staff had a very limited understanding of Catherine's drugs; for example- they thought 'nozinam' in the syringe driver was for the epilepsy [in fact a broad-spectrum anti-emetic]. It was making Catherine sleepy. Catherine said she wanted to go home. She said this in front of Gary when he arrived. I sensed the conflict between them.

CJ:　'Could you have responded in other ways?'

TS:　*'I'm unsure.... perhaps ask the GP to speak with the hospital doctors?'*

CJ:　'I sense your anxiety that Catherine's desire to come home should be respected. Look at Gary's perspective and ask yourself whose needs are we responding to? Do you understand and respond to Gary on his emotional level or your own? Can he cope with Catherine's illness? Perhaps his difficulty with coping and emotional distress explains why arranging a support package to support Catherine at home was not enough to persuade him to have her home?'
Trudy is uncomfortable. I sense my challenge has Trudy slightly on her back foot.
TS *'I feel the hospital is colluding with Gary in terms of his own needs rather than Catherine's – as if Catherine had become some object to talk about and do things with.'*
We explore Trudy's options and potential consequences. One option was to involve Clare, the Macmillan nurse, more actively in Catherine's care. It felt like bringing in reinforcements to battle Gary.

CJ:　'Do you want Clare to confront Gary?'

TS:　*'Clare doesn't know the family well whereas I do. I don't know how Catherine would feel if Clare came in.'*

CJ:　'What you're really saying is that you don't know how you will feel if Clare comes in – will you feel pushed out? Is that your fear? Is it time to confront Gary with the conflict of needs on an emotional level? Could you do that is you felt it appropriate?'

TS:　*'Say more.'*

CJ:　'For example, 'I can see this is tough for you Gary.' He might be feeling guilty about not having his wife at home, so such a response might help him face his guilt? It is not merely a stark choice of either hospital or home to die but to take each day as it comes, to leave the doors open. The cathartic response would make it easier to confront Gary – 'What does Catherine want?' 'Should you respect her wishes?'

TS:　*'If she came home she could always go back into hospital or the hospice if things deteriorate badly. I haven't really talked with him. I feel concerned that I should be manipulating him toward my views. I accept my sympathies and interests have lain primarily with Catherine.'*

CJ:　'I sense a major issue for Catherine is being in control of her own dying, ensuring that those she leaves behind can cope without her. Issues about her two sons and why she needs to be at home.'

TS nods:　*'This session helped me to see things differently, most notably paying attention to Gary's needs and how this is central to getting Catherine home. It has influenced my future actions and helped me anticipate what Gary may be thinking. I will arrange to meet him again! Thank you.'*

Session 3

Forty-one days later, Trudy picked up the threads of her unfolding experience with Catherine and Gary:

> *I did visit and confront him with the prospect of Catherine coming home. He was uptight. He said 'I know I am being selfish but I've got a life to lead, and the boys as well. If Catherine is coming home then someone has to be here all the time.' He was adamant and said that he had to return imminently to work in Indonesia. I didn't pursue it because I could see it was making him more uptight. I contacted the hospital. They said Catherine could be kept on insurance funding because she had a syringe driver which counted as treatment. I offered to look after her if she came home. But after that I didn't hear from them or Gary. I became despondent about it. Then, this week, she was sent home for the day. Gary informed me and I went to visit her. She was downstairs sitting at the kitchen table. She looked well. No syringe driver, no catheter. She was eating and drinking. Walking up and down stairs. Her legs were less swollen although her ascites remained and made her look nine months pregnant. She said 'I feel really well'. Gary interceded 'You're not well, are you?' He was challenging what she could do, getting up and down stairs. I asked her when she was coming home. She said she was working on it, pulling a face at Gary. He said that she was not ready to come home. I asked her what I could do to help when she did come home. And today I heard she is coming home on Thursday ... a phone message from Gary. The insurance funding has dried up. He has got to come to terms with it now she's returning home. I have arranged a package of care for her. She's really determined. She said that she had forced herself to eat to make herself better. There was no explanation for the epilepsy. They didn't do a brain scan and she isn't on any epileptic drugs. Perhaps it was a reaction from the nozinam? She was on dexamethasone but now there is friction between them about coming home.*

CJ: 'Trudy, how do you feel about your involvement with Catherine?'

Trudy looks me in the eye: *'I know it's going to be tough when Catherine eventually dies. Gary's comments are off-putting for Catherine. I know I need to be supportive toward Gary rather than confronting him with his persistent negative attitude because he may be feeling guilty about not wanting her home. I do feel more in tune with Gary ... sense how he's feeling more easily, and hence more available to him. After I last saw him, I let it go. I feel guilty about that. I saw him in the shops and I went off the other way rather than face him. I began to feel awkward pushing it for her. Often at home I would think how she was. I couldn't understand why they had kept the syringe driver going. Her body is covered with abscess sites from the driver – they had to change the site every day. She's on MST now ... I can see how I have been drawn into an emotional web, entangled and pulled between them. Talking it through with you I am less entangled ... I feel it differently now.'*

CJ: 'That's a good image- visualise yourself in this web and pull yourself out. Here, let me help you ...'
      I pull on an imaginary rope, pulling her free. Trudy laughs. I help Trudy frame her involvement with Catherine and Gary using the nurse–patient involvement theory of Morse[3] and Ramos.[4] Trudy identified with the Morse 'type' of 'over-involvement' – *'Yes, I've been there!'*

CJ: 'We all need to experience emotional entanglement, because only then can we recognise the place. Perhaps entanglement is an inevitable consequence of a holistic relationship because it's so hard to resist the suffering of the other. It is like a tidal wave that we must learn to surf and control yet without relinquishing its exquisite intimacy and beauty. It's okay to be vulnerable but like the expert surfer we can learn to ride it. Maybe we do get swept away sometimes but that's just another experience to learn from. That's where reflection can help us.'

TS: 'It shows how unprepared we are for emotional work and then suddenly I find myself in an emotional quagmire. Seeing the best way forward is blurred by feelings. That's so insightful.'

Session 4

Thirty days later. Trudy is late: '*Sorry … I've been to a funeral and then an urgent visit.*'

CJ: 'Not Catherine's funeral?'

TS: '*No! She's up and well. I'm seeing her twice a week. She's been having some difficulty with her son. He has problems with drugs and also a recent court appearance because of stealing.*'

Picking up the cue I inquire: 'Have you helped the sons talk about what's happening to their mother?'

TS: '*No. Gary has not returned to Indonesia yet. He's saying he has got to go next month but he's also said that someone needs to be with Catherine the whole time.*'

CJ: 'Is this necessary?'

TS: '*I don't think so, at least not 24 hours a day because if someone has 24-hour care she can't live a normal life, can she?*'

CJ: 'If you're waiting to die, can you live a "normal life"?'

TS: '*Well, she struggles to do the housework but she can wash and dress herself, etc.*'

CJ: 'You're responding to her in terms of things she can physically do, what about her responses on an emotional level? Is she coping on this level?'

TS: '*She doesn't seem want to talk on this level although she does give cues such as "living on borrowed time" … It's difficult to talk to her because her husband and sons are often there and they don't want to talk about it.*'

CJ: 'Maybe they don't know how to talk about it?'

TS: '*I have another Catherine, who is also dying yet very open to what was happening to her … she needs to resolve issues such as who was going to look after her five-year-old son. Of course, how people feel and what they think about their impending death can never be predicted. The wavelength becomes a roller-coaster!*'

CJ: 'Perhaps Catherine is ambivalent? As you said, she is not in denial. She accepts she is going to die but she also needs to cope and protect her boys. Perhaps she is trying to be brave? Imagine yourself in her shoes – what sort of things would you need to be doing?'

TS: '*Well, sort out my children, put my house in order.*'

CJ: 'Do you remember the message from "Final Gifts"?[5] That the primary task for the dying person was to ensure that those they left behind were able to cope?'

TS: '*I do, that was very powerful … The other Catherine is "coming to terms" … even things like changing internal doors in the house, things that she had wanted to do. She is now quite peaceful with everything sorted out.*'

Pursuing the point, I suggest: 'Perhaps we can see that Catherine is trying to cope with chaos. Perhaps she does need confronting in order to help her sort things out? Perhaps you are avoiding this for your discomfort and uncertainty about her ambivalence?'

TS: *'I accept your point … I just don't feel with this family that they are ready to talk about it. I don't feel her physical deterioration has become that marked where her dying has really become an issue. They are a "difficult" family, I have a number of people who are dying where talking about death is not a problem.'*

I take Trudy back to the beginning of the session: 'All this came out of me asking – Was it Catherine's funeral'!'

Trudy laughs, and then, seriously: *'We have had a lot of people dying – nine recently. It's stressful. It doesn't help having conflict with the doctors. One particular situation over drug dosage made me fume. The doctor wasn't listening to me. I didn't back down and asserted my point of view. She was short with me but she didn't bawl me out of the office.'*

CJ: 'The intimidating factor – *being short*.'

Trudy laughed: *'Some patients have commented on her manner – her New Year's resolution is to be less short!'*

CJ: 'It's promising, she has insight! Maybe she's changing. It doesn't help when work is tough to have oppressive relationships within the team. Last session I challenged you to consider the balance of being challenging and being supportive with Gary and Catherine?'

TS: *'My stance towards Gary has changed. I now see their relationship differently. I see that maybe he couldn't go to Indonesia because he couldn't leave Catherine at home and that being with her was an emotional rather than a physical thing. Could he focus on work knowing she was as she was?'*

Session 5

Twenty-one days later. Trudy says: *'Gary is letting me in now and that I'm responding to my intuition that it's now the right time to talk about dying. Catherine's in the terminal stage of her illness … I went in following a phone call from Catherine that her colostomy was obstructed. Up to this time I had been going in twice weekly. She had been self-caring so I went in to discuss what had been happening to her. On this visit she was in bed. She said she had great abdominal pain. I sought the GP's advice. The GP had prescribed a suppository but this hadn't worked and had since prescribed 'normacol'. Because of the pain I advised Catherine not to take this. I also referred her to the night nurse so she could get help if she needed it.'*

CJ: 'What treatment do you think might be best?'

After considering palliative approaches to Catherine's bowel obstruction Trudy says: *'Gary was downstairs during this visit. I had informed him that the colostomy was obstructed and that this was a sign of things worsening and hr imminent death. Gary said it wasn't fair to keep her alive. Why were we giving her all these drugs? That we needed to put an end to all this! I asked him if Catherine was talking about dying? He said that he wanted to look after her at home and not to go back into hospital. I thought he might be strapped for cash but he assured me that wasn't the reason. She didn't want to go back in and he had accepted that. The elder son didn't want to stray too far in case anything happened to mum. No talk of the younger son, he was still having his troubles. I'm now visiting every day.'*

CJ: 'Trudy why are *you* visiting every day?'

TS: '*Because my enrolled nurse is no good at counselling. She "whips in and out". Both Catherine and Gary made this observation. She's a good nurse but prefers going in and doing something physical. I need to monitor the colostomy and to respond to her symptoms on a daily basis and to help the family through the crisis.*'

CJ: 'Being there for them?'

TS: '*Yes, that's right. I had two other patients who were similar to Catherine with obstructed colostomies. One lived for three months after it had become blocked. She would vomit every day. In the end – faecal matter, not very pleasant. I have told them about such possibility. Catherine is struggling to eat just a little. She has requested some 'HiCal' drinks to keep her strength up ... I can tell by the look she gives me that she knows she has deteriorated, but she doesn't want to talk about that. She feels the lumps in her tummy ... still hoping the tumour will still go away.*'

CJ: 'It must be hard for you to see her suffer like that, her grief all bottled up inside it ... when you know it would help her to share it with you?'

It was a poignant moment to dwell in that truth, in silence for a moment. I broke the spell by challenging Trudy over her team leader responsibilities: 'What do you need to do when you know that members of your team are not responding appropriately?'

TS: '*I find it hard to tackle such issues because I don't like conflict even when I know it compromises patient care ... I want to talk more about Gary? Gary is out of control, feeling helpless, very anxious and angry. He tested out the night nurse to gauge her response – which was okay! This is going to be tough, especially when she becomes more physically dependent, vomiting, etc. I feel OK, not over-involved. I feel happy because Catherine is quite happy. Things are under control. I enjoy visiting them. Before I wasn't in control.*'

Session 6

Forty-six days later, Trudy noted how busy she was and the pressure she felt under just now. She picked up Catherine: '*Catherine.. her death. She was fighting to the end. She was on a massive dose of diamorphine – 500mg. in her syringe driver. She had another massive fit. I'll read from my diary – "I visited Catherine Monday morning early; the Marie Curie nurse had rung me to say that Catherine had a very restless night and was not responding to oral commands and there was a steady trickle of black fluid running from her mouth. I decided to assess the situation and rang the GP from Catherine's house. As I entered the bedroom I was shocked by what I saw. Catherine was groaning and rolling around the bed. Gary was trying to hold her onto the bed. She rolled from side to side, legs hanging over the edge of the bed, her catheter tube kinked and twisted around her leg, her tubing from the syringe driver had become detached. Clearly Gary was distressed. Catherine lay across the bed, her huge abdomen hard and contracting, her swollen legs looked heavy and shiny, her face, arms, and shoulders so thin that you see her bones protruding. I sat on the bed, reconnecting the syringe driver and checked the light was flashing. Gently I talked to Catherine, holding her hand. She was calm for a minute, and then she began to groan again, vomited and started to fit. Gary and I rolled Catherine onto her side in the recovery position. I called the GP to come straight away and rang the clinic, asking* the reception staff to bleep my nursing auxiliary and ask her to come to Catherine's house urgently. While we waited Gary and I talked; I admitted to Gary that I had never witnessed anything like this before in all my nursing experience.

Catherine's strength was amazing, on occasions rolling onto to her enlarged abdomen. All kinds of emotions were spinning through my head. I felt sad for Gary witnessing this, Catherine's loss of dignity- what an awful death and I was helpless to do anything. I had no valium to stop the fit and no injection available to calm Catherine. I spoke to Gary and said the only good thing about this was that Catherine doesn't know what's going on. The GP arrived – he was visibly shocked and passed me a valium enema which I inserted into Catherine's colostomy. Within a few minutes Catherine was calm. I asked the GP for another in case she fitted again and asked him if he had any midazolam 20 mg. that I could use to sedate Catherine as she was very agitated and restless. He wrote the medication and Stuart, Gary's son went to collect the prescription. Ann, my nursing auxiliary arrived, and we washed Catherine, talking gently to her, comforting her, cleansed her mouth and put a clean nightie on and clean sheets. By this time Stuart had returned and I could give the midazolam intramuscularly into her thigh. Within ten minutes she was asleep. Gary, Ann and I sat around the bed emotionally drained just looking at Catherine. I knew I could not leave Gary alone. The situation was frightening for him. Gary thanked us both and felt reassured that he was not going to be left alone. He was happier that she was asleep."'

Trudy puts her diary aside and asks herself: 'What was I trying to achieve? My main concern was for Gary who was visibly distressed. Catherine would have been horrified if she could see herself, nightie up around her breasts, legs and bottom exposed, rolling around her bed, groaning, complete loss of dignity. Gary was distraught, unable to restrain her almost falling out of bed. I was frustrated that there were no drugs prescribed that I could have given. When Catherine was asleep and calm, Gary could manage. He rarely touched Catherine – he always stood at the foot of the bed or sat in a chair. I never saw him and hold her hand although he always talked fondly of her. I came to the conclusion that he was afraid and it would be less stressful for him if Ann assisted me in all nursing duties. I've learnt so much from this but I never did get to grips with Gary. I said to him – 'It won't be long' and queried whether he wanted her family present. He said that they can come at any time but he didn't want them staying. He said –'I don't think of her death, I think of the future.' He never shed a tear. I went to the funeral. Her father was heartbroken as his wife had died of cancer as well.'

I acknowledged Trudy's feelings: 'This must have been very traumatic for you… you moved a long way to accommodate Gary within your sphere of care.'

TS: 'That's been my real learning – to see and respond to the whole family. It's true, I do normally identify with the woman in the situation, which often leaves me feeling angry at the spouses, as with Gary, because he seemed to interfere with helping me to help Catherine meet her needs.'

Skill Box

- Reflect on the value of writing and reading rich description in contrast with your own reflective writing.
- What are the strengths and weaknesses of the guide's responses to Trudy?
- How could the weaknesses be strengthened?
- Would Trudy have benefitted more from group guided reflection?
- How do you relate to Trudy's experience in terms of your own experiences?
- What insights do you draw?

- *Does such narrative have value for teaching others? In what way?*
- *In your next reflection, reflect on your use of catharsis- link this with five subsequent experiences to construct a narrative that focuses on using catharsis and emotional care. [Remind yourself of Six Category Intervention Analysis – see Chapter 5].*

Summary

My narrative of guiding Trudy illuminates reflexivity, the way one experience builds on another in such a way that enables Trudy and myself to 'look back' and see the pattern of her experience evolving through insights. It is not necessary to 'tell' these insights. They lie thick within the narrative and can be discerned by the reader alongside other insights that the reader may draw.

Endnotes

1 Trudy was undertaking the Becoming a Reflective and Effective Practitioner module – a 60-credit degree level as part of her BSc Nursing. Usually this module is delivered within the university but I was experimenting with its delivery in clinical practice.

2 I had previously given Trudy Ann Dickson's book *A woman in your own right*. The book describes the 'compassion trap' as when the practitioner gets trapped by her caring ethic. Dickson, A. (1982) *A woman in your own right*. Quartet, London.

3 Morse, J. (1991) Negotiating commitment and involvement in the nurse–patient relationship. *Journal of Advanced Nursing* 16, 552–558.

4 Ramos, M. (1992) The nurse–patient relationship: themes and variations. *Journal of Advanced Nursing* 17, 496–506.

5 Callanan, M. & Kelley, P. (1992) *Final gifts: understanding the special awareness, needs and communication of the dying*. Bantam Books, New York.

Chapter 22

Reflective Leadership

Gerald Remy

Effective leaders are mindful of living their vision

In the Beginning

Growing up in a London ghetto evokes feelings within to become a leader and triumph in adversity. I had no desire to be subordinate, so from a young age I imagined what it would be like to rule. I confess, some of my thoughts were devious, but I was a product of my surroundings, where anger, danger, despair and desolation embraced. In my ghetto, black leaders were charismatic, with physical presence and an appetite for preying on the weak and vulnerable. The street code was to control through force in the most visible way possible, as a demonstration of power and showmanship. Sociologists speak of this balance of power and it seems that all relationships have degrees of power, and its relative strength can be an aspect of one's social structure. McCornack (2009: 291) rightly suggest that to possess power one must have a type of power currency; the power currency in my society was physical strength, ruthlessness and economic prowess. I grew up in an environment that echoed, 'What can we get?' not 'What can we give?' Where leaders were feared.

However, I was raised in a religious family and though my parents instilled values of humility, forgiveness and love, I soon grew a stranger to these values, and was in this respect a carbon copy of my role model leaders. I not only found myself quite forgiving of their ruthlessness, but relished their habits, their manners and their spirit. I took every occasion to improve myself in their customs and got up to no good six days a week, and on bended knees prayed for forgiveness and took mass on one day a week.

My autobiographical experience and cultural accounting has influenced my thoughts around leadership in the past and as it stands now. Bochner and Ellis (2006) inform me that this accounting helps people to figure out what to do and how to do it. In childhood I saw leadership as coercive and acted it out as a Philistine, using my alter ego, Goliath. French and Raven (1968) identify coercive power and illuminate how this power currency allows leaders to force people to do things they don't want to do. I was comfortable with this currency in my neighbourhood, an inner city ghetto as described by Bryant (2009), where you will often find a liquor store right next to a pawnbroker, next to a betting office. The people are not sceptical, they are cynical: they have low self-esteem and negative

Becoming a Reflective Practitioner, Fifth Edition. Edited by Christopher Johns.
© 2017 John Wiley & Sons Ltd. Published 2017 by John Wiley & Sons Ltd.
Companion Website: www.wiley.com/go/johns/reflectivepractitioner

leaders; their get-up-and-go has got up and gone. So they go to the pawnbroker to forfeit their today, they go to the betting office to forfeit their tomorrow, and they go to the liquor store to forfeit their yesterday, and every day is a battle to hold onto a fragment of coercive power.

I left school with no qualifications and considered my teachers imposters who saw my kind as an underprivileged class who were on honeymoon, having escaped the hardship of slavery which my ancestors had endured. There were no black, positive leaders in England to identify with, and Margaret Thatcher was prime minister, someone who showed little empathy for the lower classes and led with an iron fist. With no prospects, no skills, and feelings of alienation, I felt that I belonged to a degraded caste. My colour was a symbol of oppression and associated with malfunction, and I had to look to America for black role models such as Martin Luther King and Malcolm X, who both had an emancipating imperative. Even now as I reflect, I am embarrassed to confess my inner thoughts, it seemed that the prophecy of the colonial masters was being fulfilled as outlined in Macleod (1974: 97), 'Negroes are degraded by nature, and when free are blacks still. They are Negroes in spite of freedom. They are poor and spiritless, because, though free, they are black. They constitute, and know, and feel that they constitute an inferior and degraded caste.'

My idea of leadership as a young man ought to be understood as my world view – the sum of my interest and sensibilities, past and present. An essential function of this ideology was to present myself as strong and physical to those around me, to portray power that was sufficiently inflexible, and obvious, to convince my subordinates of the merits of my leadership. This was a reflection of immediate self-interest, I had no soft edges, if I'd had such it would have been worse than useless, for if I yielded, it would quickly become apparent that I was human. This is why I likened myself to Goliath.

> Now the Philistines gathered together their armies to battle, and were gathered together at …Judah.
>
> And there went out a champion out of the camp of the Philistines, named Goliath, of Gath, whose height was six cubits and a span.
>
> And he had an helmet of brass upon his head, and he was armed with a coat of mail; and the weight of the coat was five thousand shekels of brass.
>
> And he had greaves of brass upon his legs, and a target of brass between his shoulders.
>
> And the staff of his spear was like a weaver's beam; and his spear's head weighed six hundred shekels of iron …
>
> And he stood and cried unto the armies of Israel, and said unto them, Why are ye come out to set your battle in array?
> (I Samuel 17:1, 4-8)

Was I not a Philistine!

Can you imagine the dilemma I was confronted with on my first lecture on the MSc course on leadership in healthcare, when the programme leader tasked the group to write a leadership vision statement that we found desirable. I was quite content with Goliath, and desired his many traits, but I didn't want to confess this. Wheatley (1999: 20) suggests that we survive only as we learn. On that basis most of us are zombies, because we only share our nice self and resist sharing our dark self. I was ill-prepared to share my love of Goliath so did not engage in genuine participative openness, and failed to speak out. I convinced myself that we are all different and after the course will all go our separate ways and turn back to what we know. I now accept the explicit assumption that the way to accelerate our learning is by sharing our implicit views and that in early lectures I avoided reflexive openness. Senge (1990: 227) describes reflexive openness, as 'the willingness to challenge our own thinking, to recognize that any certainty we ever have is, at best, a hypothesis about the world and is always subject to test and improvement'.

I had never come across the term transformational leadership; all my childhood leaders were clearly transactional and seductively so, I even had a secret admiration for Margaret Thatcher, who transmitted fear and cold-bloodedness. Tension brewed within me: would I reveal my Philistine complex, or play it safe? However, in considering transformational leadership, I liked what Burns (1978) had to say – that the transformational leader engages with others in such a way that leaders and followers raise one another to higher levels of motivation and morality. I also liked what Johns (2009: 224) wrote, 'leadership is being authentic, vulnerable, present, humble and available to others, yet it is also being tough, focussed and challenging'.

Assuming that Burns and Johns were right I decided to test their assumptions and guarded my alter ego Goliath, but during my investigation of a transformational leader I began to find meaning.

Adapting Wheatley's words (1999: 25), What if we could reframe the search? What if we stopped looking for control and began, in earnest, the search for meaning? Meaning we will find in places we never thought to look before – all around us in nature's living, dynamic systems. In fact, once we begin to look with new eyes, teachers are everywhere.

I held onto the creative tension between the vision of myself as Goliath and a new vision of myself as a transformational leader throughout the MSc course. The more I researched leadership, the more I became convinced that coercive power is born from a sense of powerlessness and the desire to feel important. There is a deep sensibility within all of us to belong to something and find meaning for our lives – who are we? why are we here? and what is our purpose? The more I considered leadership the more comfortable I became with the concept of a servant leader, as characterised by Greenleaf's (2002: 50) thoughts, in that we all seek some sort of healing from a fractured past, and there is something implicit in the compact between servant and leader for they both share and search for wholeness. Leading by power became a thing of distortion to me, and the MSc course challenged me to move out of spaces that restricted me. In all probability throughout my life I replaced love with domination and now the journey was to claw it back. In this emancipation of self, I was confronted with a statement from Beck, cited by Johns (2009: 57): 'For a time our life may feel worse than before, as what we have concealed becomes clear.' How could I liberate a team of people as a leader, if I did not liberate myself first?

In view of this, I decided to be courageous. I was really left with no choice but to reveal Goliath and pitch that great Philistine against David, the shepherd boy who destroyed him. In retrospect, I didn't truly realise what I was doing when I used the biblical theme of David and Goliath, but now, as I consider it, I realise I was holding creative tension, I was pitching myself against myself, I was weighing up the Goliath within against the David within, my transactional side against my transformational side. The quest was to test the merits of both. This allowed me to review my patterns of thinking, enabling me to lift the mundane into something more significant. I did stumble, but this is a necessary experience connected with learning, and made me more available to myself, and centred me for reflection.

While David was a shepherd boy he tended his father's sheep and endured many trials in the trenches in an attempt to protect his animals. One could argue that these earlier experiences of warding off lions and bears placed him in a good position to be fearless and have faith in his ability to defend and protect. David clearly saw himself as a servant first, and it has been said that people freely respond to individuals who are chosen as leaders because they have been proven as trusted servants (Greenleaf 2002: 24). An emerging leader must also endure the trenches and rely on past experiences of courage and failure to prepare for what is to come.

My past experiences had given me a desire to lead and I felt especially favoured to be chosen as a manager. I had pleased my superiors up the chain and was more than happy to bear their armour. As I scaled the ranks of the hospital hierarchy, I flirted with the transactional world. I was maintaining the power equilibrium, but I should have known better. Wheatley (1999: 108) urges managers to be equilibrium-busters, no longer the caretakers of control, but to stir things up. However, Instead of exposing the transactional nature of the organisation to provoke positive change, I provoked my staff instead. I had a tendency to respond badly to situations of criticism – with conflict, which I attributed to my Goliath complex. Like a Philistine, I defied those that rose up against me, and preferred to fight rather than sit down in dialogue. Coser (1956: 151–156) proposes that conflicts are a normal and inevitable consequence of all organisational life, but while Coser may be right, if Goliath is involved, it leads to personal, interpersonal and organisational disaster. Kelly (1970: 151–156) and Litterer (1966: 178–186) contend that conflict should be completely purged from the organisational setting, and while Kelly and Litterer's imperative may be overly ambitious I began an attempt to reverse conflict energy, or at least reduce the negative drain, to turn conflict energy towards a positive enterprise both for myself and the staff I managed and whom I wished to lead. But at every opportunity when I relieved myself of patience, courage and persistence, Goliath's ancestors would whisper in my ear,

> And he stood and cried unto the armies of Israel, and said unto them, Why are ye come out to set your battle in array? am not I a Philistine, and ye servants to Saul? choose you a man for you, and let him come down to me.
>
> If he be able to fight with me, and to kill me, then will we be your servants: but if I prevail against him, and kill him, then shall ye be our servants, and serve us.
>
> And the Philistine said, I defy the armies of Israel this day; give me a man, that we may fight together.
> (I Samuel 17: 8-10)

I had to become a harpist and learn to become one with the harp and the motion of a transformational world. The biblical story tells us that whenever an evil spirit came on King Saul, David would take up his harp and play. Then relief would come to Saul; he would feel better, and the evil spirit would leave him (I Samuel 16: 23). I had to lift this evil spirit that hovered over the transactional organisation and over me, but before I could achieve this I had to tune my harp, expel my frustration and create a psalm:

My leadership despair

When I am transactional my mouth is like an open tomb
Where only death and desolation reside.
When I am transformational I begin to breathe
I begin to know and am poised to lead.
When I am transactional, I say to myself 'Oh wretched man that thou art';
When I am transformational I can slay dragons.
When I am transactional the invisible world is hidden from me;
When I am transformational the seamless fabric of possibilities comes into existence.

If being transformational is so emancipating
Why then am I still polluted with the dark seduction of the transactional world?
It might be to do with my childhood?
It might be to do with my ego?

And the illusion of being all-powerful and all knowing.
But, if I continue to nourish my ego
My tower of Babel will come tumbling down.
So I owe it to myself to free myself
And embrace the idea of humility to release humanity
So I can glide motionless towards the envisioned land.

Using David and Goliath to hold creative tension was risky, as some could view this metaphor as nonsense. I willingly offered up this dilemma for the reader and put my neck on line because without risk there is no transgression. Okri writes (1997). 'Without transgression there is no danger, no risk, no *frisson*, no experiment, no discovery, and no creativity'. With respect to the storytelling aspect of my narrative I would echo the words of Fritz (1989), 'Throughout history, almost every culture has had art, music, dance, architecture, poetry, storytelling, pottery, and sculpture. The desire to create is not limited by beliefs, nationality, creed, educational background, or era. The urge resides in all of us (it) is not limited to the arts, but can encompass all of life, from the mundane to the profound'.

The battle of David and Goliath is quite similar to many skirmishes that take place up and down the country between ordinary men and women in hospital settings. I argue that all organizations have a David, and a Goliath that needs slaying. However, when we try to defeat Goliath on his terms with his weapons we lose. It is my hypothesis that Goliath can be defeated, but only with more superior weapons.

In the hospital setting the attacks on staff and practitioners are cleverly calculated and conspired, acted out through what French and Raven (1968) and Bryant (2010) describe as coercive power, which overpowers individuals, strips the practitioner of autonomy and destroys their ability to learn anything meaningful, resulting in a failing organization. Greenleaf's (2002: 98) thoughts on coercive power are, 'it is used principally to destroy. Not much that endures can be built with it. Even presumably autocratic institutions like businesses are learning that the value of coercive power is inverse to its use.'

When I reflect on my leadership, there is no place for coercion. It is pointless to use the same armour and weapons as Goliath, because he is much more skilled and accustomed to them than I. It is better to disarm him with weapons, what I would term smooth stones, that represent a smile, humanness, morality, ethics, spirituality and the most powerful weapon of all, care and love. Not romanticised love, but the type of love that Senge (1990: 285) refers to, which is *agape*, that has nothing to do with emotions and romance but is the type of love that is filled with intentions.

Five Smooth Stones

David was the youngest of seven brothers and took care of his father's sheep in the fields around Bethlehem. Sometimes wild animals would try to steal and eat the young lambs. David fought the wild animals with just a sling and a stone (I Samuel 17: 34–36). A good shepherd watches, protects and love his sheep, as does a good leader. Wheatley (1999: 131) suggest that we need leaders to help us develop the clear identity that lights the dark moments of confusion, leaders who support us as we learn to live by our values, leaders who understand that we are best controlled by concepts that invite our participation.

In my capacity as leader and shepherd I desperately want to care for my lambs, but every now and then I come across a wolf in sheep's clothing. These wolves jeopardise my plan as it sometimes takes a long time to detect them, convert them or keep them away. I refer here to members of staff who are unwilling to change, unwilling to learn and convey transactional tendencies in an attempt to appease their benefactors, the hierarchy of the organisation. I understand to an extent why they are like this because there is the persistent demand by Goliath to condition practitioners and embed them in the culture of transactional thinking and these transactional tendencies are often compounded by the effects of the baggage of one's own background, taking mine as an example.

In the long evenings before the flickering firelight David played his harp and sang songs that he made up as he watched over his sleeping sheep. He thought about the greatness of God who had created all things. He knew how he loved his sheep and how he was willing to risk his life to protect them (I & II Samuel). Though I love my sheep (my staff), I am wary about risking my career for them. I am not as loyal or fearless as David. What I do know, is everything in this world is somehow connected and this strange attractor of connectedness means that I have to connect with my allies as well as my enemies. Connecting with my enemies, the transactional masters who purposefully despise me and plot against me, is hard to adopt, hard to apply. Greene and Elffers (1998: 1) propose that we should always make those above us feel comfortably superior and not overly display our talents unless we provoke fear, that we should in essence make our masters appear more brilliant than they are in order to harness our own power. Until I am better able to connect with my enemies I will tentatively continue to play my 'political' harp, to appeal to their transactional world, with the hope that the melodies soothe them away from the dark side, towards transformation. I am hopeful.

David relied on a spiritual connection, as do I. David was often inspired, and many of his thoughts are found in the book of Psalms, which means 'songs' of praise, gratitude and introspection. As I parallel my journey with that of an emerging David, I too have a collection of psalms, more formally referred to as 'reflections' which I keep in a journal. My favourite journal entry is entitled 'Psalm of Victory',

Psalm of Victory

As I position myself in front of Goliath the earth trembles,
Hills are moved from their place and mountains quake in anticipation,
Fire from his nostrils kindles the coals at my feet, my brightness dims,
His mighty pavilion is set on dark waters smothered by thick grey clouds.
I waver.
His armies release their arrows but they fall at my feet,
I run into his troops and leap over his fortresses,
I know my way is perfect,
Armed with just 'five stones'. My enemies begin to retreat.
They cried out a loud noise but there was none to save them,
They scattered like dust.
Great deliverance was given unto me.
I thank God for anointing me,
But with great deliverance comes great responsibility,
And with great leadership there must be transgression!

David knew that God would help him, so he went before King Saul and said, 'I will go against this heathen Philistine who defies the armies of the living God.' King Saul answered,

'You are not able to go against this Philistine, for you are a young man, and this giant has been a trained soldier all of his life.' David had faith and a belief that he could achieve the impossible. As leaders we must have faith and realise that the enemy is both internal and external. That enemy within us is maybe more dangerous as it holds back our movements to creating a better society, the enemy within is responsible for our mediocre performance. In short, as Greenleaf (2002: 59) puts it: 'the enemy has strong natural servants who have the potential to lead but do not!' There is the hope that we can remove the blinkers and reconnect to become whole. I am hopeful.

Since no other soldier was willing to fight the giant Goliath, King Saul decided to allow little David to fight. Without any armour, David stooped at the brook in the valley, gathered five smooth stones and placed them in his shepherd's pouch. These are the five stones to which I pin my entire leadership framework on: Morality, Spirituality, Ethics, Values and Love. These are the weapons I choose to slay Goliath and cut off his head and feed his rotting corpse to the fowls of the air.

When I confront my organization with my sling and five smooth stones, no doubt they will laugh at me and like the Philistine giant will shout, 'Am I a dog that you come against me with stones?' But I will breathe gently take my footing, choose the appropriate stone and place it in my sling, draw back and take aim. As each stone takes flight and makes contact with that great giant (the transactional world), I will slowly disarm him; he will stumble and eventually he will fall.

I will rescue myself and my beloved sheep and we will shout and sing for joy because of our victories over Goliath, and I will be able to play a new tune with my harp and sing a new song and dance to a new beat. During the battles I will sojourn above the trenches and ballet and boogie regardless of the sharp rocks beneath my feet, I am prepared to tread on coals of fire knowing that my way is sure and my approach is filled with meaning. But until I reach the promise land, I will continually retune my harp.

Four Years On: What is the Condition of My Harp?

When I consider my role model leaders of the past, I am embarrassed. When I consider my new role models I see activists such as Martin Luther King, Malcolm X, Nelson Mandela and the biblical characters of King David and Jesus Christ. It should come as no surprise that I choose leaders who I could identify with racially and religiously, which relates to my cultural accounting. My obvious dilemma was that both Martin Luther King and Malcolm were assassinated for their efforts, Mandela was a political prisoner for over 27 years and Jesus Christ was crucified. Is this the fate of a great leader, I wonder? In view of this should I just put away my harp and be satisfied with being a 'good' but not a 'great' leader?

In addressing this dilemma, I have come to the conclusion that a great leader is prepared to sacrifice much, even his or her life, it would seem. I fear that I am too vain to sacrifice my own life or even my career for leadership, and this is perhaps my Achilles heel. I see moments where I need to speak out or even shout out, but I hold back. Great anguish overcomes me when I observe injustice or transactional behaviour, but I bury myself in the trenches and play a soothing tune with my harp to justify my failure to act. If I am being honest, my harp serves both an emancipatory and a cowardly role. I realise that I am still forming my five stones as I often lack the courage, persistence and conviction of my new role models. But they are still my inspiration, I have no intention to revert back to my childhood role models.

Distinguishing the Sheep from the Wolves

In my capacity as leader and shepherd of a team of health professionals, I desperately want to care for my lambs and sheep, but every now and then I come across a wolf in sheep's clothing, who jeopardises my plans and who is often hard to detect. When I am faced with wolves in sheep's clothing I bring to memory one of my psalms:

> *Wolf: Abandon your wicked ways*
>
> Beware of their style and gold plated smile
> Sharp teeth, slippery tongue and sugar-coated lies.
> They suck the blood of the weak and befriend the coward,
> Sneak around in the dark for whom they can devour.
> They play a good game, and disguise their shame,
> Causing mischief, folly, fear and pain.
> But can they be tamed?
> Who am I kidding?
> They will never stop feeding
> Until they accept the need for healing.

As I said, I am constantly polishing my five soft stones, but applying the theories of transformational leadership into everyday practice does not come as easy as writing a psalm, and this is where the art of creative tension comes to life. I would like to share one experience where I attempted to sharpen my skills in detecting the wolves in sheep clothing, with the intention to convert them and reverse their learning disability.

Two members of my team just can't get along. They are both mature and senior members of the department and in their own right contribute much to the service that we provide. They both feel that the other has a hidden agenda for power and an appetite for leadership. When they sit before me to complain, they provide me with ample examples of how the other is divisive and manipulative and unconnected to care. They put me in the awkward position of choosing whom I should keep and whom I should dismiss. Often, when I am in situations like this I think to myself what would my new role models do, and as I listen, I begin to hear voices of reason and start to calculate the various responses that will disarm the frustration and resolve the feud. But each time I come up with a suggestion, they both reject it. Then I am left asking 'What would you like me to do about this?' to which they reply 'I don't know, you are the manager, you sort it out'. On hearing these words, I feel that my leadership is being criticised and get a little frosty, and think to myself, 'You're the one with the problem, not me!' I then feel compelled to respond with an immediate reply or solution. But I have realised that solutions should not be contrived, reactive, or based on anger or feeling vulnerable but on what is best. So I send them away and say 'I need to reflect on this, let me think about this and come back to you', to which they roll their eyes, shrug their shoulders and leave my office unfulfilled. When they have left, I think to myself Whom do I believe? What does the evidence suggest? How do I judge who is the wolf and who the sheep? I then silently vent my frustration at their criticism of my leadership and coil up, but before I become bent and twisted out of shape, I recall one of my psalms:

> *Taking off my armour*
>
> As I sit and build my empire I can do no wrong,
> But what if I am challenged on how I lead?

Will I pretend to listen? Or
Will I listen and be prepared to enter into dialogue?
At the heart of my leadership I want to build a learning environment,
But I now realise that I first must learn!
Starting with learning to deal with criticism.
This means I must take off my bronze helmet,
My coat of amour, and place my javelin at my feet.
This will be hard for me, because when I am wearing my armour
I feel so comfortable.
I am probably still wearing it now.

In considering my reflexivity, I call the two members of staff to meet me once more. I feel that to learn we must share, we must listen we must dig down to the roots. As the leader my greatest role in this is to exercise wisdom, or what I would call knowing without knowing. Clinical competence, knowledge, expertise, rationality and experience are all attributes that provide us with a kind of knowing in a situation. However, wisdom is the gift that tells us what to do with these attributes, right now for the greater good! And superior wisdom, or 'knowing without knowing', propels us to pave the way – to lead. A leader must possess this gift, to enable others to believe that the leader knows what to do, how to do it and to act in the now for the best.

Wisdom is ethical and purposeful and is not necessarily bestowed upon us by some great mentor, nor does it come about through education. It is more intuitive and, in my view, spiritual. But hold on: before I get too excited about the purposefulness of wisdom, I am reminded that even a fool believes he has wisdom!

There appears to be a variety of ways in which one can know or express wisdom. As a practitioner, I am considered a specialist in certain fields of nutrition. If you ask me to explain the chemical composition of a fatty acid I would dazzle you with chemistry, if you asked me to explain its function, I would give you a sequential account of ingestion, digestion, absorption, assimilation and fat mobilisation. But to a sick, dying patient all this knowledge is more than useless; what matters is the ability to connect. I needed my two members of staff to connect and this would require wisdom.

Rael writes (1993: 29):

> Wisdom we would come to find one day. Once the sacred place is discovered, we begin to open to the wisdom. It descends upon us just as it did when the beings from the spirit of life brought spirit to the people. What is interesting about wisdom is that when it happens to us, it also happens to other people who are also being lifted to the next level.

This sacred place is within if only we are open to it. It is a kind of mindfulness to see things clearly. I stumbled on it through reflection and even then didn't realise what it was. If I am wise then others touched by me will be lifted.

As I continued to listen to the individual members of staff I awaited the expectancy of a great insight, which did not rely on objective knowledge and clinical expertise. Objective knowledge and clinical expertise can only take us so far, and when we come to a dead end, we depend on a reliable insight that will guide us through the terrain of 'knowing without knowing'. We don't question whence the knowing has come, we simply accept it, believe it and are grateful for it. And what I discovered was both team members were threatened by each other. They both concentrated on what set them apart and not what aligned them. They both carried out their work to outdo the other and this trail of competitive working drained them, it took away all their energy and passion for concentrating on what was important. They were consumed by the transactional world and the sting of its tail made them resentful and spiteful. Each failed to see the contribution of the other, valued only their own achievements and overplayed their hand in trying to look the best. In front of me they expressed the persona of a sheep, but inside were ravening wolves, out to bleed each other dry and take me as hostage if need be. My imperative was to help them to direct all their negative energy towards a positive enterprise and help them to heal, to shred their wolf persona and rediscover the beautiful sheep that lay beneath.

I held a team meeting with all my team leaders, them included, and called it a team-building day. My main aim for the meeting was not to talk about the service, key performance indicators or departmental objectives, it was not to boast of how excellent we were or share our frustrations. It was to ask one question, 'What is it about our core that drives us to work with, and treat sick people?'

The group were surprised at the question. In all probability they did not register its significance, but as we started to discuss it one by one, it became obvious that we had a desire to serve, to care to meet the needs of those who are vulnerable, to be human. It was refreshing to hear the testimonies of how they had been appreciated by patients and how they had enriched patients' lives and their own by caring, and how they had assisted patients with kind and gentle words while they lay dying. This meeting was not about science or academia, it was ethical, and it was about being human. We began to weave a tapestry of all that was good about serving, and not one transactional thread could be seen. What I saw at that meeting was the revelation of that 'strange attractor' called connectedness. Greenleaf (1974) describes this as creating 'community'. One year on, the two members of staff are still not the best of friends, but they are no longer enemies, they no longer besiege me with complaints about each other and I have even had the good fortune to witness them defend each other when their work has been criticised by external agencies. In that team-building day they discovered what aligned them instead of what made them different. They became gentle sheep and I felt like a proud shepherd. We all left something behind in the meeting room that afternoon, they left behind their wolf's clothing and I left behind my helmet, shield and sword. For me this was a moment that connected the dots and in this experiment my harp was in tune. I felt that warm glow of leadership and my five smooth stones were intact.

The Future

Reflection is a word that comes up every time I enrol new students and new staff, and an objective that is undertaken by every member of my department. My team are either frustrated or amused with the frequency at which I raise this topic and its importance; they probably don't even realise that we are using it constantly to improve our practice. They are more comfortable and familiar with the term 'clinical supervision', which is where the art of reflexivity is unfolded and where my team get the time, space and opportunity to reflect. To many, reflection does not come easy. On questioning many of my new starters I find they are familiar with the concept and can even recall a few reflective models, but I am well aware that they attach little importance to it and I know for certain that the large majority are not keeping reflective journals or diaries. As a leader who documents my reflections in the form of psalms, I can occasionally get depressed with the discovery that my staff are not role modelling my efforts in regard to reflexivity, and at times I am tempted to get transactional and force them to show me a weekly reflexive journal, in a vain attempt to force them to know what's good for them, but when I get these transactional tremors I remember that infamous Philistine, that giant called Goliath, and shudder at the thought of what brought him down to his knees – a small smooth stone. With that thought, I will continue to play my harp, I will continue to experiment with leadership strategies, and I will continue to brag about the purposefulness of reflection, and its sweet sound will harness my team toward the Promised Land.

References

Bochner, A, P. and Ellis S.C. (2006) Communication as autoethnography. In Gregory J. Shepherd, Jeffrey St. John and Ted Striphas (eds.), *Communication as ... perspectives on Theory*. Sage, Thousand Oaks, CA.

Bryant, J. H. (2009) *Love leadership: the new way to lead in a fear-based world*. Jossey-Bass, San Francisco.

Burns, J. M. (1978) *Leadership*. New York, Harper & Row.

Coser, L. A. (1956) *The functions of social conflict*. Free Press, Glencoe, IL.

French, J. and Raven, B. (1968) The basis of social power, In D. Cartwright and A. Zander (eds.), *Group dynamics*. Row Peterson, Evanston, IL.

Fritz, R. (1989) *The path of least resistance*. Fawcett-Columbine, New York.

Greene, R. and Elffers, J. (1998) *The 48 laws of power*. Penguin Putnam, New York.

Greenleaf, R. (2002) *Servant leadership: a journey into the nature of legitimate power & greatness*. Paulist Press, New York.

Holy Bible. Authorised (Kings James) Version.

Johns, C. (2009) *Becoming a reflective practitioner* [3rd edition]. Wiley-Blackwell, Oxford.

Kelly, J. (1970) Make conflict work for you. *Harvard Business Review* 48, 103–113

Litterer, J. A. (1966) Conflict in organizations: a re-examination. *Academy of Management Journal* 9, 178–186

Macleod, D. J. (1974) *Slavery, race and the American Revolution*. Cambridge University Press, Cambridge.

McCornack, S. (2009) *Reflect and relate, an introduction to interpersonal communication*. Bedford/St. Martin's, Boston.

Okri, B. (1997) *A way of being free*. Phoenix House, London.

Rael, J. (1993) *Being and vibration*. Council Oak Books, Tulsa, OK.

Senge, P. (1990) *The fifth discipline: the art and practice of the learning organization*. Century Business, London.

Wheatley, J. M. (1999) *Leadership and the new science: discovering order in a chaotic world*. Berrett, San Francisco.

Chapter 23

'People are not Numbers to Crunch'

Christopher Johns and Otter Rose-Johns

> I am not a number, I am not a number, I am not a number.
> I am a human being. Please don't crunch me.

Introduction

Hi. I'm Beady-Eye, so called because I like to keep my eye on what's going on in healthcare, especially at a time of deep public unrest with the quality of care in the shadow of the Mid Staffs report. It is deeper than that, as the *Sunday Times* reported 'one in five hospitals fail to meet care standards leaving patients to endure a catalogue of neglect' (*Sunday Times* 27 April 2014, p. 13).

My local paper headlines 'Patients Happier With Care At Bedford Hospital Following A Care Quality Commission Survey. 91% of patients [$N = 420$] reported that their overall quality of care was excellent, very good or good, 86% said they were treated with dignity and respect at all times.' (*Bedfordshire Times & Citizen*, February 18 2012). I wonder about the difference between excellent, very good and good. I also wonder about the 14% who didn't say they were treated with dignity and respect. That's one person in every seven. Reading on, '83% felt they were definitely given enough privacy when discussing their condition or treatment. 76% said they definitely had confidence and trust in the doctor examining or treating them, whilst 63% felt they were definitely involved in decisions about their care and treatment. Hospital Chief Executive, Jo Harrison, said she was delighted that patient satisfaction was so high.'

I'm wondering, is she reading the same report? What do these statistics actually mean? What stories and truths do they hide?

In June 2008, the Royal College of Nursing (RCN) was so concerned with the lack of dignity given to patients that it launched its own dignity campaign, including 'The Dignity Toolkit' as a mechanism for progressing its 'Dignity in Care' campaign.

As Tim Baggs, RCN, East and West Midlands, notes 'With the help of some very useful tools and guidance, the RCN's dignity campaign has inspired changes in healthcare practice

Becoming a Reflective Practitioner, Fifth Edition. Edited by Christopher Johns.
© 2017 John Wiley & Sons Ltd. Published 2017 by John Wiley & Sons Ltd.
Companion Website: www.wiley.com/go/johns/reflectivepractitioner

and environments that put the needs of the patient first. It has also empowered nurses to feel confident about prioritising the delivery of high quality, dignified care and influencing for practical solutions where they feel they are distracted or diverted from doing this.'[1] What has happened that has caused nurses not to treat patients with dignity? I sense they do not see the person. It is a shocking indictment of nursing and health care. And can a toolkit really empower nurses?

Walking to the station some time ago I pass the Virgin Money poster 'People are not numbers to crunch.' The advert is a claim for humanised banking. It seems to me that is just what health care has become, number crunching, reflected in such statistical approaches to measuring the quality of care. It is all about numbers. Caring seems to exist only in the shadowy margins, only rearing its head as significant when complaints roll in.

I wonder – what is quality of care? One thing I do think is important is that people introduce themselves when meeting new people. I think this is especially true for health practitioners when meeting vulnerable patients. Would you agree? Lets reflect on that through engaging in a performance narrative.

Performance narrative is a method of communicating insights, especially about current disturbing social issues, to both inform and engage others towards creating better worlds. Narrative performers intend to influence people to see the world differently, especially a world that has been normalised and rendered unproblematic.[2] They intend to disturb or interrupt complacency and the taken-for-granted, to inspire reflection and provoke action. Denzin writes:[3]

> Such interruptions are meant to unsettle and challenge taken-for-granted assumptions concerning problematic issues in public life. They create a space for dialogue and questions, giving voice to positions previously silenced or ignored.

In the following performance narrative I accompanied Otter, my partner, for an angiogram. Our experience left much to be desired.

So, switch on your reflective sense, and, as you read this narrative, open your imagination, reflect on your own experiences, and draw your insights.

The Story of Three Blind Mice and the Movie Star

The car park dismal this July day. Otter and I follow the signs. We take the lift to the second floor. Hands firmly clenched, not quite knowing what to expect. We arrive at the cardiac clinic 15 minutes before 9. Otter booked for an angiogram. She hands in the pre-assessment questionnaire. Stuff like next of kin and religion. I wonder if the answers are glanced at. The obligatory overnight bag packed 'just in case'. Just in case things do not go well. Otter could die. The receptionist perfunctory – 'Please take a seat in the waiting room.'

Rows of seats face us. Other people congregated. Nervous hellos punctuate the awkward silence waiting, waiting for the chime of 9.

A familiar face. I know Peter from Badminton. He hadn't been recently. He tells his story, revealing the precarious edge of life. Booked in for a cardio-version.

Waiting. We wait anxiously as if extras in the film *High Anxiety*.[4] My mouth dry. A glass of water would be helpful. I glance about – no water machine. A budget cut or simply no-one had thought about it?

Waiting. Drumming of fingers. Flicking through the neatly stacked car mags disturbing order. No one else is reading.

Squeeze Otter's hand, more for my benefit than hers. It hasn't been an easy journey; chest pain and breathlessness, sapping at her energy and mood. I imagine her heart straining against the odds through blocked arteries.

'How are you feeling love?'

'Like a red ball of wool unravelling with threads hanging down.'

We are on edge, not knowing what's in store beyond the closed door.

The chime of 9. I shift expectantly. A minute later someone in blues appears from behind the closed door. No introduction just the command 'Follow me' and like timid sheep rounded up we obey herded through the door. Peter and the others shepherded into the 'Cardio-version Bay'.

I say 'Good luck Peter.'

'You too' he replies.

A human touch. Otter is shepherded into an adjacent four-bedded bay. I tag along carrying the bag. The first bed on the right indicated. I wonder the nurse's response if I had asked for the window view? No time for flippancy. Serious stuff this. But then shouldn't all serious stuff be approached with a smile in the soul?[5]

We are the only occupants. A gown on the bed. The anonymous person in blues says 'Please change and someone will be with you shortly'. The liminal transfer from person to patient. Leave your autonomy at the door. At least the gown covers the body, unlike many I have seen with open back held tenuously together with a tie, that is, if you are lucky. If not, bare bum exposed for all to recoil with horror or knickers left on in protest. But then you've become a patient. What price dignity?

We wait. We twiddle our thumbs. Slowly, the minutes tick by.

Enter the First Blind Mouse

She saunters into the bay dressed in blues, clipboard in hand. She positions herself at the end of the bed as if keeping her distance surveying the work to be done. No introduction. No recognition of me. 'Hello – I'm here' I say to myself.

She wears a name badge on her chest. The writing is too small to read from where I'm sitting. My eyes strain to make out her name … No, I can't make it out. I cast my eyes aside. God forgive -she might think I'm staring at her breasts. I imagine her comment 'Right pervert in there'; but I want to know her name. I strain again to no avail. My eyes turn away fearful of judgement. Maybe I should simply ask 'What is your name nurse?

But I don't. Why am I rendered silent? Am I merely a bystander outside her gaze?

She does the talking, firing questions, scribbling on her clipboard. In response to each answer she exclaims 'fantastic'.

Check your date of birth? Fantastic!

When was the last time you had anything to eat or drink? Fantastic!

Have you had your medicines this morning? Fantastic!

Did you bring your medicines in with you? Fantastic!

Are you allergic to anything? Fantastic!

Patient identity confirmed. The name bracelet fixed. A final fantastic and then she goes, no doubt pleased she has been both efficient and friendly. I look at Otter. She looks at me.

'Fanbloodytastic!' I laugh.

I name her 'Little Miss Fantastic'. Roger Hargreaves eat your heart out.

'Shooosh,' Otter says anxiously, 'they'll hear you. We might get thrown out'.

Otter anxious not to make a fuss, to be the good patient.

My laugh turns to a frown.

No empathy for someone admitted for an angiogram and possible stent insertion
No inquiry how Otter is feeling or if she is anxious about anything.
No information of what to expect.

Otter is simply an object being processed. But surely, this is a specialist cardiac unit. There is something very wrong here. No Oscar for her performance, unless of course, it's a horror movie.

I am a bystander outside your gaze.

> Outside your gaze
> You do not see me.
> Yes, me, sitting over here
> anxious about my partner
> life on edge.
> Tell me your name at least,
> greet me with a smile,
> ask me how I am;
> not a lot to ask really,
> or perhaps it is,
> wrapped up, as you are, in the machine.
> Perfunctory responses
> *fantastic, fantastic, fantastic*!
> I wonder how you would respond
> if I had said
> 'Excuse me – what is your name nurse?'
> or 'Hello, I'm Chris,' and stood to shake your hand.
> I didn't so I don't know.

Readers – imagine how you would feel going for an angiogram or being the partner of someone who is? Perhaps you have had other hospital experiences that resonate.

Enter the Second Blind Mouse

Again without a name. Again no recognition of me. Again my eyes strain but I cannot read the name on her badge. Again my eyes avert. She is armed with a premed. The sight of the needle, Otter protests, her anxiety spilling over – 'I need more than that.'

The nurse insists -'This will be enough.'

Still Otter protests.

'This will be enough,' the mouse reiterates.

She does not ask about the anxiety. Better to keep her distance than get involved? Me too – but I want to shout at her – LISTEN! But again, my voice is silent. Task done she exits. 'Carry on nurse,' I flip, but there is nothing amusing in this farce.

Enter the Movie Star

He pulls the curtain round. Big smile, friendly manner, open-necked shirt. Stethoscope positioned along his collar.

'Hi, I'm Ray Bishop, I'm doing the angiogram.'

Shakes my hand. Explains in his friendly manner – 'An angiogram has 1 in 1,000 mortality. Proceed to a stent, which I would like if appropriate, mortality rises to 1 in 100.

He pauses momentarily. Gauges our reaction. Otter grimaces.

We feel the charisma. It's infectious. It helps to ease the fear. Morale lifted. Otter signs the paper in her consenting scrawl. Otter more relaxed as if God had passed by and spread magic dust. Spit out the bad taste left by the two blind mice with no names. We've met the real movie star. George Clooney eat your heart out.

[Otter sings wearing her movie star glasses 'A movie star, a movie star, you think you are a movie star' .... [6]]

[Pause]

Suddenly, the curtains are pulled back. Two people dressed in blues enter. No introduction. Banter as they take Otter in the bed. I sit in the void alone. I am a bystander outside their gaze. I must find my own way. What if I make a fuss? 'See me, see me. I have needs too!'

Such potential drama averted by my passivity. A good relative is barely seen and unheard. Don't they know that not acknowledging anxiety increases it?

How much longer waiting? It seems forever. I try to read but my mind is plagued. Mind swirling. Imagining the worse.

Otter returns.

'How are you?'

'Not good,' she whispers 'they went in through my groin – they couldn't get in at the wrist.' Grimace of embarrassment with all on show. A plug to hold firmly to stem the flow.

Enter the Third Blind Mouse

Again with no name. Again no recognition of me. Not even a name badge!

She begins a cycle of observation- blood pressure and pulse and the insistent demand – 'drink as much as possible'. No inquiry into how Otter is feeling beyond 'OK?'

Otter not one to make a fuss. Why the haste? Perhaps targets to be met? Clear the decks by 5 or hell to pay? Otter needs a wee.

She asks 'Can I get up?'

The nurse tuts- 'Are you sure you can't wait?'

'No' Otter says.

The nurse tuts again and reluctantly brings the pan.

'Try and keep your legs straight' she instructs.

Otter retorts 'Have you tried pissing with your legs straight?'

No reply but needless to say the bed's now wet. The nurse has to change the sheet.

Otter- 'Oh dear, I am a nuisance.'

[You are a nuisance.]

Ray returns, his charisma bubbling. News about the angiogram – 'The main arteries are clear and hence no stent inserted.'

The 'not so good news' – 'It seems the minor arteries are blocked ... difficult to treat.'

Ominous words- what does 'difficult to treat' mean? A heart attack waiting for you? Death around the corner? Yet his concern feels genuine. Indeed I have confidence in this man. I could drink with him in a pub. The bad news is then not so bad simply because it is he who is saying it. He adds 'Treatment with drugs as best we can.' As best we can rings hollow. Not so optimistic. He leaves us spinning with the news.

Otter's Poem

My heart is on the blink
like a clogged sink,
accumulated muck
that has narrowed the flow.
Heart muscle groans,

pushing hard,
cells moan,
the tight pain,
despair – where has my energy gone?
Legs ache,
not even a stent will do the trick
with syndrome *X*.
Perhaps a wire brush
To clear the debris?
Easier said than done.
The spray dilates.
one, two, three, puffs,
small relief.
Can I live like this when I have been so fit?

Periodically, the third blind mouse returns. Not once does she inquire how we are feeling after such news. Instead her constant demand 'Drink, drink'. 'Yes – drink and be merry,' I think. Pushing the pace – 'Sit up and get out of bed as quickly as possible.' We are being shoved along a conveyor belt. I imagine her thought – 'Come, come: others are worse off than you,' and perhaps that's true but it doesn't alter our predicament. Otter buckles to the demand but doesn't feel so good.

Across the bay we now have a neighbour who talks and talks. His anxiety spilling out, no doubt glad to have an ear denied to him by the blind mice. He informs us he is having stent replacements. We get the full history of his heart attack and treatments. Driving his car in Cambridge or somewhere. He is alone, frightened. His words pass over me for I am wrapped in my own concerns. But he doesn't stop talking. His anxiety spilling out. I can touch his fear. I say to myself, 'Why don't you shut the fuck up? I've enough on my plate,' whilst nodding my head sympathetically. Eventually they come and take him and, for a moment, we have some peace.

Otter continues to drink and drink. Pushing herself. Sitting up gradually as demanded.

Being a good patient, the compliant child. Now she needs another pee. No more wet beds.

'Get me to the loo!' she cries.

Gingerly, bare-footed, we make it slowly to the WC across the corridor. Gush of pee. Relief!

Otter- 'I feel light headed.'

A stream of watery vomit gushes from her mouth. I catch her as she faints and slide her to the floor. Doctors spill from the doctors' room. It is Ray who holds her, comforts her. He is the hero, the movie star. It could be Clark Gable and Vivian Leigh. Nurses congregate. He castigates them for pushing too hard – I hum, *'three blind mice… the farmer's wife, who cut of their tails with a carving knife'*. Will they love him less with their tails trimmed or is it vomit off a mouse's back?

After ten minutes or so Otter feels a bit better. A wheelchair fetched to make it the few yards back to bed. The demand put on hold.

In the Bay, we have more neighbours. The one in the corner doesn't look so good.

They take him but he doesn't return. The bay loaded with potential death. The bed directly opposite overflowing with a huge man. I imagine his arteries clogged with fat.

His anxious wife next to him. A litany of complaint spews from him. He isn't comfortable – blah blah blah blah blah. His complaints unrelenting, inexorable.

The nurses get an ear-bashing. I want to shout 'Shut the fuck up! We need some quiet in the aftermath. The nurses have enough to do.' Perhaps that is why they 'shut off' and keep their distance. Wear their suits of armour to protect from all the emotional and psychological muck thrown at them. So called professional detachment.[7]

But why should I sympathise with them? Surely, such anxiety must be expected on death's precipice? I wonder (yet again) – What is nursing? Of course they should engage on both an emotional and psychological level but they seem ill-prepared for such a role. Trapped in the mice run they have no room to turn. Being blind they cannot see.

> Three blind mice,
> three blind mice,
> see how they run,
> see how they run.
> They've lost their sight in the healthcare machine,
> their ability to care has been wiped quite clean,
> have you ever seen anything so sad in your life
> as three blind mice,
> three blind mice.

Another hour passes. Pressure off, but Otter is restless. So am I. We've both had enough of this healthcare machine. I pull the curtains round. Clothes pulled on. We move through to the waiting room, pass by the nurses' station where congregated nurses do not lift their heads. But that is not the end. We have to wait for drugs. Delay [what a surprise] but still an echocardiogram to be squeezed in. Ray would like this done before we go. A male radiographer anonymous in blues pulls Otter away. Again I am left in the void.

Otter returns and tells the story – 'I was all wired up with my breasts exposed, and Ray walked in! What price my dignity!'

[What price dignity]

Sardonically, I joust, 'But you are just a patient. Not even that, a statistic – 'One of 14% or 59, who did not say they were treated with respect and dignity at all times.'

Waiting. Waiting. My anger brewing. My exasperation breaks out 'How much longer?!'

Otter shrugs 'I'm going to make a fuss.' No result. We are being processed within the machine. Otter slinks back into the uncomfortable chair. At last the drugs arrive.

Sarcastically, I quip 'We were just about to roll out our sleeping bags.' The nurse looks at me blankly. The sarcasm fallen on stony ground. 'Never mind' I bleakly lament. We leave. The car park still dismal in July.

I say, 'I feel as if I've been through a wringer.'

Otter, 'Me too, squeezed dry in the healthcare machine'

But then was it so bad? What should we expect? Perhaps nothing more from nurses. They used to be the ones who cared while the doctor focused on the disease. Now it seems that all has changed. Maybe the CQC should know the human story behind the statistic that hides the truth, seeing only what it sees. As a relative I'm not even a statistic, not even a number to crunch. Do they ask relatives about their experience or are relatives merely bystanders outside their gaze?

I pull away the Chief Executive's mask of delight and confront: 'Do you know this is one area in desperate need of repair? Surely, one vital measure of the quality of care is that all professionals should introduce themselves to create at least the potential for human relationship? Knowing how fearful people are with heart problems, I also expect each nurse to express some empathy, to ask how the patient is feeling, to create the potential for the person to express his or her anxiety. The manner of the nurses we came into contact with exacerbated our anxiety rather than lessening it, deflating us rather than lifting us. Why is that? Is it because they too have become numbers in a machine that has lost its ability to care? Is it because they have lamentable leadership from the top down?'

In a *Guardian* article (Campbell 2013) entitled 'Hospitals to Reduce Needless Collection of Information', Health Secretary Jeremy Hunt is quoted, following the Mid Staffordshire NHS inquiry (Francis 2013), as saying that 'creating a culture of care, not bureaucracy in the NHS is essential… doctors and nurses went into their professions to help patients, not number crunch'.

Perhaps Hunt, too, had read the Virgin poster and slipped its rhetoric into political spiel? Yet how do we turn rhetoric into reality? There's the rub.

So, I must poke a finger in the ribs. Startle your complacency and connect you to the great sea of human suffering when you might prefer to turn your head away. If so, then nothing gets changed and the world slips greater into moral decay and where quality measures blur the truth. Which leaves me with two questions – Why was I so silent? and Could I have responded differently to make the situation better? I recognise throughout my nursing career a weight of hospital authority that silences relatives until a point of outrage is reached. Being a recipient of healthcare I sense this oppressive weight. It is as if people have been conditioned to be good patients and relatives, stemming back to capitalist idea of healthcare – that in exchange for healthcare people will submit to medical authority in the now-questionable belief that the hospital will do you no harm and act for the best.[8] No room for patient autonomy despite the rhetoric.

Here I draw upon compelling research whereby relatives naïvely trust that health care practitioners to care for them.[9] When this is not manifest, as in my experience, such naïve trust turns to disillusionment and breakdown of trust. How easy would it have been for all nurses to acknowledge Otter's and my need from the outset? Well, probably not so easy, when an uncaring attitude becomes normal and hence the problem is not acknowledged, or when it is, rationalised as due to difficult patients. RCN campaigns such as 'Dignity'[10] are knee-jerk reactions to crisis. Inevitably they fizzle out. Lack of dignity is a failure of leadership to ensure dignity. Maybe another time I will find my voice to confront the machine and assert that we are not numbers to crunch before outrage kicks in. Imagine the nurses' response.

Acknowledgement

An edited version of the narrative was published by the *British Journal of Cardiac Nursing*[11] to invoke social action.

Endnotes

1   Endnotes http://www.ulh.nhs.uk/for_patients/dignity_in_care/rcn_toolkit.asp
2   (Goffman, E. (1959) *The presentation of self in everyday life.* Doubleday, new York (p. 15), cited in Schechhner, R. (2006) *Performance studies: an introduction* [2nd edition] Routledge, New York (p. 29).
3   Denzin, N. (2003) *Performance ethnography: critical pedagogy and the politics of culture.* Sage, Thousand Oaks, CA (p. 111).
4   Mel Brooks movie [1978]
5   Okri, B. (1997) *A way of being free.* Phoenix House, London.
6   '*Moviestar*' is a popular 1975 song, written and performed by Swedish pop singer Harpo. The single was produced and arranged by Bengt Palmers.

7   Menzies-Lyth writes 'The core of the anxiety situation for the nurse lies in her relationship with the patient. The closer and more concentrated this relationship, the more the nurse is likely to experience this anxiety ... a necessary psychological task for the entrant into any profession that works with people is the development of adequate professional detachment' [pp. 51, 54]. Menzies- Lyth I. (1988) A case study in the functioning of social systems as a defence against anxiety. In *Containing anxiety in institutions: selected essays*. Free Association Books, London.

8   Parsons, T. (1951) Illness and the role of the physician: a sociological analysis. *American Journal of Orthopsychiatry* 21, 452–460.

9   Thorne, S. & Robinson, S. (1988) Reciprocal trust in health care relationships. *Journal of Advanced Nursing* 13, 782–789.

10 RCN's definition of dignity:

> This definition of dignity was published by the Royal College of Nursing in 2008. It is also available to download at The RCN's definition of dignity (PDF 77.2KB) [https://www2.rcn.org.uk/__data/assets/pdf_file/0003/191730/003298.pdf].
>
> Dignity is concerned with how people feel, think and behave in relation to the worth or value of themselves and others. To treat someone with dignity is to treat them as being of worth, in a way that is respectful of them as valued individuals.
>
> In care situations, dignity may be promoted or diminished by:
>
> o the physical environment
> o organisational culture
> o the attitudes and behaviour of the nursing team and others
> o the way in which care activities are carried out.
>
> When dignity is present people feel in control, valued, confident, comfortable and able to make decisions for themselves. When dignity is absent people feel devalued, lacking control and comfort. They may lack confidence and be unable to make decisions for themselves. They may feel humiliated, embarrassed or ashamed.
>
> Dignity applies equally to those who have capacity and to those who lack it. Everyone has equal worth as human beings and must be treated as if they are able to feel, think and behave in relation to their own worth or value.
>
> The nursing team should, therefore, treat all people in all settings and of any health status with dignity, and dignified care should continue after death (RCN 2008).

11 Johns, C. (2014) The importance of empathy: people are not numbers. *British Journal of Cardiac Nursing*, 8.10, 466.

Chapter 24

Smoking Kills

Christopher Johns and Otter Rose-Johns

Tough men do not die easily

Some thoughts on narrative performance

As a reflective practitioner I feel the need to share my insights to a wider world because they are significant in creating a better healthcare world. It seems pointless to write narrative without performing it to an audience – what I term the sixth dialogical movement. Creating narrative performance is the means to achieve this. Perhaps the creative urge is the nature of reflective practice. As Loori writes,[1] 'through our art we bring into existence something that previously did not exist. We enlarge the universe'.

Performance also enables creative feedback to fuel my creativity as I seek ever more creative ways to perform, to answer my own questions – 'Do I communicate my insights effectively through performance'? 'What messages does the audience get'? Again, as Loori writes,[2] 'creative feedback offers artists an opportunity to get a sense of the impact of their work: the visceral, direct effect that they are having on their audience'.

Smoking kills

Smoking kills is a performance narrative centred around my hospice practice as a complementary therapist working with three men with lung cancer. Its message is stark – smoking kills and dying from lung cancer for *tough* men is not easy. Yet is the hospice approach right? Lets disturb that idea. Rattle the comfy cage. The performance also intends to confront smoking as a social habit – hopefully disturbing people who smoke or who are tempted to smoke. I extended the performance to include a critique of supervision as developmental and support mechanism for 'tough work'.

Note: it is not possible to publish the images – these can be viewed on the Wiley-Blackwell website.[3] PP refers to PowerPoint as used within the performance to accompany the words.

[Please refer the website for PP2 on Smoking skills]

Becoming a Reflective Practitioner, Fifth Edition. Edited by Christopher Johns.
© 2017 John Wiley & Sons Ltd. Published 2017 by John Wiley & Sons Ltd.
Companion Website: www.wiley.com/go/johns/reflectivepractitioner

Men dying of lung cancer
Imagine lungs full of tumour
Dying is not easy work
No, not easy at all
Not easy for any of us.

The hospice a place of dying
No place for tough men
Or perhaps it is
Soften you up
So dying is easier
A job well done?
But is it?

Heh kiddo
Put that fag down
It ain't macho
It's full of shit.

Context

Everything I do, everything we do, is always an interpretation of context.

As Wheatley puts it *[Please refer the website for PP3 on Smoking skills]*:

The new physics cogently explains that there is no objective reality out there waiting to reveal its secrets. There are no recipes or formulas, no checklists or expert advice that describe 'reality'. If context is as crucial as the science explains, then nothing really transfers; everything is always new and different and unique to each of us. We must engage with each other, experiment to find what works for us, and support one another as the true inventors we are'.[4]

[Please refer the website for PP4 on Smoking skills]

I am an oddball.
I collect stories
A curriculum revolutionary
turning it upside down
shaking it out
Scrapping against the technical rational
grain.
Stories are about listening.
I construct narrative.

Narratives are transgressive,[5] confronting complacency, normal practice, assumptions and hegemonic structures, ripping out bullies and sacred cows. It does this quietly or brutally.

Listen.

I mean *really* listen.

Make a note of at least one thing to dialogue with.

Part 1

The year 1981. I was the only Morris dancer in the side who smoked. Peer pressure. Nick said 'Why do you smoke?'

I can appreciate that those who do not smoke do not like smoke from others. Makes your breath and clothes smell.

Why did I smoke? Habit I guess. Something to do with my mouth, my hand, pleasure. I gave up just like that.

I just ate more until Nick said one day patting my belly – 'You're getting fat'.

Part 2

[Please refer the website for PP5 on Smoking skills]

Walking down West End, a poster in a community centre window catches my eye. It reads, 'The worst day of Steve's life was when he had to tell his 12 year old daughter he had lung cancer. The message – if you think giving up smoking is difficult try telling your children you have lung cancer.'

Gritty stuff.

Yet I sense this message is largely passed by. Just another anti-smoking poster stuck in a window. Surely, anyone with any sense wouldn't smoke? Would they?

But then death is over there not here.[6]

[Please refer the website for PP6 and PP7 on Smoking skills]

The smoker turns away from the message.

Death is over there not here.

Each time the smoker reaches for the cigarette packet or to roll a fag, they are confronted with the health risks graphically displayed on the cigarette packets that litter the street like monuments to those who have died or are dying of smoking-related diseases.

[Please refer the website for PP8-15 on Smoking skills]

I imagine the cost of skin care products spent for the premature ageing of skin due to smoking. No doubt cigarette companies have a commercial interest in skin products and private medical clinics. I imagine their slogan 'We cause the problem and we can solve the problem.' Good business acumen!

[Please refer the website for PP16 on Smoking skills]

At the psychiatric hospital we sat around rolling and smoking our baccie. It was social bonding and enjoyable. It was good to smoke, to fill the lungs and blow smoke rings. No one seemed to think about the health risks but then cigarette packets were not blazoned by such graphic reminders.

But would that have mattered? We were young and immortal. Death is for old people. It didn't seem to bother us that our breath and clothes reeked of fags ... yet I wonder now, looking back, what message did that give young people on the adolescent unit?

[Please refer the website for PP17 on Smoking skills]

It is not easy to witness the woman smoking in her car with children sitting in the rear seats. I want to rip the cigarette from her mouth, or more punitively, take her children away. They deserve better.

[Please refer the website for PP18 on Smoking skills]
Does this child have a choice?

[Please refer the website for PP19 on Smoking skills]
Do her parents not hear the message -smoking seriously harms you and others around you . . . .

[Please refer the website for PP20 and 21 on Smoking skills]
… No matter what language you speak.

[Please refer the website for PP22 on Smoking skills]
Whilst all the displayed images are shocking, the one image that resonates most is the image of diseased lungs and the message 'Smoking causes fatal lung cancer'.

I work with men dying from lung cancer. It is not easy to journey alongside and witness their suffering.

Part 3

[Please refer the website for PP23 on Smoking skills]
Walking along Lowestoft beach I watch the waves moving in and moving out. Rhythmic movement. The tide turning.

Refer the website for PP24 on Smoking skills. > Becker writes,[7] 'Throughout the whole body we can sense an overall tidal movement of the whole body, a coming in and ebbing out. It is as if the whole body, functioning as a unit, is responding to a force similar to that moving the tides of the ocean. It is a rhythmic movement within all the fluids of the body that gives primary life to the body.'

My skill as a therapist is to tune into these tides and move them into healthier patterns. Harnessing the body's energy for transformation.

[Please refer the website for PP25 on Smoking skills]
At the hospice. Corin, one of the consultants, pulls me aside. She asks if I will talk with Luke. He has lung cancer. She says that he turns away, will not engage with anyone. I had met him briefly last week.

But first I call on Ken. He is a softly spoken Irishman also diagnosed with lung cancer. Entering his room, he is hooked up on oxygen, breathless. He has soft eyes and speaks with a beautiful Irish lilt.

I have not met him before but adopt a dubious familiar manner.

'Good morning Ken. How are you this morning?'

He looks at me and doesn't reply as if words are hard work.

'I'm here today if you would like any therapy.'

'I will let the nurses know if I want one later.' Perhaps said more to get rid of me than actual intent.

I say 'No pressure' knowing full well that my presence is pressure.

I sense he is more concerned with the oxygen pressure sustaining his breath than my dilemma with putting pressure on him regards a therapy. I imagine breathlessness as a constant struggle to get enough oxygen to the tissues starved blue. The brain fuzzed with the effort.

I am a surfer and the waves are high and messy.

Down the corridor I knock and enter Luke's room. He is alone. Last week Ben, his grandson, had sat by his side. Ben had said to Luke in response to his agreeing to have reflexology 'You wouldn't have had that before.'

Ben explained that Luke had been a tough man all his life. In other words, accepting something like reflexology was soft, unmanly, as if Luke had turned soft in his dying.

Luke is silent. I wonder what he thinks listening to Ben. I imagine his mind in chaos.

[Please refer the website for PP26 on Smoking skills]

Sometimes the patient presents with finely chiselled, clearly delineated symptoms ... At other times he conveys a baffling sense of the swirling, inchoate, undifferentiated affective surge, he uses many words to try and describe this sense of turbulence, but chaos often seems to get nearest the mark. The [psycho]therapist lives at the point of his patient's disclosure and has a persistent sense of being 'on the brink' of something more, as though he is a surf-rider who always wonders if the next wave will carry him further still, he is poised at the unfolding invitational edge of experience that flows out of previous experience. The 'here and now' and the 'there and then' are inextricably interdependent, and the therapist's task is to facilitate the patient's increasing self-awareness, so that their sense of inner chaos changes and what was originally perceived as inexplicable and capricious, gradually becomes coherent and purposeful.[8]

[Please refer the website for PP27 on Smoking skills]

Today, we are alone. I sit with him. I simply ask 'How are you Luke?'

He looks at me and lucidly says, 'I have no fear of dying just about the way I will die.' I imagine him lying here churning over this idea.

Kearney writes,[9] 'For most of us the focus of this fear is the actual dying process itself, what it is going to be like as we are going through it, rather than what might, or might not, happen afterward.'

Words that ring caution – 'for most of us'. Words always need interpretation within the particular moment and yet they resonate with Luke's experience. Expressing his fear reveals his vulnerable and deeper self surfacing from beneath defensive egoic layers. Fear reduces a man. It needs careful attention, perhaps guidance to lift it into the light so it might be worked through, otherwise the terrified ego will torment him as it does.

I say 'In my experience many people share your fear.'

I say that not to normalise his fear, but to suggest he is not alone. I suspect he has many weeks yet to live although I know the way things can turn quickly.

I ask 'Do you want to talk about this fear?'

Silence. The fear hovers between us.

I add 'The hospice will make you comfortable and staff are always available if you want to talk.'

Silence.

I continue, 'Not easy for a tough man.' picking up on Ben's words.

He sighs, 'No.'

How do you reassure someone fearful of the dying but not of death itself?

Perhaps reassure is the wrong word that sets me down the wrong track.

Perhaps simply to acknowledge the fear without flinching. Perhaps I should not interfere. He is alone, the liminality of dying betwixt and between.[10]

Elias writes,[11] 'For some of the dying it might be right to be alone. Perhaps they are able to dream and not want to be disturbed. One must sense what they need.'

One must sense what they need. I imagine an army of women march to put him right, anxious, like Corin, because he will not give himself to them, will not surrender himself. I can feel the pressure to submit.

I mix oils that give a strong earthy aroma; frankincense, patchouli and juniper. Yang oils, masculine oils. Nothing soft about these oils. I explain them, reinforcing their yang quality.

I place my hands along each foot. Listening. Sensing the tides. I do not try and force this sensation but let his body speak to me. Yet the tidal rhythm alludes me.

I have been told these tides are more difficult to sense with cancer patients, if in fact they can be heard at all.[12] I sense I must listen from a wider perspective, sensing the energy moving beneath each hand. Luke drifts into sleep. He stirs and smiles as if woken from a dream before closing his eyes again. I surf the messy waves.

I turn my head and gaze outside the window. I am distracted as I watch Ken sitting in the sunshine outside his room with two women at the patio table. A light breeze faintly stirs the background trees. He pulls hard on a cigarette. He pulls hard and with each exhalation he pauses to take deep breaths before the next drag; the first fag smoked and then another.

The women too pull hard on their cigarettes. It seems all are intent on this moment's guilty pleasure knowing the damage done, and now, not much to be done, at least for him. Between drags he engages in conversation; and then the final drag. The fag is stubbed. He dons again the oxygen mask.

Luke is asleep. I wash my hands and quietly leave him. I imagine the knot looser.

Later I tell Corin, the doctor, I had seen Luke. She says it is good I am a man, that some men need other men, beyond comfort into understanding perhaps only known between men. Men amongst men who can tough it out, adapting as necessary from the unfolding drama. Like chameleons.

Later, I ask myself -could I have responded differently, in particular my response 'In my experience many people share your fear.'

Did I say that for my benefit as something to say or for his benefit so he felt less alone with his fear? Using 'Six Category Intervention Analysis' as a reflective framework[13] I frame my response as 'supportive' and 'giving information'.

I imagine other responses:

Cathartic – 'I sense it is difficult for you to express your fear'

Catalytic – 'Tell me about your fears'

Giving advice – 'Why not talk to the doctor about it [knowing Corin had tried] or maybe someone else you can relate to?'

Confrontational – 'Holding in your fear won't help deal with it.'

Perhaps to create space I could have said 'Let's think about what you've just said.'

What would have been the consequences of these different responses? I sense the cathartic may have worked well. Yet I imagine he would have said 'yes' or else just turned his head away. Saying 'yes' might have opened a catalytic space but that might have been too soon. I rule out the confrontational and giving-advice responses.

It's helpful to consider these. Seeds planted in my mind. I sense there are no prescriptions.

I think about Luke in the context of the 'good death'.

Reading *Death's dominion* I am caught on the idea of 'coherence' – that a good death is related to dying in a coherent way with the way someone has lived.

Woods writes,[14] 'For Dworkin (1993),[15] the idea of coherence is closely tied to personal autonomy.'

Woods quotes Dworkin 'making someone die in a way that others approve, but he believes a horrifying contradiction of his life, is a devastating, odious form of tyranny' [p. 217].

The counter-argument is that the terminal phase of an illness changes things.[16]

I sense the significance of Dworkin's words for Luke. Lying in a hospice bed at the mercy of women does not cohere with a tough life. Perhaps Luke feels the incoherence and struggles against it. No doubt dying is complex. We observers struggle to tune in. Yet I see also the way the hospice adopts a normative approach that may fail to see the patient.

Next week. Luke's name is missing from the list of names on the whiteboard. I immediately fear the worse but no, he has gone home. It might have gone either way in the unpredictability of hospice as if precarious fulcrums bend and shift.

The phone rings. Luke is coming back in. Things haven't gone so well. Tide's turning. Ken has died.

Part 4

[Please refer the website for PP28 on Smoking skills]

I come in for group supervision[17] with the other therapists. The supervision is mandatory. The group is facilitated by Dora, the senior clinical psychologist. I am also accountable to her. She has a manner that makes me uncomfortable as if I am being judged. I think she sees supervision as a form of quality control rather than a personal space for me to reflect.

I say I would like to talk about my experience with Luke. It doesn't go well.

Dora asks pointedly, 'Why do you think male patients need men to talk to?'

'I don't know whether they particularly do. I was asked to see him by Corin.'

'Did Corin have a problem with him?'

'She mentioned difficulty engaging with him. I would have gone to visit him in the natural flow of things anyway. However, Corin's comment made me see him differently– more as a man to man thing.'

'Do you think female staff have a problem with him?'

'I don't know. He might find it easier talking to a man but not necessarily about dying.'

' I don't accept that but let's move on. It's not really your role either.'

I feel unheard and 'put in my place'.[18] How should I respond? I resist the emotional pull into child mode in response to Dora's critical parent. I sense she feels threatened by this conversation – as if being a woman her competence has been challenged, or that Luke might respond more easily to me being a man. As the psychologist, 'talking' is her remit. Maybe I've trodden on her toes. The hospice is very female-oriented- all the clinicians are women except for two male therapists, but then we are marginal anyway.

I risk 'Do I tread on your toes talking to Luke?'

'Perhaps you interfere with our approach, leaving him confused.'

I want to argue that I have no particular approach. That I just talk with him. Perhaps it is they who create confusion in Luke's head? Pressure building. No point in digging my grave any deeper! Instead I ask 'If you were in my shoes how would you have responded to Luke?'

A pregnant pause before Zenda, one of the other therapists who has been at the hospice many years and sees herself as the lead therapist, challenges my decision to use 'yang' oils: 'It is good practice to balance yin and yang oils. If we want to help people like Luke then balancing the oils we use will help him to find balance, won't it?'

I reply 'Well, I have no evidence to support your supposition, although I was taught in much the same way. Given that these oils do have yin and yang qualities- then my rationale is to strengthen his yang, firm up his toughness to face out his predicament. Logic suggests that yin oils will soften his toughness make him more vulnerable.'

Zenda retorts 'I don't agree.'

'OK, we beg to differ but it is an important aspect of therapy to consider. Have you given him a therapy?'

Zenda is hesitant 'No … he declined when I offered.'

Dora retorts in her inimitable 'critical parent' manner,[19] 'Such matters are not the remit of complementary therapists. Skilled psychologists will pick up this issue. I imagine he felt even more alone when you said that. He needn't tough it out, he has experienced and skilled support to help him.'

I am browbeaten. Better to yield.[20] I know they want to soften Luke up so he will talk about his fears. In doing so he can release them and feel calmer. But maybe that's not his style. He needs to be in control – so we should strengthen his defences not break them down and leave him more vulnerable. At least that's my perspective. Maybe I'm wrong? Maybe there is no right or wrong. That implies some objective reality to judge against. I must interpret the situation as I find it, although the assumptions I bring to the situation are clearly significant in governing my responses. I sink into the swampy lowlands[21] without a helping hand.

Zenda says she wants to talk about her upset when a young mother recently died. Dora licks her lips with glee. Yet again I am left frustrated with my supervision. I need to change this arrangement. Perhaps the word supervision is wrong in the wrong hands as if those hands are intent on shaping your practice to conform rather than being creative. Guided reflection sounds better. Whatever, it should be fecund.[22]

Part 5

Along Lowestoft beach I take pictures of groynes – vivid images that remind me of the destruction of lung cancer. Dear smoker – imagine your lungs cracked, split open, covered in green and black gunge. In hospice we see the end-result. Perhaps I should show these images to young people. Ask them to imagine. Tell them they have a choice.

[Please refer the website for PP29 on Smoking skills]

Part 6

The week after next I am again at the hospice. Luke has been discharged to a nursing home. I wish I had seen him. Corin says he wouldn't talk about his fears.

I say 'he toughed it out then.'

Corin looks at me and says, 'I guess he did in his own way. You might drop in on Max. He's another one we're having difficulty[23] with.'

Should I say 'What does Dora think?'

But Dora seems distant, out of the picture.

[Please refer the website for PP30-45 on Smoking skills]

Max, your grey moustache and trimmed grey beard reminiscent of Frank Zappa, that worn face. Your demeanour laid back yet open. I do not say 'I was asked to see you because you were having difficulty.'

'Hi Max, I'm Chris. I'm the Tuesday therapist. Just popping by to say hello and I'm around today.'

He is very welcoming 'Come in, take a seat.'

I pull up the seat. I am not the therapist standing over. I say 'Tell me what's been happening.'

Max articulately relates his story. 'I was diagnosed with lung cancer 18 months ago. We were managing the pain with co-codamol but now that's not enough. The pain bites deeper. Yet I feel strange on morphine and now a chest infection complicates things. I was in the USA with my family … I know it was a risk going … but we needed the holiday. Something inside seemed to snap. I knew I was in trouble so we came back and I got admitted to the hospice. Great place.'

Max, you show me the swollen lymph nodes, grey lumps stretching, yet you play down the idea of fear about them invading you.

Max laughs, 'Best to put me down?'

'How do I do that?' I ask.

Max laughs again. He has no answer but I sense his fear bubbling through his protective veneer.

'So what can you offer?' he says.

He chooses reflexology. 'I've had it before. It was good.'

I feel a strong vibe with Max. He was a roadie for many years. Indeed he had met his Italian wife as a roadie in Italy 'Couldn't speak a word of the language, but she was beautiful. Our eyes met and that was that.'

I mix the same yang oils I had used with Luke. Max comments favourably on their pungent earthiness. Patchouli is the old hippy incense he much appreciates.

My hands listen along the soles of his feet. The left foot is dead, cold like marble. No sense of the tides. I open my perception wider. Maybe after five minutes, energy stirs.

A similar pattern with the right foot. I sense the energy has been blocked for some time; channels that have petrified in the cancer-ridden wilderness. With each stroke of my hands I imagine the accumulated gunge of lung tumour being washed out with the tide.

Your wife enters and sits quietly in meditative pose. Her phone intermittently bleeps in her bag on an adjacent chair. She does not stir; at least until you cough and cough again. Stricken lungs straining; she is up passing you a sputum pot for you to spit your phlegm. Images of groynes comes to mind. Lung cancer is not pleasant.

Afterwards Max is grateful. I leave them in peace.

How might Max view it?

Part 7 Max's song

[Please refer the website for PP46 on Smoking skills]

I'm Max. I'm dying of lung cancer. The fucking fags have done me. Gina, my lovely wife sits by my side. Her presence makes me suffer, feelings of guilt pull at me. The fucking fags and now I'm fucked. Of course you never expect it to hit you … and even when it did, that it could be dealt with …

How should I die, as a man? What counts as masculinity? I try not show my feelings, thoughts or behaviours that might be interpreted by the observer as 'unmanly'. Yet I have a softer side wrapped within the macho. Perhaps my 'unmanly' feelings, thoughts and behaviours leak out in other, more subliminal ways, know doubt keenly observed by the voyeuristic personnel who demand my engagement with death. All such talk feels pointless. I try and be a good husband, perhaps an even better husband, comforting Gina is easier than she comforting me. My boys now young men. Their 'manly' behaviour being cool containing the hurt.

How do I compensate for my denial of feelings?

A knock on the door.

'Come in,' I rasp.

Chris walks in. A rare man amongst all the women here. Jim, the maintenance guy, sometimes drops by for a chat. Can talk to him. Old hippies. A wavelength thing.

Chris asks how am I? His eyes do to not deviate and I have nowhere to hide. His talk casual and ordinary, as if he somehow knows what it is like for me. My head full of stuff but how to say it without crumbling? He draws me in and I spill it out. It is a relief. I suspect unmanly behaviour is threatening especially to those who hold rigid perceptions of how men should behave when facing death. All the docs and nurses are women. Caring, but I sense they struggle with my gruffness, my denial of feelings, my dismissiveness and general resistance to their help. Any whiff of spiritual stuff I'm off. Why do people try so hard to be nice? But I am fragile. My masculine identity has been about control. Now, I am not in control. The wounded and perishing hunter-gatherer. Perhaps that's why I exaggerate my resistance to their control. Even my wife fussing irritates me. Men have historically oppressed women and now the tide turns.

Part 8

Scene 1

[Please refer the website for PP47 on Smoking skills]

Walking home from the station. I pass by the Italian café. A man sweeps cigarette butts from the pavement; hundreds of them litter; the gutter overflowing with them.

I imagine rows of men standing outside pulling at cigarettes. With each inhalation the drop of tar condenses from the smoke to line and irritate the lung. Perhaps Max and Luke and Ken and all the others stand amongst them, laughing in the quiet afternoon; drop by drop accumulating, until the lungs are dark with tar; clogged alveoli; stricken walls breaking down. Signs of emphysema; breathless; ankles swelling. That irritating cough and cough and stained sputum …

> Max pauses from the therapy and coughs
> Spits his blackened phlegm into the sputum pot …

Cell changes; tumours form; and the cancer has you … and maybe if you are lucky the surgeon's blade will cut it out. If not the grim reaper sharpens his blade.

[Please refer the website for PP48 on Smoking skills]

Scene 2

The man pauses to light his cigarette butt. The first drag. The tip burns brightly. Deep inhalation. That first hit as nicotine hits the blood stream. Another pull. He looks at me. My eyes avert. Everywhere I turn people are lighting up. And still fag packets litter the street with their graphic messages of death. Smoking kills. The lanes are killing fields; and yet, we try and avoid death; death is embarrassing, to be hidden, even in a hospice. We always have a choice but sometimes when something is so addictive and destructive we need help.

[Please refer the website for PP49 on Smoking skills]

Part 9

I continue to see Max over the next three weeks getting to know Gina and his two sons. Ideas of coherence spin. It transcends the idea of men need men to talk with. That seems only a part of it. And then one morning he is dead. I need to talk about this more in supervision.

Dead flowers for your grave [Open Hamlet packet]
[Please refer the website for PP50 on Smoking skills]

> I won't forget to put roses on your grave
> She said, one sad day.
> Roses that have withered in the passing of time,
> Dead flowers a requiem to your life cut short;
> She crushes the empty fag packet,
> She tosses it into a bin.
> Like life itself, crushed and tossed away.

Dying is not easy for tough men. I know this but that doesn't make it easy. Yet for the first time I have reflected on the idea of masculinity in patients and my own in response. I am a male. I am not a female. Hence my masculinity is a significant aspect of presenting myself to the patient. Do I manage my presentation? Do I adapt to the person as I find them? I certainly endeavoured to tune into Ken's, Luke's and Max's wavelength and flow with them, with the intention of helping to ease suffering.

Suffering is not a symptom to manage. Easing their suffering is not a task to be done.

I do not claim I was effective, but then how might effectiveness be measured?

Being a chameleon comes to mind. I remember a paper written about that.[24]

Something about a chameleon adapting to its environment like tuning into their wavelengths and flowing with them. Is being a chameleon being authentic? I am not a stereotype.

Fisher[25] writes:

[Please refer the website for PP51 on Smoking skills] 'The ability of male nurses to do bodywork and provide care is dependent on the way they "do" gender, that is, they have to be perceived to be performing the masculine identity that best represents the individual patient's ideology of what it is to be a man, which is set in a particular location and time.'

[Please refer the website for PP52 on Smoking skills]

I ask myself- 'what did Max want from me?' It seems a reasonable question if therapy is outcome focused. However, if therapy is process focused then the outcomes will naturally unfold. It's getting the process right! Pattern appreciation and response Richard Cowling[26] and Margaret Newman[27] come to mind. Minnesota wisdom!

More homework, more dialogue, more juxtaposition, more synthesis. Putting it all together, adding detail to the broad canvas. Of course, I might predict that Max will be more relaxed and comfortable after therapy but it is a prediction fraught with danger within the unpredictability of the moment. Good bonding stuff. What would I measure along that scale? [28]

Part 10

Two months since the last therapists' group supervision session. I am uneasy. Visions of Dora haunt. What to do about it? I could raise my uneasiness within the group itself – 'I need to talk about my concerns with our current supervision arrangement.' That would be the most responsible and assertive way to go about it although I feel anxious about this, sensing I would get little sympathy from either Dora or my peers, who are more conventional than me and reluctant to disturb things.

It goes badly as I feared. Dora says 'The group is not the place to discuss this. Supervision is provided for your benefit so you should take a more positive and responsible approach. If you make an appointment we can discuss your work here.'

I am the problem. I say 'I want to talk about coherence and the idea of the good death.'

Dora reminds me that it is not my turn to share. I am silenced.

Next week I arrange to discuss supervision with Carol, the medical director. We have a good relationship. She, like Corin, appreciates my dynamic approach to therapy even though it might tread on the toes of others. 'Let's have lunch next time you're in – next Tuesday.'

'So Chris, I guess supervision isn't going well?'

'No. I don't like to complain to you. I have tried dealing with it in the group but to no avail. Dora is intent on imposing her values, roles and responsibilities on the group-putting us in a place she defines rather than enabling us to grow and find our own place.[29] Her psychologist persona takes over, blurring a distinction between what is therapy and what is supervision.'

I point out eight issues with the current supervision arrangement:

[Please refer the website for PP53 on Smoking skills]

1 Dora stands outside the group as a facilitator.
2 She is ultimately the therapists' manager.
3 She views supervision as a form of quality control reflected in her judgemental and confrontational style, with her focus on outcome rather than on process.
4 Her style borders on psychotherapy, as if supervision is a form of therapy blurring distinction between supervision and therapy.
5 The group is a ghetto of therapists.
6 It is mandatory to attend – indeed, missing more than one session in six can lead to a termination of work at the hospice.
7 Sessions every two months make it difficult to maintain a sense of continuity.
8 Lack of contract.

'What is your solution?' Carol asks seemingly not fazed. I appreciate the style – don't simply post problems but post solutions.

I pull out my list and say I would prefer:

[Please refer the website for PP54 on Smoking skills]

1 A system whereby the facilitator is part of the group rather than posing as an 'expert' and whereby facilitation is rotated, with the remit of developing facilitation skills.
2 A system whereby each session is evaluated at the end of each session to summarise what we have learnt about practice and the supervision process.
3 A non-judgemental approach whereby people can share difficult issues with trust.
4 A focus on growth and practice development, not a focus on quality control — where what counts as quality is set by the facilitator / organisation.
5 Mixed groups spanning the breadth of professionals who work at the hospice – this would enable cross-fertilization of ideas and build up professional relationships that would flow out into practice.
6 Voluntary attendance – this would be a mark of professional commitment to self-development, perhaps encouraging people to keep a portfolio useful for any Continuing Professional Development (CPD) accountability.
7 Sessions offered weekly. Perhaps no more than eight people per group. I am uncertain about the same people meeting in the same group.
8 An agreed working contract, subject to regular review.

[Please refer the website for PP55 on Smoking skills]
Carol responds, 'I can see you have really given this some thought. I appreciate that. It's easy to set up systems that then become routine without critique. Indeed critique can seem personal, as I'm sure Dora would agree. Practicalities always seem tricky – making good ideas pragmatic yet effective. I will put 'supervision review' on the agenda for the next senior team away day. Would you like to attend for the supervision slot to make the case?'

'Yes I would. I hope we can dialogue about this rather than get caught up in emotional tension.'

As if to soften my critique I add, 'I do value the organisation creating supervision space for the voluntary therapists. It is so easy to feel marginalised, on the edge of care where what we do is often simply regarded as "relaxation" rather than a meaningful therapeutic approach.'

The moral being if you aren't paid then it can't be worth much. However I feel a tinge of anxiety anticipating confronting Dora. I do not like conflict but sometimes, ethically, we have to make a stand. Practice is political. I will not yield.

Denouement

The meeting is postponed. Dora is sick. I wonder – is that avoidance?

Luke did not die well. He had a lot of pain and needed much medication. I imagine his soul pain bubbling up, disturbing.

I resonate with the idea of coherence.

The way theory opens the shutters. Maybe Corin and others just couldn't get on Luke and Max's wavelengths, wrapped up, as they are, in the 'hospice' model.

Maybe Luke would have preferred a diet of Clint Eastwood and Charles Bronson films than 'psycho-babble'.

> The hospice a place of death,
> No place for tough men.
> Or perhaps it is.
> Soften you up
> So dying is easier,
> A job well done.
> But is it?

Part 11

Dialogue with audience.

Endnotes

1 Endnotes Loori, J. D. (2005) *The Zen of creativity: cultivating your artistic life.* Ballantine Books, New York, p. 84.
2 Loori op. cit. p. 98.
3 Wiley-Blackwell website
4 Wheatley, M. J. (1999) *Leadership and the new science.* Berrett-Koehler, San Francisco.
5 Okri, B. (1997) *A way of being free.* Phoenix House, London. Okri writes – 'in storytelling there is always transgression, and in all art. Without trangression, without the red boundary, there is no danger, no risk, no *frisson*, no experiment, no discovery, and no creativity. Without extending some hidden or visible frontier of the possible, without disturbing something of the incomplete order of things, there is no challenge … [taken from *The joys of storytelling 2*, pp. 63–66.
6 The words 'death is over there not here' are taken from a Murakami novel.
7 Becker, R. (1997) *Life in motion.* Stillness Press, Portland, p. 27.
8 Cox, M. (1988) *Structuring the therapeutic process: compromise with chaos* [revised edition]. Jessica Kingsley, London.
9 Kearney M (1997) *Mortally wounded: stories of soul pain, death and healing.* Touchstone, New York, p. 15.
10 I take the term liminality as related to performance from Turner – the idea of crossing a threshold from one state into a liminal space 'betwixt and between' before entering another state. The expression 'in limbo' stems from the same idea. Turner also drew on van Gennep's notion of rites of passage — as if a passage is a liminal state between one thing and another. Turner, V. (1988) *The anthropology of performance.* PAJ Publications, New York, pp. 25, 26.
11 Elias, N. (1985) *The loneliness of dying.* Basil Blackwell, Oxford, p. 84.
12 Becker, R. (1997) op. cit.
13 Heron, J. (1975) *Six category intervention analysis.* Human Potential Research Group, University of Surrey, Guildford.
14 Woods, S. (2007) *Death's dominion: ethics at the end of life.* Open University Press, Maidenhead.
15 Dworkin, R. (1993) *Life's dominion: an argument about abortion., euthanasia and individual freedom.* Alfred A Knopf, New York.
16 Sandman, L. (2005) *A good death: on the value of death and dying.* Open University Press, Maidenhead.

17 See pages 250-1 for a discussion on clinical supervision.
18 Mayeroff, M. (1971) *On caring*. Harper Perennial, New York.
19 See pages 158, 198 for a discussion on Transactional Analysis.
20 'better to yield' refers to the idea that it is better to yield than to perish without a sense of failure. It is the top rung of the assertiveness ladder [see pages 197-201]. The idea stems from Jones, R. and Jones, G. (1996) *Earth dance drum*. Commune-E-Key, Salt Lake City, p. 281.
21 'swampy lowlands' refers to the idea that much of professional practice is like swampy lowlands as opposed to the hard high ground of technical rationality. Schon, D. (1987) *Educating the reflective practitioner*. Jossey-Bass, San Francisco.
22 Fecund: producing or capable of producing an abundance of offspring or new growth; highly fertile. [Google search.]
23 But what is difficult? Simply someone who for whatever reason makes the practitioner anxious. Hence the practitioner responds to manage his anxiety, for example by labelling and marginal-ising the person as 'difficult'. See Johnson, M. and Webb, C. (1995) Rediscovering unpopular patients : the concept of social judgment. *Journal of Advanced Nursing* 21, 466–475.
24 Aranda, K. and Street, A. (1999) Being authentic and being a chameleon: nurse–patient inter-action revisited. *Nursing Inquiry* 6.2, 75–82.
25 Fisher, M. J. (1999) Being a chameleon: labour processes of male nurses performing bodywork. *Journal of Advanced Nursing* 65, 2668–2677.
26 Cowling, W. R. (2000) Healing as appreciating wholeness. *Advances in Nursing Science* 22.3, 16–32.
27 Newman, M. (1999) The rhythm of relating in a paradigm of wholeness. *Image: Journal of Nursing Scholarship* 31.3, 227–230.
28 Tajero developed a scale for measuring patient–nurse bonding – as if such a thing might be measurable. It reflects the absurdity of a technical rational approach. I write it tongue in cheek! Tejero, L. M. S. (2010) Development and validation of an instrument to measure nurse patient bonding. *International Journal of Nursing Studies* 47.5, 608–615.
29 Mayeroff, M. (1971) *On caring*. Harper Perennial, New York.

Chapter 25

Anthea: An Inquiry into Dignity

Christopher Johns and Otter Rose-Johns

The performance turn implodes the curriculum

Introduction

The experience that forms the performance narrative 'Anthea: An Inquiry into Dignity' was shared by a staff nurse in guided reflection as part of a BSc Nursing programme for post-registration nurses. The post-discharge experience to her home is fiction, constructed to raise and problematise contemporary issues in end of life care. The reflection by Murphy in Part 3 is based on personal experience.

Performance opens a dialogical space with the audience and performance participants towards social action. As Denzin (2003: 41) writes:[1]

> Each performance event becomes an occasion for the imagination of a world where things can be different, a radical utopian space where a politics of hope can be experienced.

And yet the performance must adequately communicate its critique of those social conditions that are unsatisfactory, giving authentic voice to voices that have been marginalised or silenced.

The performance is accompanied by a sequence of paintings intuitively produced by Otter as a dialogue with the words. Indeed the performance was originally conceived and performed to enable 'painting pauses' whereby an audience can intuitively dialogue through painting with the words.[2] For publishing reasons, it is not possible to show the accompanying paintings marked* in the text. However, the full set of paintings are available on Wiley-Blackwell's website.[3] Music may enhance the performance, although one must be careful of copyright breach.

The performance contains a number of 'empathic poems'[4] I wrote to represent the voices of different players to contrast with Anthea's voice. In a similar vein to painting images, the audience could be asked to write these poems at suitable moments to put themselves in the shoes of the various players. For example, the audience could be asked, 'How does Kate feel about this experience?' whilst the performance is paused.

Such activity draws the audience deeper into the performance as they focus creatively on emerging issues whilst naturally reflecting on their own experiences.

'Anthea: An Inquiry into Dignity' has been performed to nurses, therapists and General Practitioner trainees The intention, as with all performance narratives, is to open a dialogical space to stir social action towards creating a better world for patients and practitioners.

When performed with therapists at the Christie Hospital in Manchester, we invited audience members to participate, briefing and giving volunteers written texts. Similarly, you may perform your own version of 'Anthea: An Inquiry into Dignity'. Or you can write your own performance.

Cast

Beady Eye
Anthea/ Maisey
Kate [nurse]
The GP locum
Olive [Hospital chaplain]
Carol [Clinical Nurse Specialist]
Murphy [Anthea's husband]
Rachel }
Jaimee } Anthea's children
Lizzie [Friend of Anthea's]
Helen [Health Visitor]

[Please refer the website for PP1 on Anthea].

Part 1

Beady Eye: 'Hi. I'm beady eye. I keep my beady eye on things. It is a lamentable fact that people are not always treated with dignity. Why is that? Without doubt managers get wrapped up in bureaucracy and targets. Resources are strapped. Practitioners are stressed, have low morale. As a consequence they lose sight of values. Work becomes a chore. People become numbers to crunch. I am going to stick my beady eye out and say that a failure to ensure dignity is a failure of leadership.

Let's say that one perspective on leadership is to enable every practitioner to take responsibility for their performance within a community of shared values.

Yet in the transactional organisation such aspiration becomes blurred in norms and anxiety. Indeed, real leadership may be resisted because it threatens the status quo.

Stories are wake-up calls to challenge unsatisfactory practice, norms and complacency. Listen to and reflect on Anthea's story of suffering in the face of dying.

I wonder if people remember these words by Cicely Saunders:

[Please refer the website for PP2 on Anthea]. 'You matter because you are you, and you matter to the end of your life. We will do all we can not only to help you die peacefully, but also to live until you die.'[5]

Performance is a call for dialogue and action. To dialogue we must first listen carefully. As you engage with this performance be curious, for nothing can be taken for granted. After the performance we invite you to dialogue and explore how the world might become a better place as a consequence. Make a note of at least one idea to dialogue with.'

[Please refer the website for PP3 on Anthea].

[Anthea sits on chair centre stage in dressing gown. Hazard tape around the chair.]

Anthea: Three days confined in this room. I have become a prisoner, alone and afraid. The door firmly shut.

I know I am dying. Treatment can only buy me time but at what cost? Hanging on as quality peels away. But I hang on. Do I have a choice? My ego resists the slide into death. The mortal coil twists. As a mother of young children it is harder to let go.

I will miss my kids growing up and those grandchildren as yet unborn. That's tough to contemplate. My burden on others burdens me. Others do not understand. Worse they think they do.

Dying is not easy. I need people to be sensitive. My suffering when that fails.

My words make my suffering visible. My words are resistance. Claiming agency even at this late stage. Words to open dialogue. Words to find self.[6] I imagine each woman responds differently.[7] We are not numbers to crunch.

My name is Anthea. I've never liked that name. I prefer Maisey, my middle name. I am 45 years old. Two years ago my life was normal, largely taken for granted. Married with three kids. I worked as an accountant. My hobby is painting. And then I got breast cancer. I don't know what caused it. My mum died of it. Maybe smoking when I was younger? Being a good mother I gave up when pregnant.

It was treated. First a lumpectomy and removal of glands then chemo – that awful FEC regime where all my hair fell out and my guts puked up no matter what anti-emetics they gave me, had me going loopy climbing walls.

[Please refer the website for PP4 on Anthea].

Red poison in my veins. *I shudder* remembering.
Then radiotherapy and then hormones. The full ticket.
I thought I was OK, In the pink so to speak.
Life could almost return to normal where I could wear the 'normal-me' mask and then everyone is OK. Wear a 'cancer-mask' and people shrink away. I say normal but it left a fear of relapse. I am always looking over my shoulder.

And then *it* did come back. *It* spread through my body. The 'normal-me' mask slipped. More chemo, more sickness. My life pumped full of holes through which I leaked and drained away. Despair leaked through the smile.

Outbursts of poor me.

[Please refer the website for PP5 on Anthea].

Now they come wearing gowns and cheery masks, looming large from the grey. Like spectres emerging from a dense mist; no doubt recoiling in terror, only approaching when necessary. They observe me from a distance as if indifferent to my plight. Their strained tolerance as I push that call-bell yet again. And then no-one came, leaving me alone when I was so upset and in pain. They must think I am a pain. I guess they see many poor sods like me that any empathy or compassion they might have had has drained away.

Perhaps they fear me – 'Get too close you might catch it!' Maybe I'll grab one and see how they react!

One nurse, doing my observations, asks 'Do you have any pain Anthea?'

I grimace. Being called Anthea riles.

Bite my tongue. She doesn't introduce herself. I should inquire 'What's your name?' but I have become passive.

I say 'Yes, I ache all over.'

Sounding like a textbook she inquires, 'How would you describe your pain?'

I look into her eyes but they turn away.

What words might capture my pain?

Trip through the alphabet: Alone, anguish, abandoned, alienated; Black, boxed, burdened, betrayed; Confused, chaotic, crap; Dog-tired, disembodied, desperate, despair...

'Dog-tired' reminds me of Nietzsche who said, 'I have given a name to my pain and call it dog.'[8] Not that I know much about philosophy.

Empty; Frightened, fragmented, filthy... all that diarrhoea; Leper, lost; Mute, mangled, mugged, mangy; Panic, punished, pitiful, powerless; Squashed, shunned, suffering, shell-shocked... cancer a shell exploding; Terrible, trapped, tortured; Yuk ...yuk is so evocative.

[Please refer the website for PP6 on Anthea].

I say 'my pain is like torture'.

At first, she doesn't know what to say. Then she says 'I mean what type of pain – sharp, dull, spasmodic..?'

She doesn't get it!

Frustrated I reply 'I'm fine really, it's only a slight niggle. Two paracetamol should do it'.

I wear my 'I'm fine' mask, not wanting to open a can of worms

She said 'Are you sure?'

'Yes, yes.'

I need some morphine but her manner makes me defiant. I sense my pain splashes off her suit of armour.

Everything is chaos. I spin out of control

Give me a paint brush and it would look like this:

[Please refer the website for PP7 on Anthea].
(Kate [nurse] moves on to stage pushing a dressing trolley with catheter)

Kate [cheerily]: 'Hi, Anthea, I'm Kate, I've just come on duty. How are you?'

Anthea: Amazed that she introduced herself, I can almost forgive her for calling me Anthea.

Before I can answer, she continues 'We need to catheterise you so we can maintain a strict fluid balance'.

The catheter wrapped in its transparent sheath taunts me.

'Look, my name is Maisey!

Kate blushes as if I've hit a nerve.

Guilt bites 'Sorry, but you've caught me at a bad moment but no way you're sticking that thing in me. Take it away!'

The wave of anger rises from my gut.

Her 'cheery mask' slips.

My 'I'm fine' mask slips.

Anger gives way to self-pity, I blurt 'I didn't come here to be tortured.'

Awkwardly she replies 'I'm sorry, I hadn't realised. Look, inserting the catheter and the barrier nursing is just routine, it will help us to treat you more effectively. There's no need to take it personally.'

'But I do take it personally!' I shout. Something breaks inside. Tears flood me.

(Anthea picks up the catheter and throws it defiantly onto the floor)

[Please refer the website for PP8 on Anthea]. How is it that one person can be in the presence of another person in pain and not know it, not knowing it to the point where she herself inflicts it, and goes on inflicting it.[9]

[Please refer the website for PP9 on Anthea].

Kate is shocked at my outburst. She moves away, taking the trolley with her. For the moment, I am spared.

About 20 minutes later she returns. Now she wants to insert some suppositories! Evidently, they now think the diarrhoea is overflow from the constipation. No more catheter talk thank goodness!

Resistance is not, then, so futile!

I have been through so much that nothing could ever be embarrassing again.

Or could it?

My bottom exposed. Her fingers insert the small hard capsules. A moment's pain ...

'Ouch, that wasn't pleasant'.

She laughs- 'No as long as they do their job, eh?'

I hate this cheery banter. A few minutes later I feel this urge to shit. It just comes away from me. I am buried in shit.

Layers of paper stained in shit are monuments to my despair.

I apologise about the smell. It can't be nice work for her. Her gloved fingers buried in my shit. I imagine she must detach herself to bear it. I wonder how she sees me?

Mixed images I expect – a poor cow and a bloody nuisance.

[Please refer the website for PP10 on Anthea]. I must let this pain flow through me and pass on. If I resist or try and stop it, it will detonate inside me, shatter me, splatter my pieces against every wall and person that I touch.[10]

[Please refer the website for PP11 on Anthea].

Kate stands above me. Gently she asks 'Tell me, what has been happening?' But no words come. She pulls up a chair. I sense her concern. I spill my story – 'Three days ago I got very sick at home. The pain had been getting worse. My GP increased the morphine. I couldn't go to the toilet. I was vomiting. I must have become delirious. I remember the smell of the diarrhoea ... how awful I felt making such a mess. It just poured from me. Murphy, that's my husband, was at his wits' end. My daughter Rachel, she's only 15, I remember her crying 'Dad, dad, what's happening with mum?' Jaimee, that's my son was out somewhere. He's 17. He finds it difficult to stay in the home with all this going on. Murphy panicked and called the GP. A locum visited. He didn't know me from Eve.

He must have called the ambulance. I didn't want to come into hospital. I tried to tell him. Poor Murphy must have felt helpless. They said the single room was necessary in case my diarrhoea was infectious.

I told them I had breast cancer and that the cancer has spread to my liver and bones but I don't think they really acknowledged that. They didn't see *me*.

Kate is silent, as if she doesn't know what to say.

Kate's song

Late shift.
Woman with d and v, history of cancer.
Barrier nursed in a single room waiting test results. She needs to be catheterised.
Doctors have ordered strict fluid balance
Entering her room all gowned up, my face masked.
She looks fed up, lonely. Touchy. Anger spills from her.
I was told she was difficult, always ringing the bell for attention as if we've not got enough on our plate!
She resists me.
My anger rising.
What's her problem? [*confrontational*]
What's her problem? [*inquisitive*]
And then I saw her, a suffering woman in this single room when she didn't even want to be admitted.
If that was me … how would I feel?
We're not good at this stuff
Suffering, compassion, empathy.
Lose sight of the person.
Makes me feel helpless.
Makes me feel guilty.
Maybe tomorrow I can help her better.

Kate exits

[*Please refer the website for PP12 on Anthea*].
[*Kate enters stage*]
Anthea: Oh it's you again. How do you intend to torture me today?
(However her energy is different. Eye contact.)
Kate: How are you today Maisey?
Anthea: I blink. Someone listening at last.
It lifts me.[11] I manage a thin smile.
'OK, but I'm still stuck in this room.'
Kate responds 'Hopefully we'll get the results later this morning.'
Hopefully – I want certainty.
We both know I'm not infectious but I must remain here 'just in case'. The ball set in motion must play out its medical game.
'I'm so tired. I just want to go home.'
And then, out of the blue, Kate asks 'Do you have a religion?'
Caught on the hop I stutter 'No, well I am a Christian'.
She asks 'Would you like to see the chaplain?'
Perhaps she thinks I'm dying. Or maybe that's her solution to fix my despair? To be honest, I don't really care so I say 'OK'. I've always thought my faith matters but then

does it? In the dark night it seems to bring little solace when fear grips tighter. I know deep down that I do not have long for this earth even as I turn away from death's dark face.

The chaplain is a woman. Her dog collar caught my eye beneath the protective gown.
She says 'Hi, Maisey? I'm Olive, the chaplain. Just popping by to say hello. How are you feeling?'
I note her defensive ploy – 'just popping by', as if her presence is not always welcome.
I say 'I feel suffocated by a darkness'.
Blimey where did that come from!
It's her cue – she says '"God's love is light sprung up" – from Matthew 4 verse 16.'
These words take me by surprise. I feel an immediate surge of hope, a hope I had lost in the void of darkness. I cry and she comforts me. Poor pitiful me.

Later, Kate informs me that they have met to talk about me. I wonder about the 'they'. I imagine 'they' huddled around a table chatting about me as if I am some object. I wonder if they ever think about the way they present themselves; their patronising talk, passing judgement, planning torture, spilling pity. God I'm cynical.
A new women enters. 'Anthea?'
'No, Maisey'
'Oh I'm sorry, I'm Carol, the clinical nurse specialist for breast care. Do you mind if I sit down?'
'Go ahead,' I say
'Thanks. I hear things haven't been easy?'
All smiles but I sense she has an agenda. She continues 'I hear you weren't happy being admitted.'
'No' I reply.
'Your results are fine. You can go home. I will liaise with your GP to ensure future seamless care.'
She rambles on, the gist of which is lost on me.
'Just get me out of here' I plead, 'And make certain I don't get admitted to hospital again. I can't through this again!'
'Murphy' I had cried, 'don't let them take me'. But he did.'

[Anthea changes behind screen into home clothes]

Locum's song

Anthea was a victim of a healthcare system that threw us together within an emotional home crisis. Victim? Why do I use that word?
Listening to her, confused, babbling, the husband pleading for me to do something, the children distraught? I didn't know them. On reflection I don't feel good about the situation but could I have done better?
I can't see how. Maybe if a seamless care plan existed I could have made a different decision? I'll take it to the next GP's supervision group and explore it. Maybe something can be learned.

[Anthea moves to new chair.
Installation – Chest with drawers with vase of white flowers]

[Please refer the website for PP13 on Anthea]. I do not wish my anger and pain and fear about cancer to fossilise into yet another silence, nor to rob me of whatever strength can lie at the core of this experience, openly acknowledged and examined.

[Please refer the website for PP14 on Anthea].

Anthea: Home again. I wonder if my GP knows? I'm angry at them for letting me down. I know, I know … it's just the system but how would anyone of them like it!?

No word from them. Perhaps it's up to me to make contact but that Carol said a plan would be put in place. I don't trust them.

Murphy was reluctant for me to come home so soon. He thinks I need hospice care but that's tantamount to giving up.

I won't contemplate that move!

I know it's not easy for them.

It's not easy for any of us.

Murphy avoids my eyes when I need him to hold me. He's guilty and fearful. The children are anxious. 'Mum,' they say and then don't know what to say. No, it isn't easy for any of us. We can't talk about these things. If only we could … if only we could tell each our stories I feel our torture would lessen.[12]

[Rachel, Jaimee and Murphy tell their songs]

Rachel's poem

Upstairs in my room,
Homework piled high,
My head buried in books.
A safer place to be than downstairs
Where the air is thick with tension.
I don't know what to say to mum to make it OK
I'm scared.
Will I get it too?
Do I have that to look forward to?
Suppose I am angry at her for having that thing,
For bringing it into the house.
Why can't things be as they were?
OK, they weren't perfect in many ways,
She doesn't understand me at times.
But I love my mum.
I don't want her to die.
My friend Tracy's mum died last year,
The same thing.
It was so sad.
Upstairs, behind closed doors she doesn't see me cry.

Jaimee's poem

Mum puked up this morning.
Ugh the noise, the smell.
Thought that had all stopped?
Hope she's OK …
Things aren't spoken about in this house.
But then I don't know what to say,
Probably best to say nothing?
Mum and dad been shouting again.
He's struggling a bit …
Letting little things wind him up.
He's been a tough man all his life,

No need to take it out on me though.
She'll get better soon too I'm sure.
Yeah.
Where are my football boots?
School match today.
Got a date with Gillie on Friday night.
Be great when I pass my driving test,
Umm this body spray smells good.
Mum, mum, please get better!
Upstairs she doesn't see me cry.

Murphy's song

My precious Maisey is dying.
Time is running out,
Almost visible like a sand clock,
Yet she soldiers on,
Yoga and this and that, never stopping,
Gotta keep fit, she says.
Build up my strength.
Pretending that all is well,
Not wanting to bother us.
She keeps most things to herself.
I want to help her more.
Her irritation when I try,
'You don't understand,' she says.
I can't concentrate at work.
Worrying.
I can't face life without her.
The future is a painful mist.
She holds me when I should hold her.
Wipes my tear away when I should wipe hers.
I need to be strong, but in truth I'm falling apart.
She says it will be OK,
Her smile strained.
She has lost so much weight.
I wanted her to stay in hospital so she can be
comfortable,
But oh no, not her, stubborn to the end.
What to do for the best?
It's so hard to know,
So hard.
I feel helpless.[13]

Music – Gloomy Sunday, Billie Holiday

[Please refer the website for PP15 on Anthea]. And I began to recognize a source of power within myself that comes from the knowledge that while it is most desirable not to be afraid, learning to put fear in perspective gave me great strength.

[Anthea leads group embrace
Anthea returns to chair]

[Please refer the website for PP16 on Anthea].

Anthea

Gloomy Sunday.
I love the music of Billie Holiday.
Captures my mood.
Gloomy skies oppress me,
How I like the sun to shine.
Sombre thoughts of death haunt me.
I feel betwixt and between
in a liminal space where identity blurs.[14]

[Anthea opens one drawer and pulls out packets of antidepressants]

Anti-depressants numb me. I feel such a failure that I can't cope without them. Part of me says I must be positive and get on with life. Life is so precious. The other, darker part opens the reaper's gate.

I'm not eating much. Food doesn't taste right. I still have a bitter taste in my mouth from the chemotherapy. Thin as a rake. I'm probably size zero by now! Maybe I can get a job as a model? Funny, I've always wanted to lose weight but not like this, not that I've ever been fat although more cuddly as Murphy reminds me. No appetite for that either!

[Anthea pulls out a memory letter from her mother written shortly before she died]

My mum left me this memory letter to read after her death from breast cancer 14 years ago. How I miss her now. How I wish she were here.
[reads from the letter]

Darling Anthea
I want you to know how much I love you. I am looking down on you each day. Don't be sad but think of me smiling at you. I am at peace, free from the pain and suffering. I want you to be brave and remember me to my lovely grandchildren I barely had time to know.
Love
Mum xxxxx

She pressed lavender into the letter, her favourite smell. The way aromas hold memories. Maybe I will write letters to my family.

Talk about being positive. I've been swimming. Nothing too strenuous mind you. I tire so easily, yet, it gets me out of the house, doing something for me. I saw a notice up at the pool for yoga classes. I signed up. Sign up for anything that helps.

Even had a fag again. I stubbed it out after a few drags. My head went dizzy. The ciggie packet said 'Smoking kills'.

'Right on' I said.

Had a laugh with my friend Lizzy. I have this poach pod to poach eggs. Well, Lizzy put it on like a bra – like this.

[puts on bra]

We wondered if we could leave the egg in it as a substitute for the implant. How we laughed. Then Lizzy said the word 'poached' as if someone had 'poached' my breast.

Pun on the word poached. Geddit? Well, we thought it was funny. Black humour I suppose but better then crying. Thank God for Lizzy.

Murphy told me the other day, when I was bad tempered, 'Be a happy egg.' It reminded me of egg boxes; the one with biggies made me smile [*holds egg box*] as my breasts have always been small. I made a mask from the happy egg egg-box.

[*puts on happy egg box mask*]

Another bit of black humour but I think he saw the funny side of it. He's a good man but he's not good with the emotional stuff. All tight inside.

The Macmillan nurse came calling. She phoned and invited herself to visit, 'Just to see how things are,' as she put it.

I expect the GP sent her round. Helen's her name. Sitting there, sipping tea, observing me with a suitable gravitas-cum-cheery mask, processing me, the well-rehearsed words. Reaching towards me, my slight recoil. Don't touch me! I am not an object of pity! Her presence felt like another, more subtle form of torture. She suggested that I had work to do 'to come through cancer' into acceptance and healing;[15] the difference between a victim and being a survivor. What the fuck was she going on about! Made me feel a failure. Excuse my language.

And then, out of the blue she asked 'Where would you like to die?'

I looked at her dumbfounded. She said 'I need to ask so we can plan your care.' Talk about rubbing your face in it! I couldn't answer. Eventually I blurted 'On a beach in the Caribbean with soft yellow sand filtering between my fingers, a pina colada in reach.' She laughed awkwardly and said 'Come on Anthea, you've got to be realistic...'

'Oh come on Helen you've got to have a sense of humour.' But I didn't say that.

I said 'I suppose it depends on the circumstances?'

She said 'I'll visit again soon.'

I said defiantly 'I'll call you if I need you.'

I hadn't wanted to see a Mac nurse. They are harbingers of death. The thought of dying petrifies me. I know I have to face it, but I'm scared. Perhaps if you can push something away for long enough it will go away? I wanted to say something to Murphy but I know it will upset him. I rationalise she could help Murphy and the kids a bit. My kids, I say kids but they grow up so quickly. Jaimee looked at me this morning as if wanting to say something.

'What is it?' I said

'Oh nothing mum. See you later.'

Off to school. In his final year and then university. He's a bright kid. Caught between boy and man – what does he say to his dying mother?

Got an appointment with the oncologist tomorrow. Review treatment options. I lost my confidence in health services after the last admission. I'm undecided whether to have further chemotherapy. It didn't help in the long run, did it! And the side effects. That's scary to stop chemo! Like giving up. Death moves closer. Maybe yoga and meditation is a better approach. Help me find some stillness? I did try some meditation but my mind went into turmoil. I read something about it that made sense but Murphy said it was just New Age twaddle. I was so annoyed with him.

I read on the internet that raw carrot juice was good for cancer. What to believe in? I know some women try everything going, which reminds me of Ruth Picardie's book *Before I say goodbye* that I found immensely funny and tragic. I wet myself reading her account of what she describes as complementary medicine panic.[16]

One positive thing Helen did say was 'I can arrange for you to go to hospice day care.'

'Why?' I asked.

'Get support.' She said.

'Support for what? I don't want to sit around with other people dying of cancer like a leper colony.'

[Please refer the website for PP17 on Anthea].

'You might like some complementary therapy. It's very relaxing.' She said.

'My friend Lucy said she enjoyed some so, yes, OK, I'll give it a try just for the therapy mind you, not the other stuff thank you. I don't need public exposure.'

I didn't like visiting the hospice. Made me very self-conscious as if everyone knew why I was there. People seemed kind but the air of death about the place was disconcerting. The therapist was good at relaxing me. My feet wouldn't relax at first. I don't like my feet being touched and my nails are such a mess.

The therapy released something in me. Afterwards, it felt as if the room was completely different as if I had moved into a more still place. Outside I could hear a solitary bird singing. It was so poignant I cried.

(Anthea sits at easel, begins to paint)

I also did some artwork at the hospice. I was in my element, painting is so expressive. Like playing again. It opened the way to my heart and perhaps my soul even if some of the images appeared deeply dark! Hospices must be living places not dying places.

(Anthea returns to canvas)

[Please refer the website for PP18 on Anthea]. Get your box of crayons out and begin to colour in your vision of your heart. Let the dark-coloured memories accentuate the bright colours of your self. Trust the shadows to direct you to the light beyond. The hurtful memories will not bite so much, the good memories will lick your wounds.[17]

[Please refer the website for PP19 on Anthea].

Kate: Somewhere I read 'We must love and accept our own reflection before we can gaze into the heart of another'.[18] Many people turn away from reflection, uncomfortable with facing themselves whilst rationalising that it's all navel gazing and a waste of time.

But I know if I am to take myself seriously as a health practitioner I must first turn towards my reflection and accept it for what it is, as a platform to move towards greater authenticity and caring. That is my commitment, that is my responsibility, for my, our, patients deserve nothing less.

I took my story to the newly formed supervision group. I am informed that is the third time over the past ten years they have tried to establish such a group. Now the CQC demand such activity. We are fortunate the new grade 6 is an accomplished facilitator. My story told in a few minutes. Make a long story short. He opened up the dialogue asking how could Anthea or Maisey have been cared for more effectively, more person-centred, in tune with our newly developed vision? Other staff, some reluctant to be there, shifted uneasily. Confronting our own lack of caring is not easy work. He was insistent, yet not judgemental and gradually the group found their voice and in my opinion opened their hearts and minds. It will take time for the group to work well but with good leadership it's possible. That night I slept better, not disturbed by deceitful sleep.[19] Supervision helps me clean the smudges so I can see myself clearly, even if it is painful. But it is OK to be vulnerable in the face of the other's suffering. We just need to be skilled and poised to deal with it so we remain present in our humanness to the other in their humanness. The next day at work I felt more awake, more tuned into myself, my colleagues and most significantly, my patients. I just saw them in their suffering and was more available to them. I was inspired reading about the Burford model[20] its approach to pattern appreciation with its first cue- 'Who is this person'? a cue inviting their story … something to remind us when we lose sight of dignity.

[Please refer the website for PP20 on Anthea].
Tom's story

My first managerial role. Already I feel the transactional demand on me to run a tight ship. Yet I am resolute to be a true servant-leader, to create a practice community based on service, mutual responsibility and support.[21] Only if I respect my staff as humans doing a tough job can I expect them to treat patients with dignity as humans in their suffering. No blame and shame. We learn as a learning community. Not easy when the quality finger is pointed at me. Jabbing away in its anxiety.

[Please refer the website for PP20 on Anthea].
Murphy's story

I'm at the end of my tether.
It's not easy watching your loved one wither away as if a rotting grape on a vine.
I suppose I'm feeling sorry for myself, but also stoic not wanting to burden anyone.
Just like Maisey.
All seemed well at home for a few weeks and then she lost her appetite.
Lost weight and became very tired.
Then, one morning she said something had snapped inside her.
I knew she was dying.
I contacted Helen behind Maisey's back.
She visited and said she could arrange a hospice admission.
Maisey was angry, defiant, but I eventually persuaded her it was for the best – that they could help get her back on her feet.
I know this was a deception but it seemed to reassure her.

She died with her mouth open.
I saw a few teeth.
Made me think that I don't want people coming to see me when I die.
They tried to clamp it shut.
What is worse – open or closed?
Horrific from whatever angle.
Death is not pretty.
You can't wrap it up neatly.

When she died she was struggling to say something.
Puking green smelly bile.
She sat forward.
I held her gently.
She was trying to say something.
Words not properly formed
she couldn't see anything.

Did I imagine she said 'I love you. I love you'.
Her words slurred.
A nurse came in. 'Doesn't get much better than that' she cheerily said.
Maisey's dying she meant.
It was horrid.
I could have slapped her.
I sensed they only saw her as dying not living.
She probably needed to convince herself so she could sleep more easily. Choked, I just wanted to get out of there

[Please refer the website for PP20 on Anthea].

Rachel's song

Dad buried in his grief.'Come on Dad, dig yourself out of it.'
But he doesn't know how. The house a shrine. Morbid. My mum's
face everywhere. I miss my mum. We are going to have a memorial
service at the hospice. Perhaps the trigger for moving on. Maybe then
the house can breathe again.
Elvis has not yet left the building.

Summary

Performance narrative opens a dialogical space to engage with an audience as social action towards creating a better world – the sixth dialogical movement.[22] The audience are invited to engage with the performance with open hearts and minds, given that performance is often experienced as a whole-body phenomenon rather than a cognitive one. Without doubt, the performance stirs the audience's own experiences and inner dialogue between these experiences and the performance. Perhaps everything about palliative or end of life care is encapsulated within this performance narrative and with skilled guidance can be teased out for dialogue. Alternatively, the audience can be asked at the beginning to identify at least one issue to dialogue. The scope for performance narrative integral to curriculum, both prepared narratives such as 'An Inquiry into Dignity' and 'Smoking Kills', and ones practitioners can construct from their own experiences,[23] is vast with immense creative learning potential.

Endnotes

1   Denzin, N. (2003) *Performance ethnography: critical pedagogy and the politics of culture*. Sage., Thousand Oaks, CA, p. 41.
2   This exercise was included in the MSc Leadership in Health Care programme to promote right brain play and creativity.
3   Wiley-Blackwell website …
4   See Chapter 5.
5   http://www.azquotes.com/quote/521987
6   The self meaning 'a person's essential being that distinguishes them from other people'. [*Concise OED*, p. 934]

7   Consider – each woman responds to the crisis that breast cancer brings to her life out of a whole pattern, which is the design of who she is and how her life has been lived. Lorde, A. (1980) *The cancer journals*. Spinsters, INK. Argyle, NY, p. 9.

8   Nietzsche, F. W. and Kaufmann, W. A. (1974) *The gay science*. Random House, New York.

9   Scarry, E. (1985) *The body in pain: the making and unmaking of the world*. Oxford University Press, Oxford. p. 12.

10 Audre Lorde, op. cit., p. 12.

11 Reference to Rael:

> When a new idea calls our attention to its reality, what is going on is that energy wants to lift us. It starts to lift us to a higher place where we can become what we are going to be next. When it begins to lift to a higher level something dramatic can happen. What is interesting about this lifting energy is that when it happens to us, it also happens to other people who are also being lifted to the next level. (Rael, J. (1993) *Being and vibration*. Tulsa: Council Oak Books, see pp. 88, 89.)

12 Lindholm, I., Rehnsfeldt, A., Arman, M. and Hamrin, E. (2002) Significant others' experiences of suffering when living with women with breast cancer. *Scandinavian Journal of Caring Science* 16, 248–255.

13 Lindholm et al., op.cit., p. 250.

14 'betwixt and between' – Anthea's narrative can be viewed as representing a liminal space betwixt and between (Turner 1969). At first she is put in a position of extreme vulnerability, stripped of former identities and position in the social world – she enters a time/ place where they are not that, or not this, neither here or there, in the midst of a social journey from one social self to another – for the time being they are [seemingly] powerless and blurred identity. Secondly, she is inscribed with a new identity despite her desire to hold onto her old identity. She is seemingly powerless to halt this inevitable transition.
Turner, V. (1969) *The ritual process: structure and anti-structure*. Aldine, Chicago, p. 95.

15 Perrault, A. and Bourbannais, F. G. (2005) The experience of suffering as lived by woman with breast cancer. *International Journal of Palliative Nursing* 11.10, 510–519.

16 Ruth Picardie (1998) *Before I say goodbye*. Penguin Books, London; see pp. 76–79.

17 Jones, R. and Jones, G .(1996) *Earth dance drum*. Commune-E-Key, Salt Lake City, p. 72.

18 Jones and Jones, op. cit., p. 148.

19 Okri writes, 'Quietly, or dramatically, storytellers are reorganisers of accepted reality, dreamers of alternative histories, disturbers of deceitful sleep.' Okri, B. (1997) *A way of being free*. Phoenix House, London, p. 63. Cited in Johns. C. (2004) *Being mindful, easing suffering; reflections on palliative care*. Jessica Kingsley, London, pp. 60–63.

20 The Burford model was developed at Burford hospital in 1989 as a reflective and person-centred approach to clinical practice. Johns, C. (1994) *The Burford NDU Model: caring in practice*. Blackwell Scientific, Oxford; Johns, C. (2013) *Becoming a reflective practitioner*. Wiley-Blackwell, Oxford; see Chapter **19**.

21 The idea of servant leadership is inspired by Robert Greenleaf's book *Servant-leadership*: Greenleaf, R. (1977/2002) *Servant leadership: a journey into the nature of legitimate power and greatness*. Paulist Press, New York. See also *Mindful leadership* for an analysis of realizing genuine leadership in a transactional culture. Johns, C. (2015) *Mindful leadership: a guide for the health care professions*. Palgrave Macmillan, London.

22 See Chapter 5, 'Six dialogical movements of narrative construction'.

23 See Chapters 9 and 16.

Appendices

Becoming a Reflective Practitioner, Fifth Edition. Edited by Christopher Johns.
© 2017 John Wiley & Sons Ltd. Published 2017 by John Wiley & Sons Ltd.
Companion Website: www.wiley.com/go/johns/reflectivepractitioner

Appendix 1

BSc Becoming a reflective and effective practitioner programme

This is a level 3, 60 credit programme, delivered over two semesters as part of the BSc Nursing studies degree enabling qualified practitioners to obtain a degree. The programme is open to 16 practitioners divided into two groups, each group facilitated by a teacher. The groups switch over guides for the second semester to broaden the learning experience.

Each semester comprised 15 weeks interspersed with a number of workshops = 20 guided reflection sessions + 10 workshops. Each session is 3 hours.

Workshops:

- Contracting guided reflection
- Reflection through art × 2
- Developing a vision of practice
- Ethics
- Managing self
- Conflict management
- Leadership
- Critiquing theory
- Evaluating guided reflection [see appendix 4]

Appendix 2

Guided reflection evaluation tool

Introduction

It is imperative to evaluate the effectiveness of guided reflection, both in terms of process and learning outcome to open a dialogical space to explore with guides and peers how guided reflection can become more effective. Clearly this requires an openness by both practitioners and guides – itself a reflection of the guidance relationship.

Guided reflection evaluation tool

This tool has been designed to enable you to reflect on the quality of your individual or group guided reflection/ clinical supervision. The information will facilitate giving feed-back to your guide/ supervisor concerning the effectiveness of supervision.

How long have you been in supervision with your current supervisor?	
Is your supervisor [please circle]	Line manager Non-line manager within the organisation Outside the organisation
What is your grade?	
What is the grade/ position of your supervisor?	
How frequently did you contract supervision?	Every ……………….. days
How frequently [on average] do you actually have supervision?	Every ……………….. days

Whilst completing the tool is perhaps time-consuming, please complete it carefully and honestly. *In particular, please comment on your scores with specific examples.*

Mark along each scale the extent you agree with each statement:

5   most strongly agree
1   least agree

1	I felt safe to disclose my experiences	5	4	3	2	1

Comment

2	It was easy to identify experiences to reflect on	5	4	3	2	1

Comment

| 3 | I always came to each session prepared to share an experience | 5 | 4 | 3 | 2 | 1 |

Comment

| 4 | I never cancelled sessions | 5 | 4 | 3 | 2 | 1 |

Comment

| 5 | The balance of challenge and support was excellent [I didn't feel too threatened or comfortable] | 5 | 4 | 3 | 2 | 1 |

Comment

| 6 | Guidance has inspired me | 5 | 4 | 3 | 2 | 1 |

Comment

| 7 | Guidance helped me clarify key issues and gain new insights into my practice | 5 | 4 | 3 | 2 | 1 |

Comment

| 8 | I have become very reflective | 5 | 4 | 3 | 2 | 1 |

Comment

| 9 | I have become more open and curious about my practice | 5 | 4 | 3 | 2 | 1 |

Comment

| 10 | I felt I was being moulded into becoming the guide's 'clone' | 5 | 4 | 3 | 2 | 1 |

Comment

| 11 | I have become aware of the factors that influence the way I think, feel and respond within situations | 5 | 4 | 3 | 2 | 1 |

Comment

| 12 | I am more aware/ focused on my role responsibility , authority, and autonomy | 5 | 4 | 3 | 2 | 1 |

Comment

| 13 | The input of theory was both relevant and substantial | 5 | 4 | 3 | 2 | 1 |

Comment

| 14 | Work has become more meaningful and interesting | 5 | 4 | 3 | 2 | 1 |

Comment

| 15 | Guidance picked me up when I felt overwhelmed | 5 | 4 | 3 | 2 | 1 |

Comment

| 16 | Reflection has helped me to express my ideas, opinions, and feelings | 5 | 4 | 3 | 2 | 1 |

Comment

| 17 | Guidance enabled me to tackle issues that I might otherwise would have avoided | 5 | 4 | 3 | 2 | 1 |

Comment

| 18 | Guidance helped me deal with negative emotions [such as anger, failure, outrage, guilt, distress, resentment] | 5 | 4 | 3 | 2 | 1 |

Comment

| 19 | I am more in control of 'who I am' | 5 | 4 | 3 | 2 | 1 |

Comment

| 20 | My guide really listened to me | 5 | 4 | 3 | 2 | 1 |

Comment

| 21 | I was happy with my guide | 5 | 4 | 3 | 2 | 1 |

Comment

| 22 | I never felt judged by my guide | 5 | 4 | 3 | 2 | 1 |

Comment

23	We constantly reviewed the way guidance has enabled me to develop and sustain my practice	5	4	3	2	1

Comment

24	We always commenced each session by reviewing the previous session and picking up issues	5	4	3	2	1

Comment

25	Guided reflection sessions were never interrupted	5	4	3	2	1

Comment

26	I always knew what I needed to do at the end of each session	5	4	3	2	1

Comment

27	My Guide always wanted 'to fix' the problem for me	5	4	3	2	1

Comment

28	My supervisor was overly parental and patronising	5	4	3	2	1

Comment

29	The environment for guided reflection was excellent	5	4	3	2	1

Comment

Use this space to make any further comment

Guided reflection evaluation tool /f - revised March 2002.

Appendix 3

The classroom critical incident questionnaire (Brookfield 1996: 115)

The Guide invites the student to submit these anonymously. He analyses the responses and gives feedback next session and invites dialogue. Brookfield recognises the benefits of this approach to build trust, alert the group to problems before a disaster occurs, and to give the guide feedback about ways he might develop his facilitation.

- At what moment in the class this week did you feel most engaged with what was happening?
- At what moment in the class this week did you feel most distanced from what was happening?
- What action that anyone [teacher or student) took in class did you find most affirming or helpful?
- What action that anyone (teacher or student) took in class this week did you find the most puzzling?
- What about the class surprised you the most? (This could be something about your own reactions to what went on, or something that someone did, or anything else that occurs to you).

Reference

Brookfield S (1996) *Becoming a Critically reflective teacher*. Josey-Bass, San Francisco.

Index